THE
CERTIFIED OCCUPATIONAL
THERAPY ASSISTANT

Principles, Concepts and Techniques

2nd Edition

THE
CERTIFIED OCCUPATIONAL
THERAPY ASSISTANT

Principles, Concepts and Techniques

2nd Edition

Editor

Sally E. Ryan, COTA, ROH

Faculty Assistant and Instructor
The College of St. Catherine
Department of Occupational Therapy
St. Paul, Minnesota

SLACK Incorporated, 6900 Grove Road, Thorofare, NJ 08086-9447

SLACK International Book Distributors

Japan
  Igaku-Shoin, Ltd.
  Tokyo International P.O. Box 5063
  1-28-36 Hongo, Bunkyo-Ku
  Tokyo 113
  Japan

Australia
  McGraw-Hill Book Company
  4 Barcoo Street
  Roseville East 2069
  New South Wales
  Australia

Canada
  McGraw-Hill Ryerson Limited
  300 Water Street
  Whitby, Ontario
  L1N 9B6
  Canada

United Kingdom
  McGraw-Hill Book Company
  Shoppenhangers Road
  Maidenhead, Berkshire SL6 2QL
  England

In all other regions throughout the world, SLACK professional reference books are available through offices and affiliates of McGraw-Hill, Inc. For the name and address of the office serving your area, please correspond to

McGraw-Hill, Inc.
Medical Publishing Group
Attn: International Marketing Director
1221 Avenue of the Americas —28th Floor
New York, NY 10020
(212)-512-3955 (phone)
(212)-512-4717 (fax)

Editorial Director: Cheryl D. Willoughby
Publisher: Harry C. Benson

Previously published as *The Certified Occupational Therapy Assistant: Roles and Responsibilities*.

The Certified occupational therapy assistant: principles, concepts, and techniques / Sally E. Ryan, Editor. -- 2nd ed.
  p. cm.
  Includes bibliographical references and index.
  Contents: v. 1. Foundations.
  ISBN 1-55642-178-8 (pbk.)
  1. Occupational therapy.   2. Occupational therapy—practice
  3. Occupational therapy assistants. I. Ryan, Sally E.
  RM735.C47 1993   615.8'515--dc20   90-50395

Printed in the United States of America

Published by: SLACK Incorporated
               6900 Grove Road
               Thorofare, NJ 08086-9447

Last digit is print number: 10   9   8   7   6   5   4   3   2   1

*Dedicated to the Advancement of the Profession of
Occupational Therapy
and to
Colonel Ruth A. Robinson, OTR
who, in an interview before her death in 1989,
stated that she felt her greatest contribution to the
profession of occupational therapy was the
development of the program and curriculum to train
occupational therapy assistants.*

Contents

Expanded Contents

SECTION III
Technology

About the Editor

A graduate of the first occupational therapy assistant program at Duluth, Minnesota, in 1964, Sally Ryan has just entered her 28th year as a certified occupational therapy assistant and member of the profession. She has taken extensive coursework at the University of Minnesota as a James Wright Hunt Scholar, and at the College of St. Catherine, St. Paul. Her background includes experience in practice, clinical education supervision, and management in long-term care; consultation; and teaching in the professional occupational therapy program at the College of St. Catherine.

In the past, Ms. Ryan has served in a variety of leadership positions at the local, state and national levels. She has served as representative to the American Occupational Therapy Association (AOTA) Representative Assembly from Minnesota; chair of the Representative Assembly Nominating Committee; a member-at-large of the AOTA Executive Board; member and on-site evaluator of the AOTA Accreditation Committee; and member and secretary of the AOTA Standards and Ethics Commission. She has also served the AOTA as a member of the Philosophical Base Task Force and the 1981 Role Delineation Steering Committee, and as a consultant to the COTA Task Force. She is currently the Treasurer and Chair of the Fiscal Advisory Board of the American Occupational Therapy Certification Board.

Ms. Ryan is the recipient of numerous state and national awards. She is the first COTA to receive the AOTA Award of Excellence, has been recognized as an Outstanding Young Woman of America, and was among the first recipients of the AOTA Roster of Honor.

Ms. Ryan has been invited to present numerous keynote addresses, presentations, and workshops, both nationally and internationally. Frequently her topics focus on COTA roles and relationships and intraprofessional team building.

Contributing Authors

Ben Atchison is an Assistant Professor of Occupational Therapy at Eastern Michigan University in Ypsilanti, Michigan. He received his undergraduate degree in occupational therapy at Western Michigan University in Kalamazoo and a Master's Degree in Education from Georgia State University in Atlanta. He is pursuing a doctoral degree in instructional technology at Eastern Michigan University. Professor Atchison is currently serving as Chair of the Physical Disabilities Special Interest Section of the American Occupational Therapy Association. As an Army officer, he holds the position of Assistant Chief, Occupational Therapy Section for the 323rd General Hospital of the United States Army Reserve Medical Department. Professor Atchison has extensive experience in a wide variety of practice areas, including pediatrics, adult outpatient rehabilitation, and home health care. His scholarly contributions have included publications and presentations regarding the elderly, homeless, AIDS, the assessment and management of visual perceptual disorders, and educational design. He has been recognized in *Outstanding Young Men in America* and is the recipient of the Excellence in Teaching Award from Eastern Michigan University and has been designated as a Fellow by the American Occupational Therapy Association.

Harriet Backhaus received her certificate from the occupational therapy assistant program at Westminister College in Fulton, Missouri, and an undergraduate degree in education from Harris College in St. Louis. She is currently employed at the Program in Occupational Therapy at Washington University in St. Louis where she is involved in both clinical practice and undergraduate teaching. Ms. Backhaus is a member of the advisory committee for the occupational therapy assistant program at St. Louis Community College at Meramec, and recently completed a term as a member of the Certification Examination Development Committee of the American Occupational Therapy Certification Board. Her interest in therapeutic media and skills in selecting purposeful activities through activity analysis are widely recognized.

B. Joan Bellman earned a Bachelor of Science degree in occupational therapy from Virginia Commonwealth University in Richmond, Virginia. She held the positions of clinician, clinical education supervisor, and chief of occupational therapy at District of Columbia General Hospital for 29 years, before retiring from government service in 1988. Ms. Bellman has served as a member of the Certification Committee of the American Occupational Therapy Association and as President of the District of Columbia Occupational Therapy Association. Her professional experience has been primarily in the area of adult physical dysfunction, with a special interest and expertise in the fabrication of hand splints and assistive devices. She is currently employed part-time by the Visiting Nurse Association of the District of Columbia and Adventist Home Health Services, Inc. for Northern Prince George's County, Maryland.

Robert K. Bing is Professor Emeritus of Occupational Therapy at the University of Texas School of Allied Health Sciences at Galveston, Texas. He received his undergraduate degree in occupational therapy from the University of Illinois and his Master of Arts and Doctor of Education degrees were conferred by the University of Maryland. His varied clinical experiences include the United States Army, Norwich State Hospital in Connecticut, Nebraska Psychiatric Institute, Illinois Psychiatric Institute, and the University of Texas Medical Branch Hospitals, where he served as the founding dean, School of Allied Health Sciences, and professor of occupational therapy. He has also served as a member of the faculty in occupational therapy departments of six universities. Dr. Bing was elected President of the Maryland and Texas Occupational Therapy Associations and President of the American Occupational Therapy Association. He is the recipient of the Award of Merit and the Eleanor Clarke Slagle Lectureship and was designated as a Fellow of the American Occupational Therapy Association. Dr. Bing was also recently named a Galveston Unsung Hero for his volunteer work and service as a liaison officer for the East Texas AIDS Project. Currently, he is retired and devoting much of his time to professional writing.

Toné F. Blechert received an Associate in Arts degree as an occupational therapy assistant from St. Mary's Junior College and a baccalaureate degree in communications from Metropolitan State University in Minneapolis, Minnesota. She is currently pursuing a master's degree in organizational leadership from the College of St. Catherine in St. Paul. Throughout her career, she has held a number of leadership positions, which have included chair of the American Occupational Therapy Association COTA Task Force and member of the faculty and the steering committee for the Professional and Technical Role Analysis Project (PATRA). Ms. Blechert recently completed a term as a member of the Board of Directors of the American Occupational Therapy Foundation. She has served as a faculty member in the occupational therapy assistant program at the St. Mary's Campus of the College of St. Catherine since 1984. She also serves as the Coordinator of Academic Advising for that campus. In recognition of her numerous professional publications and presentations, she received the Communication Award from the Minnesota Occupational Therapy Association. Ms. Blechert is also a recipient of the Award of Excellence, the Roster of Honor, and the Service Award given by the American Occupational Therapy Association.

Bonnie Brooks earned her undergradute degree in occupational therapy at Indiana University in Indianapolis and also completed a Master of Science Degree in Education at Loyola University in Chicago. Early in her career, she was instrumental in the development of several occupational therapy assistant programs and also served as a faculty member in both technical and professional education. As the Assistant Director of Education at the American Occupational Therapy Association, Ms. Brooks was responsible for assisting in the development of new technical programs and for ongoing activities and initiatives in occupational therapy assistant education. She also served as the liaison to the COTA Task Force and the COTA Advisory Committee, and she was instrumental in providing the COTA perspective for all major AOTA committees and projects. She was also responsible for implementing the first national COTA network. Ms. Brooks has been recognized as a Fellow by the American Occupational Therapy Association, and currently is employed by RehabWorks of Florida in Sarasota where she provides direct service and consultation to long-term care facilities.

Shirley Holland Carr, at the time of her death in 1992, was employed as an occupational therapist at the Pupil Appraisal Service for the East Baton Rouge Parish School in Louisiana, a position she held for more than eight years. Ms. Carr earned her undergraduate degree in education at Tufts University in Boston and received a diploma from the Boston School of Occupational Therapy. Later, she completed her Master of Science degree in psychology at Auburn University. Her many years of practice were community-oriented and included experience in child development, mental health, management, and professional and technical education. In the latter capacity, she was instrumental in planning as well as serving as the director of several occupational therapy assistant programs. Ms. Carr was a recipient of the Award of Excellence for "outstanding performance in professional development" given by the Missouri Occupational Therapy Association, and she was

also been designated as a Fellow by the American Occupational Therapy Association.

Mary K. Cowan is an Associate Professor of Occupational Therapy at Eastern Kentucky University, where she has held a faculty appointment since 1989. Professor Cowan earned her undergraduate degree in occupational therapy at the University of Minnesota and later completed a Master of Arts program in educational psychology at the same institution. She has worked clinically with children with all types of handicapping conditions, particularly in public education settings. Her present study and research focuses on postural stability as it relates to educational performance. She is certified in the Bobath Approach to the treatment of children with cerebral palsy and the administration and interpretation of the Southern California Sensory Integration Tests. Professor Cowan has been recognized as a Fellow of the American Occupational Therapy Association.

Sister Genevieve Cummings is an Associate Professor and Chair of the Occupational Therapy Department at the College of St. Catherine in St. Paul, Minnesota, where she has held a faculty appointment since 1960. She received her undergraduate degree in occupational therapy from that institution and later earned a Master of Arts degree in child development from the University of Minnesota. Throughout her career, Professor Cummings has been recognized as an outstanding leader, and has served in a number of capacities in the American Occupational Therapy Association, including a member of the Executive Board, Chair of the Standards and Ethics Commission, and Representative from the State of Minnesota to the Representative Assembly. She has been the recipient of many honors, which include recognition by the Association as one of the first Fellows. She has also been the recipient of the Occupational Therapist of the Year and the Communication Awards given by the Minnesota Occupational Therapy Association.

Mary Ellen Lange Dunford is an Assistant Professor and Coordinator for the Occupational Therapy Assistant Program at Kirkwood Community College in Cedar Rapids, Iowa. Professor Dunford received her baccalaureate degree in occupational therapy from the College of St. Catherine in St. Paul, Minnesota, and she is currently pusuing a master's degree in education at the University of Iowa. As a practitioner, she specialized in pediatrics and did pioneering work in the development of methods for adapting and using electronic devices for treatment. An active member of the Iowa Occupational Therapy Association, she held various leadership positions within the organization. Her contributions to the education of certified occupational therapy assistants has had a significant impact on the roles and responsibilities of COTAs practicing in Iowa.

Azela Gohl-Giese is an Associate Professor of Occupational Therapy at the College of St. Catherine in St. Paul, Minnnesota, where she has held a faculty appointment since 1962. Professor Gohl-Giese earned her undergraduate degree in occupational therapy from the College of St. Catherine and later completed a Master of Science degree in management at Cardinal Stritch College. During her tenure at the College her teaching responsibilities have had a primary focus in the areas of psychiatry and group dynamics, where she has placed a strong emphasis on the importance of the therapeutic use of activity in collaboration with team members, especially the certified occupational therapy assistant. Currently she serves as the fieldwork coordinator, working closely with clinical educators in designing learning experiences for students, many of whom are practicing COTAs working toward a baccalaureate degree. A number of these students are enrolled in the Weekend College Occupational Therapy Program, where Ms. Gohl-Giese served as the first coordinator.

Nancy Kari is an Associate Professor of Occupational Therapy at the College of St. Catherine in St. Paul, Minnesota, where she has been a faculty member since 1978. She received her baccalaureate degree in occupational therapy from the University of Wisconsin at Madison and a Master's Degree in public health from the University of Minnesota. Pursuing her interests in organizational governance and institutional change, she also serves as adjunct faculty with Project Public Life, a national initiative to reengage citizens in public life, at the Humphrey Institute of Public Affairs at the University of Minnesota. Associated with this work, she co-directs the Lazarus Project, an action-research pilot program that investigates issues of empowerment within nursing homes. The goal of her pioneering work is to create a community model, which is an alternative to the traditional medical and therapeutic models of governance. Professor Kari has published papers on team building and on the politics of empowerment and is a recent recipient of the Communication Award given by the Minnesota Occupational Therapy Association. She is also a recipient of the Cordelia Meyers Writer's Award, given by the American Occupational Therapy Association.

M. Jeanne Madigan has been Professor and Chair of the Department of Occupational Therapy at Virginia Commonwealth University in Richmond, Virginia, since 1984. She received her undergraduate degree in occupational therapy from the College of St. Catherine in St. Paul, Minnesota; her Master of Arts degree in occupational therapy from the University of Southern California; and her Doctorate in Education, with an emphasis in curriculum and instruction, from Loyola University in Chicago. Dr. Madigan has served on numerous education and evaluation-related committees and task forces of the American Occupational Therapy

Association, including Chair of the Certification and Program Advisory Committees, Essentials Review Committee, and the Role Delineation Committee; and she has been designated as a Fellow by the Association. She has served as a consultant and a member of advisory committees of several occupational therapy assistant educational programs, and she is currently serving as a member of the advisory committee of the first occupational therapy assistant program in Virginia at J. Sargent Reynolds College.

LaDonn People is an instructor in the Department of Occupational Therapy at Eastern Michigan University in Ypsilanti where she has held a faculty appointment since 1990. Formerly, she was employed for 18 years as an instructor in the occupational therapy assistant program at Wayne County Community College in Detroit and as the fieldwork coordinator in that institution for ten years. Ms. People earned her undergraduate degree in occupational therapy from Eastern Michigan University and later completed a Master of Arts degree in occupational education at the University of Michigan in Ann Arbor. She is presently pursuing a doctoral degree in instructional technology at Wayne State University in Detroit. Her professional interest and expertise are in the areas of physical dysfunction and gerontology.

Brian J. Ryan received his Bachelor of Science degree in electrical engineering from the University of Minnesota in Minneapolis. His interest in computers grew out of a need to collect and analyze large data sets in relation to his work in failure analysis, parts control and quality control. As a private pilot, he also found numerous computer applications for navigation and communication. Mr. Ryan currently serves as a Principle Engineer at Alliant Tech Systems in Hopkins, Minnesota, in the Reliability, Maintainability and Safety Departments. He also serves as a consultant to the Pavek Wireless Museum in Minneapolis and the Experimental Aircraft Association Museum in Oshkosh, Wisconsin, where he has been instrumental in research and development of new electronic communications exhibits. His interest in occupational therapy was brought about through marriage to a COTA.

Patrice Schober-Branigan is an occupational therapist at the Minnesota Center for Health and Rehabilitation in Minneapolis, Minnesota. Ms. Schober-Branigan earned her Bachelor of Arts degree in occupational therapy from the College of St. Catherine in St. Paul, Minnesota. She has completed considerable advanced study and training in hand rehabilitation and was previously an active member of the American Society of Hand Therapists. Ms. Schober-Branigan has lectured on the topic of hand rehabilitation and splinting to occupational therapists, occupational therapy assistants, physicians, nurses and students. She has also published, and has designed and presented programs to industry on prevention of cumulative trauma. In her clinical work in a hand surgery practice, she has trained and supervised a COTA in static splinting techniques. Her specialization has broadened to the larger field of industrial rehabilitation and ergonomics, and she especially enjoys her work in a holistic, multidisciplinary rehabilitation center.

Phillip D. Shannon is the Coordinator of the Community Health Education and Medicaid Access Enhancement Project, co-sponsored by the Cameron County Health Department in San Benito, Texas, and by Project HOPE in Millwood, Virginia. His undergraduate degree in occupational therapy from California State University at San Jose was followed by two graduate degrees from the University of Southern California, a Master of Arts degree in occupational therapy and a Master of Public Administration degree. He has served as a program director in both technical and professional occupational therapy educational programs and is a retired officer of the United States Army. Mr. Shannon has published extensively in professional journals, primarily on the philosophy and theory of occupational therapy, and he has published chapters in three books as well. In addition to developing and presenting numerous workshops in the United States, he developed and conducted workshops for the United States Army Seventh Medical Command in Germany from 1985-1990. He was also the principal speaker for the Sixth National Congress of the Occupational Therapy Association, Bogata, Columbia. He has been the recipient of several awards, including the Chair's Service Award from the State University of New York at Buffalo, the Service Award of the American Occupational Therapy Association, and the Retired Educator's Award from the Association's Commission on Education. He has also been recognized as a Fellow by the American Occupational Therapy Association. Mr. Shannon served as Chair of the Certification Examination Development Committee and member of the Board of Directors of the American Occupational Therapy Certification Board.

Rhonda Stewart holds an Associate of Arts degree from Wayne County Community College in Detroit, Michigan, and a Bachelor of Science degree in occupational therapy from Eastern Michigan University at Kalamazoo. She is currently pursuing a Master of Science degree in Health Administration from Central Michigan University. Ms. Stewart has practiced as both a COTA and an OTR in physical medicine and rehabilitation, mental health, and home health settings where all age groups and a variety of diagnostic problems are treated. She has taught occupational therapy assistant courses and presented workshops at Wayne County Community College and is currently employed as a staff therapist and clinical supervisor at William Beaumont Hospital in Royal Oak, Michigan, and a part-time consultant

for community rehabilitation programs. Ms. Stewart is a governor-appointed member of the Michigan Licensing and Regulation Board for Occupational Therapists and also serves as the current President of the Michigan Occupational Therapy Association. In addition, she is Chair of the Board of Directors of the Michigan Black Occupational Therapy Caucus. She has presented papers at national and state conferences on issues related to practice, management and students.

Javan E. Walker, Jr. is Director of the Division of Occupational Therapy and Associate Professor of Occupational Therapy at Florida Agricultural and Mechanical University in Tallahassee, Florida, where he developed the program. Before assuming this position he was the Director of the Occupational Therapy Assistant Program at Illinois Central College in Peoria. Professor Walker began his occupational therapy career as a COTA in the United States Army. He earned his undergraduate degree in occupational therapy from Wayne State University in Detroit and a Master of Arts degree in education from Bradley University. He is currently a doctoral candidate at Illinois State University. After 15 years of active duty as an occupational therapist, Mr. Walker currently holds the rank of Lieutenant Colonel in the United States Army Reserves. In addition to his work as an educator and a clinician, he was recently elected as the Alternate Representative to the American Occupational Therapy Association Representative Assembly for the state of Florida. Professor Walker has provided consultation to long-term care facilities and mental health programs for the past 15 years, and he is actively involved with computer technology professionally and as a leisure time pursuit.

Doris Y. Witherspoon is the Director of Industrial Technology at Henry Ford Community College in Dearborn, Michigan. Formerly she was employed at Wayne County Community College for 20 years where she held the positions of Director of the Occupational Therapy Assistant Program, Director of Allied Health, and Dean of Vocational Technology. Ms. Witherspoon developed the occupational therapy assistant program at the college and taught classes in the program for 18 years. She earned her undergraduate degree in occupational therapy from Eastern Michigan University in Ypsilanti, and later completed a Master of Science degree in occupational education from the University of Michigan. She is currently a doctoral student at Wayne State University in Detroit. As an occupational therapy assistant educator, Ms. Witherspoon served on numerous state and national committees, including the American Occupational Therapy Association Certification Committee, Chairperson of Occupational Therapy Assistant Educators for the Association's Commission on Education; she was also President of the Black Occupational Therapy Caucus.

Acknowledgments

I am indeed indebted to a number of individuals who assisted in the preparation of this book. In the early stages of planning, many occupational therapy assistant program directors, faculty members, clinicians and practitioners responded to a lengthy survey. These OTRs and COTAs provided thoughtful critiques and comments, which were of great help in determining the focus of this second edition. Special thanks is offered to Louise Fawcett who assisted with the interpretation of survey data, and to Phillip Shannon, who served as a primary reviewer and consultant during the early planning stages of this edition.

The contributions of the highly skilled contributing authors are gratefully acknowledged. Their work, individually and collectively, is the great strength of this text. Twenty-one occupational therapists and assistants have provided their extensive knowledge and expertise to this text. They come from diverse practice, education and research backgrounds; eight OTR contributors are or were occupational therapy assistant program directors. Many of the 21 authors, representing 12 states and the District of Columbia, have been actively involved in leadership roles in their state associations as well as in the American Occupational Therapy Association, the American Occupational Therapy Foundation and The American Occupational Therapy Certification Board. Nine of the authors have been recognized by AOTA as Fellows or members of the Roster of Honor. The contributions of an electrical engineer have enhanced the chapter on computers. It has been a great privilege to work with these outstanding writers, and I convey my most sincere thanks to each of them.

I would also like to offer my thanks to the reviewers who provided critiques of all of the manuscripts. Their objectivity and critical analysis of the content was most helpful in this developmental process.

Appreciation is also offered to M. Jeanne Madigan who assisted in writing a number of the related learning activities, which appear at the conclusion of each chapter.

Cheryl Willoughby, Editorial Director, and Elaine Schultz, Associate Editor, at Slack Inc., provided me with numerous resources, advice, critiques, and overall editorial assistance. Their patience, coupled with expert problem-solving skills, helped me immeasurably in this enormous task. Publication of this text would not have been possible without their expertise and assistance.

I would like to acknowledge and express my personal gratitude to Sister Genevieve Cummings, chairperson, and all of the members of the faculty of the Department of Occupational Therapy at the College of St. Catherine for their support and encouragement during the many phases of this task. Their willingness to share resources and offer critiques and support was of great help.

To the many therapists, assistants, friends and family members who provided ideas, listened to my concerns, and responded to my endless questions, I offer my most sincere appreciation. I regret that space does not allow me to list each of them individually.

My daughter Mary deserves very special thanks for assuming many tasks, which ranged from proofreading, editing, duplicating, and mailing to house cleaning, cooking, shopping and walking the dogs. Deep appreciation is offered to this versatile young woman, whose generosity of time and talent allowed me to complete a most arduous project.

Thanking my husband Brian is most difficult. He filled many supportive roles, including active listener, thoughtful reactor, consultant, reviewer, typist, illustrator, errand runner, FAX sender, telephone monitor, and household manager. Suffice it to say that this project would never have been accomplished without his sense of humor, inspiration, insight, patience, and remarkable ability to adapt. I am ever grateful.

—Sally E. Ryan

Foreword

Without a doubt, Sally Ryan is a pioneer in the professional development of the certified occupational therapy assistant, and this book is a concrete example of her many contributions. This publication is the most complete and comprehensive textbook ever compiled for the OTA, and it has become the standard for others to emulate.

Before the first edition was published, educators would have to collect information from numerous sources and create their own materials in order to instruct OTA students in their vocational responsibilities. Frequently, these materials had to be adapted to accommodate the specific needs of the occupational therapy assistant. This approach gave students the impression that there was no body of knowledge designed specifically for them. This informational deficit sent the implicit message to OTA students that they needed to know what the occupational therapist knows, only at a lower level.

The Certified Occupational Therapy Assistant: Principles, Concepts and Techniques establishes the knowledge base for the occupational therapy assistant. A more clear identification of this knowledge base will enable health care administrators to recognize the value of the COTA in helping to meet many of the staffing problems occurring in our health care settings today. Once their responsibilities have been defined, occupational therapy assistants will be able to assume the roles for which they were trained and which sometimes have been assigned to other specialists. In the national climate of managed health care costs, this appropriate use of the COTA will be an important strategy in providing cost-effective health care.

Over the past few years, Sally Ryan has focused on the concept of team building, believing that many of the current problems in our profession and health care in general are due to difficulties in team building. This lack of team work has been an impetus to incorporate team building concepts in her professional activities, and this textbook itself represents a major team-building effort. The variety and quality of the authors are outstanding, each contributor providing an essential component to the total body of knowledge, and each chapter complementing and building on the others.

The central theme of this book is occupation, the major construct of our profession. Proper emphasis is placed on purposeful activity, rather than exercises and "talk therapies," illustrating the importance of activity to the health of human beings. The use of activity as a major tool of the COTA is nicely integrated into the descriptions of functional treatment programs.

The book also emphasizes the human element of health care and the role the occupational therapy assistant performs in providing this component. Because the OTA becomes the close partner of the patient, working with the patient to facilitate an improvement in lifestyle, it is the assistant who really provides the caring and touching component that is known to be a major contributor to the healing process. This element is crucial because the human touch is too often forgotten in health care, for professionals have a tendency to do things to people without really interacting with them as human beings. This book illustrates how the quality of time the OTA spends with the patient dealing with daily life skills facilitates the provision of this necessary component.

New areas of practice are evolving for the occupational therapy assistant and they will continue to evolve. In the future, I envision areas of practice in which the OTA practices independently, with an occupational therapist available for consultation. Certainly the area of tool adaptation in industry could be such an area, as the knowledge and skills used in analyzing activities and adapting tools and equipment are basic to the practice of the OTA.

Finally, the Army is extremely proud that Sally Ryan has dedicated her book to COL Ruth Robinson, OTR (Retired). COL Robinson recognized early the critical role the assistant would play in the profession. She knew that the certified occupational therapy assistant would become a "prime mover" of the profession by allowing occupational therapists to provide health care to many more patients while increasing the quality of care. I know she would have been very proud of this textbook, its authors and its editor.

—COL Roy Swift, PhD, OTR, FAOTA
Chief, Army Medical Specialists Corps

Preface

TO THE SECOND EDITION

Work on the second edition of this text began in earnest in January of 1989. That year was particularly significant because it marked the 30th anniversary of certified occupational therapy assistants (COTAs) working in the profession.

Discussions with technical level faculty, occupational therapists and assistants serving as clinical supervisors and practitioners, as well as results of a survey directed at this audience, emphasized the need to readopt the fundamental objectives of the first edition: 1) focus on the basic principles, concepts and techniques of the profession; 2) provide both an extensive and a realistic view of the roles and functions of certified occupational therapy assistants in entry-level practice and beyond; 3) provide examples of how to successfully build intraprofessional relationships; and 4) be useful in the clinic as well as the classroom. These objectives were again used as a foundation for developing, organizing and sequencing content areas.

The content in the first edition has been greatly expanded and updated. Therefore, it was decided to publish this edition in a two-book format. This volume is an introductory text; the second volume, *Practice Issues in Occupational Therapy*, is a more advanced text, focusing on specific practice applications, as well as related knowledge and skills.

Several documents published by the American Occupational Therapy Association (AOTA) were used as primary guides for content development: The *Entry-Level Role Delineation for Registered Occupational Therapists (OTRs) and Certified Occupational Therapy Assistants (COTAs),* the *Essentials and Guidelines for an Accredited Educational Program for the Occupational Therapy Assistant, Uniform Terminology for Reporting Occupational Therapy Services,* 2nd Edition, and the *1990 Member Data Survey.* Preliminary data from the *Job Analysis Study,* conducted by the American Occupational Therapy Certification Board, was also considered.

Eight new chapters have been added to this edition, as well as a glossary and related learning activities. Other chapters have been expanded and updated. The reader will also find more photographs, illustrations, charts and forms to enhance and emphasize important points. In addition, all chapters now open with a set of key concepts and a list of essential vocabulary terms. The key concepts are designed to assist the students in focusing their study on the fundamental subjects in each chapter. The essential vocabulary words are terms important to chapter content and occupational therapy practice, and appear in bold type at first mention. Every effort has been made to define each term clearly, both in context and in the glossary.

The book is divided into five major sections. The first section focuses on historical, philosophical and theoretical perspectives, providing the reader with a basic understanding of some of the important principles that have guided the profession. The heritage of the COTA is emphasized, with prominent developmental milestones interwoven in the story.

Section II focuses on the core concepts of occupational therapy, which include principles of human development and the components of occupation that influence role performance. Another important emphasis is the occupational performance areas of activities of daily living, work and play/leisure. Following chapters point to some of the skills necessary for effective therapeutic intervention with emphasis placed on the teaching/learning process, interpersonal communication and applied group dynamics. The section concludes with a discussion of important aspects of the individualization of occupational therapy, with factors such as environment, sociocultural considerations, change and prevention stressed. Throughout this section, short case studies are included to provide the reader with examples of occupational therapy personnel working with patients of varying ages in a variety of traditional and nontraditional treatment settings.

Technology is emphasized in Section III. The use of video, small electronic toys and devices, and computers in occupational therapy evaluation and treatment are presented. The reader is provided with basic terminology and information as well as numerous applications and resources for these technologies.

Section IV is devoted to the discussion of selected contemporary media techniques. Thermoplastic splinting and adaptive equipment construction provide the reader with a variety of examples, practical applications and methods for developing skills in these important areas.

In Section V, the final segment, the focus is on purposeful activity, emphasizing the application of arts and crafts and the analysis of activities. Fundamental principles are discussed as a means for integrating many of the core concepts presented in preceding chapters. Strategies for building skill in these important aspects of practice are stressed.

When using this book, it is important for the reader to note the following:

1. In addition to the main chapter designations, all important chapter subheadings also appear in the Expanded Contents. They are titled to reflect the major objectives of the writers and the editor.

2. Every effort has been made to use gender-inclusive language throughout the book. In some instances, it was necessary to use "him or her," recognizing that this may be awkward for the reader. Exceptions to the use of gender inclusive pronouns occur in the discussion of historical material, philosophical principles and in some quotations.

3. The term *patient* has been used frequently to describe the recipient of occupational therapy services. The authors and the editor recognize that this term is not always the most appropriate; however, it is believed to be preferable to other options currently being used. Exceptions have been made in some instances where such terms as the *individual*, the *student*, the *child*, etc. have been used.

4. Related learning activities have been included at the conclusion of each chapter. Some of these were published previously in *The Certified Occupational Therapy Assistant: Roles and Responsibilites Workbook*.

5. Whenever a writing project of this magnitude is undertaken, inadvertent omissions and errors may occur. Although every attempt has been made to prevent such occurrences, it is the hope of the editor and the authors that these will be called to their attention, so that they may be corrected in the next printing.

In conclusion, it is my belief that this book and its companion volume will serve as a model and a guidepost for occupational therapy teamwork in the delivery of patient services. It will serve as an incentive for the technically and professionally educated practitioners to discover the many ways in which their skills and roles complement each other. It will also serve as a catalyst for developing new skills and roles in response to the ever-changing needs of our society.

The former President of the American Occupational Therapy Association, Carolyn Manville Baum, summed it up best in her 1980 Eleanor Clarke Slagle Address when she stated

As a profession and as professionals, let us put our resources, intelligence, and emotional commitment together and work diligently toward the ascent of our profession. The health care system, the clients (patients) we serve, and each of us individually will benefit from our commitment.

—Sally E. Ryan
1991

Preface

TO THE FIRST EDITION

Work on this text began in the spring of 1984. That year was particularly significant because it marked the 25th anniversary of certified occupational therapy assistants (COTAs) working in the profession.

The project was given impetus from the fact that there was no comprehensive book written expressly for occupational therapy assistants. Discussions with technical level faculty, occupational therapists (OTRs) serving as clinical supervisors, and assistants emphasized the need for a text that would focus on the basic principles of the profession; a book that would provide both an extensive and a realistic view of the roles and functions of certified occupational therapy assistants in entry-level practice and beyond; a book that would provide examples of how to successfully build intraprofessional relationships; and, finally, a book that could be used in the clinic as well as the classroom. These objectives were adopted as a foundation for developing, organizing and sequencing content areas.

Four documents published by the American Occupational Therapy Association (AOTA) also served as primary guides for content development: the *Entry-Level OTR and COTA Role Delineation,* the *Essentials of an Approved Educational Program for the Occupational Therapy Assistant, Uniform Terminology for Reporting Occupational Therapy Services,* and the *1982 Member Data Survey.* All but the latter are included as appendices.

The book is divided into six major sections. The first section (Historical Perspectives) introduces the themes and perspectives of the book. Section II focuses on the core knowledge of occupational therapy, which includes philosophical and theoretical material as well as principles of human development and basic influences contributing to health. The daily living skills of self-care, work, and play/leisure are also addressed as the primary foundations of the profession, along with descriptions of some of the skills necessary for effective therapeutic intervention. Emphasis is placed on the teaching/learning process, interpersonal communication, group dynamics and the occupational therapy process.

In Section III (Intervention Strategies), case studies demonstrate the roles of occupational therapy assistants and occupational therapists working with selected patients to illustrate specific ways in which the profession's role delineation can be used to provide efficient and effective health care delivery.

Section IV (Models of Practice) provides numerous examples of the team approach in working with patients of varying ages in a variety of traditional and non-traditional treatment settings. The roles of the OTR/COTA team in a hospice setting are delineated, and the roles of the COTA in work and productive occupation programs and as an activities director are addressed.

Concepts of Practice are reviewed in Section V, which includes discussions of contemporary media techniques as well as management and supervision principles and issues.

The final section (Contemporary Issues) discusses ways of enhancing intraprofessional relationships through the effective use of supervision, mentoring, and conflict management fundamentals, and reviews the maturation process of the assistant and related professional socialization elements. Principles of occupational therapy ethics are presented, and future trends for the profession are outlined.

In addition to the main chapter designations, all important chapter subheadings appear in the Table of Contents. Their titles reflect the major objectives of the writer and editor. *The Certified Occupational Therapy Assistant: Roles and Responsibilities Workbook,* also published by SLACK, Inc., provides the student with study and discussion questions and exercises, as well as additional learning resources.

Every effort has been made to use gender-inclusive language throughout the book. In some instances, it was necessary to use "him or her," recognizing that this may be awkward for the reader.

In conclusion, it is my belief that this book will serve as a model and a guidepost for occupational therapy teamwork in the delivery of patient services. It will serve as an incentive for technically and professionally educated practitioners to discover the many ways in which their skills and roles complement each other. It will also serve as a catalyst for developing new skills and roles in response to the ever-changing needs of our society.

The former President of the American Occupational Therapy Association, Carolyn Manville Baum, summed it up best in her 1980 Eleanor Clarke Slagle Address when she stated

As a profession and as professionals, let us put our resources, intelligence, and emotional commitment together and work diligently toward the ascent of our profession. The health care system, the clients (patients) we serve, and each of us individually will benefit from our commitment.

—Sally E. Ryan
1986

Section I
HISTORICAL, PHILOSOPHICAL AND THEORETICAL PRINCIPLES

Living Forward, Understanding Backward:
  A History of Occupational Therapy Principles

The COTA Heritage: Proud, Practical, Stable, Dynamic

History may be defined as a recorded narrative of events that have occurred in the past. It is a collection of information drawn from many sources that include speeches, letters, minutes of meetings, photographs, diaries, articles and interviews. In learning about history, the student is provided with an appreciation for, and understanding of, the important roots of the profession. It gives insight to the rich legacy of events, experiences and people that have shaped our past.

This first section details significant aspects of the history of occupational therapy from the perspective of the profession's principles. Lessons from our past, reflecting basic concepts, values and beliefs, continue to influence contemporary practice and will have a marked impact on our future. The developmental milestones of the certified occupational therapy assistant (COTA) are also chronicled, and the heritage of the COTA is characterized by Carr as "proud, practical, stable and dynamic."

As Bing has stated, "Fundamentally, history is experience, rather than the mere telling of quaint stories or reminiscing about past feats or failures. It is knowing enough about what has come before to know what to consider or rule out in evaluating the present, on our way to the future."

Living Forward, Understanding Backward

A HISTORY OF OCCUPATIONAL THERAPY PRINCIPLES

Robert K. Bing, EdD, OTR, FAOTA

INTRODUCTION

The renowned 19th century American philosopher, physician and psychologist, William James, is reputed to have observed that "We live forward; we understand backwards." We exist in the present, yet are future oriented. To make sense of the present or future, we must have knowledge about and an appreciation of the past.

Today, occupational therapy personnel face numerous predicaments. Educational preparation for practice is based predominantly on knowledge and skills that are marketable in a very competitive health care environment. The *what* of our art, science and technology is emphasized, often at the expense of the *why*. What is missing is the sense of what has come before, of those recurring patterns that offer legitimacy and uniqueness in the health care profession.

History is an invaluable tool to assess the present and determine future courses of action. The recording of an occupational life or medical history is a testament to the past's influence on current conditions and its ability to offer approaches to alleviate problems. Fundamentally, history is experience, rather than the mere telling of quaint stories or reminiscing about past feats or failures. It is knowing enough about what has come before to know what to consider or what to rule out in evaluating the present, on our way to the future. As Neustadt and May point out, we must learn "...how to use experience, whether remote or recent, in the process of deciding what to do today about the prospect for tomorrow."[1]

KEY CONCEPTS

Age of Enlightenment

Moral treatment

The York Retreat

Hull House and Consolation House

Invalid Occupations

National Society for the Promotion of Occupational Therapy

Habit training

Purposeful work and leisure

Interaction of mind and body

Time-honored principles

AGE OF ENLIGHTENMENT—THE 1700S

To place the history of occupational therapy in proper perspective, we could go as far back as the Garden of Eden. Dr. William Rush Dunton, Jr., one of the founders of the 20th century's occupational therapy movement, insisted that those fig leaves had to have been crocheted by Eve. She was trying to get over her troubles, which had something to do with her being "beholden" to Adam and his rib. But let us pass over all of that and begin this story in Europe over 200 years ago. This era became known as the Age of Enlightenment or, in some quarters, the Age of Reason. Those engaged in science and philosophy were known as *natural philosophers*. Nearly a century later (the late 1800s), the two disciplines separated and the term *scientist* came into the language.

In the late 1700s, Western Europe was astir with a new view of life. Social, political, economic, and religious theories promoted a general sense of human progress and perfectibility. Notions about intolerance, censorship and economic and social restraints were being abandoned and replaced by a strong faith in rational behavior. Universally valid principles governing humanity, nature and society directed people's lives and interpersonal relationships.

The changing ethic of work added a rich ingredient to this new, heady brew. Fundamental was Martin Luther's viewpoint, which declared that everyone who could work should do so. Illness and begging were unnatural. Charity should be extended only to those who could not work because of mental or physical infirmities or old age.

John Calvin added to these ideas. Although he was a theologian, he expressed a number of ideas from which contemporary capitalism sprang. Production, trade and profit were encouraged. Work was to be disciplined, rigorous, methodical and rational. There was no room for luxuries or any activities that softened the soul. deGrazia summed up this period: "Once man worked for a livelihood, to be able to live. Now he worked for something beyond his daily bread. He worked because somehow it was the right or moral thing to do."[2] By the late 1800s much of work had become a calling.

MORAL TREATMENT

Near the center of all of this invigorating change was the treatment of sick people, particularly the **mentally ill** (those with diseases and conditions causing mental impairment). Whereas long-term survivors of physical disease with physical disabilities were still rare because treatment was so inadequate, the mentally ill were a significant portion of the population.

Up to this time the insane had been housed and handled no differently than criminals and paupers and were often chained in dungeons. Moral treatment of the insane was one product of the Age of Enlightenment. It sprang from the fundamental attitudes of the day: a set of principles that govern humanity and society; faith in the ability of the human to reason; purposeful work as a moral obligation; and the supreme belief in the individual. Fast disappearing were the centuries old notions that the insane were possessed of demons; that they were no better than paupers or criminals; that crime, sin, vice and inactivity were the core of insanity.

Two men of the 18th century working in different countries, and unknown to each other, initiated the moral treatment movement. These two could not have been more dissimilar. Phillippe Pinel was a child of the French Revolution, a physician, a scholar, and a natural philosopher. William Tuke was an English merchant, wealthy, a deeply religious Quaker and a philanthropist.

Father of Moral Treatment—Phillippe Pinel

According to Pinel, moral treatment meant treating the emotions. He believed the emotionally disturbed individual was out of balance and the patient's own emotions could be used to restore equilibrium. The compassionate Pinel believed the loss of reason was the most calamatous of all human afflictions. The ability to reason, he claimed, principally separates the human from other living forms. As Pinel wrote in his famous treatise in 1806, because of mental illness, the human's "...character is always perverted, sometimes annihilated. His thoughts and actions are diverted...His personal liberty is at length taken from him...to this melancholy train of symptoms, if not early and judiciously treated...a state of most abject degradation sooner or later succeeds."[3]

Some medical historians believe Pinel was stating that moral treatment was synonymous with humane care. His writings do not bear out this assumption. He strongly believed that each patient must be critically observed and analyzed before treatment is begun. The moral method is well reasoned and carefully planned for the individual patient. Pinel's biographer, Mackler, describes moral treatment as

> ...combined gentleness with firmness. It meant giving each patient as much liberty as he could manage, but it also taught him respect for authority. Firmness was necessary at times, but no harm must come to the patient. Moral treatment meant an unvarying routine which was necessary to maintain the patient's feeling of security and respect for authority. These would help him gain control over his emotions.[4]

Occupation figured prominently in Pinel's scheme, primarily to take patients' minds away from emotional distress and to develop their abilities. Music and various forms of literature were used. Physical exercise and work were a part of institutional living. Pinel advocated patient farms on the hospital grounds. This period was largely an agricultural era, where one's life revolved around producing products necessary for survival and one's emotional content was elaborately interwoven. The care of animals and the necessary routines of growing crops provided patients with a respect for the authority of nature and yet with as much liberty as could be tolerated. The unvarying routine to maintain farming as part of the institution made a strong appeal to moral concepts, such as respect, self-esteem and dignity for the patient.

The York Retreat—William Tuke

During this same time, English society was in ferment. Gossip about King George III, who was giving the American colonies "fits," suggested that he was in similar trouble; he was said to be possessed by mania. While some questioned his right to rule, including close relatives, the general public sympathized with the king.

Part of this new humane concern was influenced by the beliefs and work of the **Society of Friends,** derisively known as the Quakers. They emerged in 17th century England and became one of the most distinctive movements of Puritanism. In the last decades of the 18th century, William Tuke and various members of his family established The York Retreat, primarily because of their religious-based concerns about the deplorable conditions in public insane **asylums.** Until this time, the term *retreat* had never been applied to an asylum. Tuke's daughter-in-law suggested the term to convey the Quaker belief that such an institution may be ". . .a place in which the unhappy might obtain refuge, a quiet haven in which (one). . .might find a means of reparation or of safety."[5]

Several fundamental principles became evident within a short time. The approach was primarily one of kindness and consideration. The patients were not thought to be devoid of reason or feelings or honor. The social environment was to be as nearly like that of a family with an atmosphere of religious sentiment and moral feeling. Tuke and Thomas Fowler, the visiting physician, believed that most insane people retain a considerable amount of self-command. The staff endeavored to gain the patient's confidence, to reinforce self-esteem, and to arrest the attention and fix it on objects that are opposite to the illusions the patient might possess.

Employment in various occupations was expected as a way for the patient to maintain control over his or her disorder. As Tuke reported

> . . .regular employment is perhaps the most efficacious; and those kinds of employment. . .to be preferred. . .are accompanied by considerable bodily actions; that are most agreeable to the patient; and

> which are most opposite to the illusions of his disease.[5]

The Retreat staff came to realize that inactivity

> . . .has a natural tendency to weaken the mind, and to induce (boredom) and discontent. . .(therefore) every kind of rational and innocent employment is encouraged. Those who are not engaged in any useful occupation, are allowed to read, write, draw, play at ball, chess, etc.[5]

Because of Quaker beliefs, patients were specifically not allowed to play for money or participate in gaming of any kind.

Occupations and amusements were prescribed to elicit emotions opposite to those of the disorder. For instance, the melancholy patient was introduced to the more active and exciting kinds of activities, and the patient with mania was encouraged to engage in sedentary tasks. The writing of poetry and essays was occasionally used; however, this activity was closely monitored so that such writings did not reinforce or continue undesirable behavior. When writing was used it was found ". . .to give the patients temporary satisfaction and make them more easily led into suitable engagements."[5]

Other activities included mathematics and natural science. These disciplines were thought to be most useful, since they had a kinship to everyday work and could be applied to other pursuits within The Retreat or after patients were released. It was believed that they helped bring back more normal patterns of thinking and attention. The **habit of attention** (Tuke's phrase) was a key element in the use of occupations. Tuke realized the various kinds of concentration required to perform a variety of tasks helped limit undesirable stimuli. Thus, work was broken into components, which were used to limit undesirable thoughts and to expand positive feelings.

The pioneer work of the Tuke family opened a new chapter in the history of the care of the insane in England and, eventually, in the United States. Mild management methods, infused with kindness and the building of self-esteem through the judicious use of occupations and amusements, brought forth more desirable behavior. Patients recovered and rarely needed to return for further care.

Pinel's major work on moral treatment was published in 1801 and Tuke's description of The Retreat appeared in 1813. These brought on a rush of reforms in institutions in Europe and, ultimately, the United States.

Sir William and Lady Ellis

Sir William Charles Ellis and his wife were in charge of newly founded county asylums in England during the first half of the 19th century. They regarded the hospital as a community—"a family," as Sir Ellis called it. He paid little attention to medical remedies and concentrated on moral treatment principles, which he believed to be difficult but most likely to result in the "gradual return to reason and happiness." Lady Ellis carried the title of *workwoman,* and she organized female patients in classes to make useful and fancy articles, which were sold at fairs and bazaars. Men were encouraged to follow their own trades or to learn new ones from tradesmen employed by the institution. As Hunter and Macalpine report:

> *Ellis and his wife. . .proved there was less danger of injury from putting the spade and hoe into the hands of a large proportion of insane persons, than from shutting them up together in idleness, under the guards of straps, strait-waistcoats, or chains.*[6]

A remarkable innovation of Sir and Lady Ellis was the establishment of **after-care houses** and night hospitals. Keenly aware of environmental and social influences on insanity, they envisioned these halfway houses ". . .as stepping-stones from the asylum to the world by which the length of patients' stay would be reduced and in many cases completed. . .to go out and mix with the world before their discharge."[6]

Moral Treatment in the United States

The roots of moral care and occupations as treatment were brought to the United States by the Quakers. They established asylums and immediately implemented the Tuke's programs. The programs were popular because they helped maintain relatively low costs by having patients perform most of the necessary work of the asylum: growing crops and vegetables, maintaining herds, and manufacturing clothing and other goods. The typical institution was a beehive of activity largely designed to help it remain as self-sufficient as possible.

Reformers were in abundance. Borrowing heavily from the York Retreat, Thomas Eddy, a member of the board of governors of the Society of the New York Hospital, proposed in 1815 the construction of a building for exclusive use by mental patients.[7] He envisioned a balanced program of exercise, entertainment and occupations. Patients

> *. . .should freely partake of bodily exercises, walking, riding, conversations, innocent sports, and a variety of other amusements. . . .Those kinds of employments are to be preferred, both on a moral and physical account which are accompanied by considerable action most aggreeable to the patient and most opposite to the illusion of his disease.*[7]

In the mid 1800s, just when it seemed that the moral movement was expected to be fully realized, unanticipated trouble came from all directions. A reform-minded humanitarian, Dorthea Lynde Dix, had been campaigning vigorously for better care of the mentally ill, including moral principles. State legislatures were responding positively by establishing public mental hospitals. By 1848 Dix decided to approach the Federal government. Her vision was the establishment of a federal system of hospitals. After six years of wearying work, Dix was rewarded when Congress passed her bill. President Franklin Pierce, however, vetoed it, claiming states' rights would be endangered if the federal government took on the care of mentally ill patients. How differently our institutional system would be today if the Dix bill had been signed.

State hospitals were experiencing great difficulties with new types of patients: immigrants from Europe who were unable to adjust to the new conditions. They became public wards, often unable to use the language, and were considered unemployable. Several hospitals attempted to introduce moral principles, even establishing English instruction. The Bloomingdale, New York, Asylum made such an attempt in 1845. Classes were also held in chemistry, geometry and the physical sciences. These classes were coupled with manual labor suitable for men and women. This approach eventually failed for many reasons. Patients often were unaccustomed to the American forms of labor. Bilingual instructors could not be found. Foreign-born mechanics and artisans could not find familiar labor. Finally, large numbers of patients were too ill to participate in the available occupations.[7]

By the mid 1800s, the American agenda largely consisted of expansionism and slavery issues. These did not bode well for improving or increasing public care of the insane. Moral treatment, including occupations, rapidly began to disappear. By the onset of the Civil War, virtually none existed in state or public-supported institutions. Custodial care continued well into the 20th century. According to Bockhoven,[8] moral treatment disappeared because 1) the founders of the US movement retired and died, leaving no disciples or successors; 2) the rapid increase in foreign-born and poor patients greatly overtaxed existing facilities and required the construction of more institutions with diminished tax support; 3) racial and religious prejudices on the part of alienists (soon to be named psychiatrists) reduced interest in humane treatment and care; 4) state legislatures became increasingly more interested in less costly custodial care; 5) trained personnel were in short supply; and 6) the incurability of insanity became a dominant belief. Deutsch quotes one eminent psychiatrist in the latter decades of the 19th century: "I have come to the conclusion that when a man becomes insane, he is about used up for this world."[9]

20TH CENTURY PROGRESSIVISM

The 20th century brought with it unparalleled exuberance. The United States had largely recovered from the Civil War and acquired considerable overseas possessions as a result of the Spanish-American War. For a few years before 1900 and for some years after, nearly all Americans had become ardent believers in progress, although they did not always agree about what the word meant. Historians generally agree that *progressivism* resulted from the realization in America of the Age of Enlightenment. Prosperity was fueled by science and technology and with a flurry of industrial inventions. Cities grew rapidly, particularly in the East and Middle West. Railroads punched their way through all kinds of barriers, and in all directions, linking the country's population. The newly invented automobile served important economic purposes and became useful in leisure pursuits, with opportunities to escape the inherent stress of change. Bates describes the era of progressivism:

> *Conditions of prosperity deeply affected the tone of American life. The hope and buoyancy were extraordinary. Indeed, the attitude of Americans on many subjects can hardly be appreciated apart from the facts of prosperity and promise of more to come. . . .Seldom in history had a country experienced so much activity, so many diversions and (apparent) opportunities.*[10]

There was more than a modest amount of zaniness during this era. Many physicians regarded increased female education as the primary cause of decreased women's health. These men felt the woman's brain simply could not assimilate a great deal of academic instruction beyond high school. Some physicians went further and claimed that women who worked were in danger of acquiring predominantly male afflictions—alcoholism, paralysis, and insanity. Women were thought to have an inborn immunity to such ills.

Drug therapy was also unusual by today's standards. The pharmaceutical firm that helped to usher in the aspirin craze introduced a new medication for bad coughs—heroin. Other across-the-counter products included cocaine tablets for the throat and general nervousness. Baby syrups were spiked with morphine, and miscarriage-producing pills, according to the ads, were a sure and great remedy for married ladies.

The Progressive Era was not always progressive. Poverty, racial injustice, ethnic unrest, sterilization of *mental defectives* (as they were known) and possible sterilization of social misfits, repression of women's rights because of leftover Victorian ideals, a marked increase in industrial accidents resulting in chronic disabilities, and a continued lack of concern about the institutionalized insane were all part of the times.

One significant feature was the emergence of an aristocracy, which came from successes in trade, industry and land acquistion. Many of the offspring of the new aristocracy, particularly women who did not marry and bear children, dedicated themselves to public service. Few of these women pursued nursing, since it was unseemly to deal with bodily fluids and excrement and the unsavory conditions surrounding illness and disease. Rather, they chose social work and, ultimately, occupational therapy because of the inherent status gained from accomplishing good work.

As one might expect from all the contradictory activity, several movements arose in this period of relative prosperity: individualism versus nationalism, racial justice versus nativism, women's rights versus men's rights, labor versus management, social justice, conservation. Bates concluded: "Much of life seemed to be changing. Somehow the old and new struggled to reach a new synthesis."[10] Two major emphases finally emerged from progressivism: a belief in freedom or the restoration of individual freedom, and the creation of a positive state wherein the government was expected to provide a variety of services to its citizens.

Chicago's Hull House

Social experiments abounded during this period, particularly in urban areas. One such experiment was Hull House, opened by Jane Addams in 1889. Hull House was intended to serve the immigrants and the poor through a variety of educational, social, and investigative programs. Along with Julia Lathrop and Florence Kelley, Addams created an environment that helped bring occupational therapy to the forefront, as a part of the restorative process of individual freedom. Eleanor Clarke Slagle, a pioneer in occupational therapy, spent two periods as a staff member at Hull House and established the first training program for occupation workers (the forerunner of occupational therapy personnel).

Invalid Occupations—Susan Tracy

The first individual in the 20th century to use occupations with acutely ill patients was Susan Tracy, a nurse. She initiated instruction in activities to student nurses as early as 1902. She coined the term **occupational nurse** to signify a specialization. By 1912 she was working full-time to apply moral treatment principles to acute medical conditions. She was convinced that remedial activities ". . .are classified according to their physiological effects as stimulants, sedatives, anesthetics. . . .Certain occupations possess like properties."[11] Tracy was also interested in experimentation and observation to enhance her practice. In 1918 she published a research paper on 25 mental tests derived from occupations. For example, by instructing the patient in using a piece of leather and a pencil, ". . .require him to make a line of dots at equal distances around the margin and at uniform distances from the edge. This constitutes a test of judgment in estimating distances."[12] Continuing with the same piece of leather, the patient is instructed to punch a hole at each dot. To do this, the patient must consider the two sides of leather and the two parts of the tool and must bring these together, thus making a *simple construction* test.[12]

Tracy determined that high-quality work was therapeutic. "It is now believed that what is worth doing at all is worth doing well and that practical, well-made articles have a greater therapeutic value than useless, poorly made articles."[13] Tracy's major work, *Studies in Invalid Occupations,* published in 1918, is a revealing compendium of her observations and experiences with different kinds of patients.[14] Among her many lasting principles, one stands out: "The patient is the product, not the article he makes."[15]

Reeducation of Convalescents— George Barton

The Progressive Era spawned a number of reformers who, although dissimilar in background, character and temperament, strove to work together on common goals. Two individuals significant to occupational therapy were George Edward Barton and William Rush Dunton, Jr. Barton, by profession an architect, contracted tuberculosis during adulthood. His constant struggle led him into a life of service to physically disabled persons.

Barton founded Consolation House in Clifton Springs, New York, in 1914, an early prototype of a rehabilitation center. Today he would be considered an entrepreneur. He was an effective speaker and writer, although often given to exaggeration. Barton's main themes were hospitals and their responsibilites to the discharged patient, the conditions the discharged patient faces, the need to return to employment after an illness, and occupations and **reeducation** of convalescents.

Barton's first published article in 1914 was based on a speech given to a group of nurses, in which he described a weakness in hospitals: "We discharge them not efficients, but inefficients. An individual leaves almost any of our institutions only to become a burden upon his family, his friends, the associated charities, or upon another institution."[16] Later in the article he warms to his subject: "I say to discharge a patient from the hospital, with his fracture healed, to be sure, but to a devestated home, to an empty desk, and to no obvious sustaining employment, is to send him out to a world cold and bleak. . ." His solution: ". . .occupation would shorten convalescence and improve the condition of many patients." He ended his oration with a rallying cry: ". . .It is time for humanity to cease regarding the hospital as a door closing upon a life which is past and to regard it henceforth as a door opening upon a life which is to come."[17]

At Consolation House, physically impaired individuals underwent a thorough review, including a social and medical history, and a consideration of their education, training, experience, successes, and failures. Barton believed that ". . .by considering these in relation to the condition (the patient) must presumably or inevitably be in for the remainder of his life, we can find some form of occupation for which he will be fitted."[18]

The word reeducation was firmly a part of Barton's terminology after World War I. He believed that hospitals should become reeducation institutions for the war-wounded to return the veteran to his rightful place in society. He declared: ". . .By a catalystic concatenation of contiguous circumstances we were forced to realize that when all is said and done, what the sick man really needed and wanted most was the restoration of his ability to work, to live independently, and to make money."[17]

Barton's major contribution to the reemergence of moral treatment principles was an awakening of physical reconstruction and reeducation through employment. Convalescence, to him was a critical time for the inclusion of something to do. Activity

> *. . .clarifies and strengthens the mind by increasing and maintaining interest in wholesome thought to the exclusion of morbid thought. . .and a proper occupation during convalescence may be made the basis. . .of a new life upon recovery. . .I mean [a job, a better job, or a job done better] than it was before.[18]*

Judicious Regimen of Activity— William Dunton

A medical school graduate of the University of Pennsylvania and a psychiatrist, William Rush Dunton, Jr., devoted his entire life to occupational therapy. A prolific writer, he published in excess of 120 books and articles related to occupational therapy and rehabilitation. He also served as treasurer and president of The National Society for the Promotion of Occupational Therapy (the forerunner of The American Occupational Therapy Association), and for 21 years he was editor of the official journal. As a physician, he spent his professional career treating psychiatric patients in an institutional setting. Key to his treatment methods was what he called a *judicious regimen of activity.* He read the works of Tuke and Pinel, as well as the efforts of significant alienists (an early term for psychiatrists) of the 19th century.

In 1895, Dunton joined the medical staff at Sheppard and Enoch Pratt Asylum in Towson, Maryland. From his readings and observations of patients there he concluded that acutely ill patients generally were not amenable to occupations because their weakened attention span would make involvement in activity fatiguing and harmful. Later, activities might be prescribed that use energies not needed for physical restoration. Stimulating attention and directing the thoughts of the patient in regular and healthful paths would ensure an early discharge from the hospital. Dunton developed a wide variety of activities from knitting and crocheting to printing, the repair of dynamos, and farm work to gain the attention and interest, as well as to meet needs, of all patients. He stated it this way: "It has been found that a patient makes more rapid progress if his attention is concentrated upon what he is making and he derives stimulating pleasure in its performance."[19] **Interest** in the activity was paramount in Dunton's thinking. He wrote:

> By "interest" is meant the state of consiousness in which the attention is attracted to a task, accompanied by a more or less pleasurable emotional state. It is believed that attention, as distinguished from interest, lacks the emotional content or accompaniment. That is, an emotion is produced by the performance of a task, motor action, or by sensory stimulus. . . .As yet there are no studies which tell us why or how certain desires or emotions are created by auditory, visual, or other stimuli.[20]

At the second annual meeting of the National Society for the Promotion of Occupational Therapy in 1918, Dunton unveiled his nine cardinal principles to guide the emerging practice of occupational therapy and to ensure that the new discipline would gain acceptance as a medical entity. These principles were the following:[21]

1. Any activity should have as its objective a cure.
2. The activity should be interesting.
3. There should be a useful purpose other than to merely gain the patient's attention and interest.
4. The activity should preferably lead to an increase in knowledge on the patient's part.
5. Activity should be carried on with others, such as a group.
6. The occupational therapist should make a careful study of the patient and attempt to meet as many needs as possible through activity.
7. Activity should cease before the onset of fatigue.
8. Genuine encouragement should be given whenever indicated.
9. Work is much to be preferred over idleness, even when the end product of the patient's labor is of poor quality or is useless.

The major purposes of occupation in the case of the mentally ill were outlined in Dunton's first book, *Occupation Therapy: A Manual for Nurses*, published in 1915.[22] The primary objective is to divert attention either from unpleasant subjects, as is true with the depressed patient, or from daydreaming or mental ruminations, as in the case of dementia praecox (schizophrenia)—that is, to divert the attention to one main subject.

Another purpose of occupation is to reeducate—to train the patient in developing mental processes through ". . .educating the hands, eyes, muscles, just as is done in the developing child."[22] Fostering an interest in hobbies is a third purpose. Hobbies serve as present and future safety valves and render a recurrence of mental illness less likely. A final purpose may be to instruct the patient in a craft until he or she has enough proficiency to take pride in the work. However, Dunton noted: "While this is proper, I fear. . .specialism is apt to cause a narrowing of one's mental outlook. . . .The individual with a knowledge of many things has more interest in the world in general."[22]

The Origin of the Term *Occupational Therapy*

There is a continuing controversy about who was initially responsible for the term *occupational therapy*—Dunton or Barton. At Sheppard and Enoch Pratt Asylum, Dunton directed the therapeutic occupations program. A special building was completed in 1902 and named The Casino. It was dedicated space for a wide variety of occupations and amusements. In 1911, Dunton initiated a training program for nurses in patient occupations, and here he first used the term *occupation therapy*. This term appeared in his handwritten lecture notes, dated October 10, 1911. This is the earliest known record of the use of this term. In later years Dunton indicated that Adolph Meyer, a renowned psychiatrist and personal and professional friend, was the first to use the term *therapy* and *therapeutic* in connection with occupations; but that he was the first person to put *occupation* and *therapy* together as one phrase.

Barton's claim to the first use of the term appeared initially in March, 1915, in *The Trained Nurse and Hospital Review*.[23] The article was based on a speech given in Massachusetts on December 28, 1914. Before then, Barton had preferred the term *occupation reeducation*, which accurately described his efforts at Consolation House. During preliminary discussions between Barton and Dunton about a national organization, during 1915 to 1916, a series of squabbles took place, mostly through correspondence. Terminology figured heavily in these differences of opinion. Barton preferred his *occupational reeducation* and Dunton held tenaciously to *occupation therapy*. Barton finally countered with *occupational therapy*, preferring the adjectival form. They did agree on the term *occupational workers*, since the word *therapist* was considered the sole property of the psychiatrist. Dunton did not change his mind until well into the 1920s.[23,24]

Habit Training—Eleanor Clarke Slagle

Eleanor Clarke Slagle is considered the most distinguished 20th century occupational therapist. One of five founders of the national professional organization, she served in every major elective office. She was also Executive Secretary for 14 years. In the first decade of this century, she was partially trained as a social worker and completed one of the early special courses in curative occupations and recreation at the Chicago School of Civics and Philanthropy, which was associated with Hull House. She worked subsequently in a number of institutions, most notably the new Henry Phipps Clinic, Johns Hopkins Hospital, in Baltimore, Maryland. There she served under the direction of the renowned psychiatrist, Adolf Meyer. At this same time, she became a devoted friend of William Dunton's family. Later, she moved to New York where she pioneered in developing occupational therapy in the State Department of Mental Hygiene.

Slagle was knowledgeable about moral treatment principles and embraced them as the core of her thinking and practice. She emphasized that occupational therapy must be a "...consciously planned, progressive program of rest, play, occupation, and exercise..."[25] She often spoke of the need for the mentally ill person to spend a fairly well-balanced day. In addition, she placed considerable emphasis on the personality of the therapist:

...the proper balance of qualities, proper physical expression, a kindly voice, gentleness, patience, ability and seeming vision, adaptability...to meet the particular needs of the individual patient in all things....Personality plus character also covers an ability to be honest and firm, with infinite kindness.[26]

Her most long-lasting contribution to the care of the mentally ill was what she entitled *habit training*. This plan was first attempted at the Rochester, New York State Hospital in 1901, but it was Slagle who developed and refined the basic principles for those patients who had been hospitalized for five to 20 years and whose behavior had steadily regressed. Habit training was 24 hours long and involved the entire ward staff. It was a reeducation program designed to overcome disorganized habits, to modify other habits, and to construct new ones, with the goal of restoring and maintaining of health. She declared: "In habit training, we show...the necessity of requiring attention, of building on the habit of attention—attention thus becomes application, voluntary and, in time, agreeable."[26]

A typical habit training schedule called for patients to arise at 6:00 A.M., wash, toilet, brush teeth, and air beds. After breakfast, they returned to the ward and made beds, and swept. Classwork followed and lasted for two hours. It consisted of a variety of simple crafts and marching exercises. After lunch, there was a rest period; continued classwork; and outdoor exercises, folk dancing, and lawn games. After supper, there was music and dancing on the ward, followed by toileting, washing, teeth brushing, and preparing for bed.[27]

After maximum benefit was achieved from habit training, the patient progressed through three phases of occupational therapy. The first was what Slagle called the *kindergarten group*. "We must show the ways of stimulating their special senses. The employment of color, music, simple exercises, games, and storytelling along with occupations, the gentle ways and means...(used) in educating the child are equally important in reeducating the adult."[26] Occupations were graded from simple to complex. The next phase was *ward classes in occupational therapy*: "...graded to the limit of accomplishment of individual patients."[28] When able to tolerate it, the patient joined in group activities. The third phase was *the occupational center*. "This promotes opportunities for more advanced projects...a complete change in environment; ...comparative freedom; ...actual responsibilities placed upon patients; the stimulation of seeing work produced; ...all these carry forward the readjustment of patients."[28]

In 1922 Slagle summarized her philosophy as follows:

Of the highest value to patients is the psychological fact that the patient is working for himself....Occupational therapy recognizes the significance of the mental attitude which the sick person takes toward illness and attempts to make that attitude more wholesome by providing activities adapted to the capacity of the individual and calculated to divert his attention from his own problems.[26]

Further, she declared: "It is directed activity, and differs from all other forms of treatment in that it is given in increasing doses as the patient improves."[29]

Figure 1-1 shows Eleanor Clarke Slagle (standing) when she was the Director of Occupational Therapy at the New York Department of Mental Hygiene. She is inspecting the weaving of a woolen rug by Mrs. Margaret Kransee, instructor at the Manhattan State Hospital, Wards Island, in 1933.

THE PHILOSOPHY OF OCCUPATION THERAPY— ADOLPH MEYER

A history of this type would not be complete without at least a brief mention of Adolph Meyer, a Swiss physician who immigrated to this country in 1892. By the end of 1910 he became professor of psychiatry at Johns Hopkins University and the first director of the Henry Phipps Clinic. Meyer "borrowed" Eleanor Clarke Slagle from Hull House for two years, during which time she founded the therapeutic occupations program in the clinic. Meyer's lasting contribution to psychiatry is the psychobiologic approach to mental illness and health. He coined this term to indicate that the human is an indivisible unit of study, rather than a composite of symptoms: "Psychobiology starts not from the mind *and* body or from elements, but from the fact that we deal with biologically organized units and groups and their functioning...the 'hes' and 'shes' of our experience—the bodies we find in action"[30] (see Chapter 6).

Meyer's commonsense approach to the problems of living was his keynote:

> *The main thing is that your point of reference should always be life itself....As long as there is life there are positive assets—action, choice, hope, not in the imagination but in the clear understanding of the situation, goals, and possibilities....To see life as it is, is one of the fundamentals of my philosophy...*[31]

Because of his friendship with Slagle and Dunton, Meyer agreed to deliver a major address at the Fifth Annual Meeting of the National Society for the Promotion of Occupational Therapy in Baltimore, October, 1921. This address has become a classic in occupational therapy literature. Meyer emphasized occupation, time, and the productive use of energy. He stated:

> *The whole of human organization has its shape in a kind of rhythm....There are many...rhythms which we must be attuned to: the larger rhythms of night and day, of sleep and waking hours...and finally the big four—work and play and rest and sleep, which our organisim must be able to balance even under difficulty. The only way to attain balance in all this is actual doing, actual practice, a program of wholesome living is the basis of wholesome feeling and thinking and fancy and interests.*[32]

In this address, Meyer successfully brought the fundamental moral treatment principles of more than a century before into contemporary occupational therapy practice, and established the foundation of what now is known as **occupational behavior,** the *Model of Human Occupation* and *occupational performance* (see Chapters 3 and 4).

FOUNDING OF THE AMERICAN OCCUPATIONAL THERAPY ASSOCIATION

The American Occupational Therapy Association (AOTA) archives hold all of the correspondence between George Barton and William Dunton and, later, Eleanor Clarke Slagle, during the era when discussions were held about creating a national organization[33] to be a mechanism for exchanging views and extending information about the fledgling "new line of medicine." The first letter in the series was from Dunton to Barton on October 15, 1915, wherein he suggested that Barton take the lead in organizing

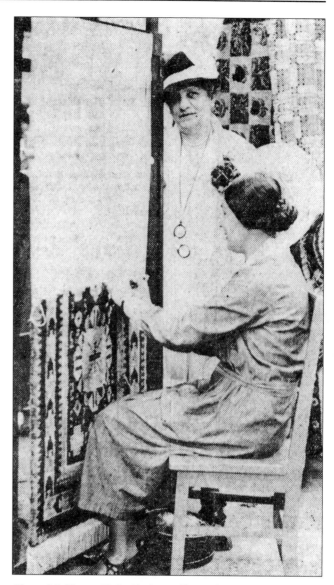

Figure 1-1. Eleanor Clarke Slagle (standing) and Margaret Kransee, 1933. (From personal archives. Robert K. Bing.)

"a central bureau for occupation workers." Barton wrote back, agreed, and suggested a title, Society for the Promotion of Occupation for Reeducation. A series of false starts ensued and Dunton became exasperated with the lack of progress. Local groups of occupation workers were forming to exchange views, and he felt they needed support and guidance from a national group. On December 7, 1916, Dunton wrote Barton again, proposing a five-member national executive committee. Disagreements between the two arose about who should be invited. They were settled on December 20, 1916, when Barton wrote Dunton with a new title, National Society for the Promotion of Occupational Therapy.

After some juggling of dates, March 15-17 were set for the organizational meeting and incorporation of the Society. Barton invited the "big five," as he called the executive committee, to use his Consolation House for the event, as he wished to be host. The invitees, other than Dunton, included Eleanor Clarke Slagle, then the General Superintendent of Occupational Therapy at Hull House; Susan Cox Johnson, the Director of Occupations, New York State Department of Public Charities; and Thomas B. Kidner, the Vocational Secretary, Canadian Military Hospital Commission. Susan E. Tracy, Instructor in Invalid Occupations, Presbyterian Hospital, Chicago, was also invited but declined because of her work schedule. Isabelle Newton, Barton's secretary at Consolation House, was invited to attend in that capacity (Figure 1-2). Barton was elected President, a position he nominated himself for a few weeks before the meeting.

The next six months proved critical. Barton became increasingly annoyed at Dunton and Slagle, who was Vice President. He suspected they were trying to overshadow his presidency. He also became involved in a heated debate about finances with Dunton, the Treasurer. Subsequently, Barton refused to attend the first annual meeting on Labor Day weekend, September, 1917, in New York City. He cited poor health. Dunton was elected the new President. There is no record that Barton attended any meetings of the national organization for the remainder of his life; however, he did remain a member.[34]

OCCUPATIONAL THERAPY'S CREED

To solidify and publicize the fundamental principles of occupational therapy a Pledge and Creed was developed in 1925 and adopted by the AOTA the next year.[35] The efforts toward developing a creed began in late 1924 when Marjorie B. Greene, Dean, Boston School of Occupational Therapy

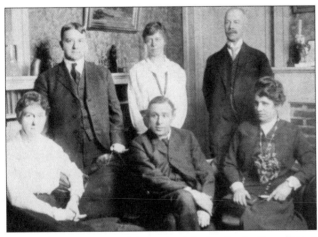

Figure 1-2. The founders of the National Society for the Promotion of Occupational Therapy. Front Row L-R: Susan Cox Johnson, George E. Barton, Eleanor Clarke Slagle. Back Row L-R: William R. Dunton, Isabel Newton, Thomas Kidner.

wrote the Association's President, Thomas B. Kidner, seeking his counsel in modifying the Pledge and Creed originally created by *Modern Hospital* and adopted by the American Hospital Association in early 1924. She indicated: "This sums up so splendidly the spirit of service and the outstanding factors of our work that we too (presumably the Boston School) are most anxious to adopt it." In due time, Dean Greene, with suggestions from Eleanor Clarke Slagle, William Dunton, and Thomas Kidner developed the desired modifications. It was adopted by AOTA at the tenth annual meeting in Atlantic City in 1926. It remains today, just as it was approved more than 60 years ago, although there have been some discussions about revising it.[36]

Pledge and Creed for Occupational Therapists

REVERENTLY AND EARNESTLY do I pledge my whole-hearted service in aiding those crippled in mind and body;

TO THIS END that my work for the sick may be successful, I will ever strive for greater knowledge, skill, and understanding in the discharge of my duties in whatsoever position I may find myself;

I SOLEMNLY DECLARE that I will hold and keep inviolate whatever I may learn of the lives of the sick;

I ACKNOWLEDGE the dignity of the cure of disease and the safeguarding of health in which no act is menial or inglorious;

I WILL WALK in upright faithfulness and obedience to those under whose guidance I am to work in the holy ministry to broken minds and bodies.

The 1925 Principles

A committee of AOTA, made up of physicians and chaired by William Rush Dunton, Jr., compiled an outline of lectures on occupational therapy for medical students and physicians.[37] The members developed a definition, objectives, statements of the use of a variety of activities with different kinds of patients, therapeutic approaches, and the qualities and qualifications of practitioners. This was the first such effort since Dunton had created his principles in 1918.[21]

The first principle states: "Occupational therapy is a method of training the sick or injured by means of instruction and employment in productive occupation."[37] One is struck by the importance of the connection between learning by doing and purposeful activity. This was the dominant theme in several of the principles. The act of doing should be seen from the patient's point of view. For example, the treatment objectives stated: "...sought are to arouse interest, courage, and confidence; to exercise mind and body on healthy activity; to overcome disability; and to re-establish capacity for industrial and social usefulness."[37]

Rules were established about the extent of activities, and attention was given to their qualities and effect on the patient. The use of crafts and work-related occupations was emphasized. Games, music and physical exercise were not to be overlooked. "Novelty, variety, individuality, and utility of the products enhance the value of an occupation as a treatment measure."[37] A warning was offered: whereas quality, quantity and salability may serve some objectives, these must not override the main purpose of the activity. Belief in the various properties of occupation is evident in the statement: "As the patient's strength and capability increase, the type and extent of occupation should be regulated and graded accordingly."[37]

The committee made a statement about the quality of work to be expected as a therapeutic approach: ". . .inferior workmanship or employment in an occupation which would be trivial for the healthy, may be (used) with the greatest benefit to the sick or injured, but standards worthy of entirely normal persons must be maintained for proper mental stimulation."[37]

The relationship between purposeful activity and the connections between the mind and body is found in this principle: "The production of a well-made. . .article, or the accomplishment of a useful task, requires healthy exercise of mind and body, gives the greatest satisfaction, and thus produces the most beneficial effects."[37] Involvement in group activity is advised ". . .because it provides exercise in social adaptation. . ."[37] The importance of occupational therapy is evident in the statement: ". . .the treatment should be prescribed and administered under constant medical advice and supervision, and correlated with the other treatment of the patient."[37] In regard to application it was stated: ". . .system and precision are as important as in other forms of treatment."[37] Evaluation rests with measuring the effect of the occupation on the patient, the extent to which objectives are being realized.

One final principle addresses the qualifications of the practitioner: "Good craftsmanship. . .ability to instruct. . .understanding, sincere interest in the patient, and an optimistic, cheerful outlook and manner. . .are essential."[37] Elsewhere in the lecture outline, the committee recommended that therapists and aides should have ". . .a therapeutic sense, the teaching instinct, and good mental balance. Personality constitutes 50 percent of the value of these workers."[37]

During this period, a number of issues were combined, including the following:

1. Purposeful work and leisure
2. The intricate involvement of the mind and body (interdependence of mental and physical aspects, also known as holism)
3. Occupational therapy as a learning process
4. The therapeutic use of one's personal qualities

The literature of the next several decades, which was a period of remarkable development in the profession, gives evidence of how these principles became operational.

Purposeful Work and Leisure. In her early endeavors as a practitioner, Clare Spackman explored the perplexing problem of engaging the patient's interests.[38] "One of the therapist's problems is in approaching the patient who refuses occupational therapy; yet, he is often the one who needs it the most. Many patients scorn occupational therapy as being child's play or beneath their dignity, or are frankly uninterested and apathetic. . ."[38] Her recommendation was to approach the patient through his or her interests. "There are few people who have not some interest and to make the right suggestion at the right time takes both experience and imagination."[38] Spackman advised: "The therapist's greatest danger in her approach is failure to make first contacts. . .sufficiently vital. Being in a hurry, and a tendency to consider only the physical motion necessary is her greatest pitfall. The need of psychological treatment. . .is as necessary as any other."[38]

Martha Gilbert, an occupational therapist at the Choctaw-Chickasaw Sanitorium in Oklahoma built her entire treatment program around purposeful work and leisure for children.[39] The sanitarium was a federal institution with 75 beds for Indian children with tuberculosis and related diseases. In 1929, times were difficult, not only because of the Great Depression, but also because Indian children were not highly valued, except by those who cared for them on a daily basis.

Gilbert developed her comprehensive program of appealing activities that activated the interest and attention of her patients. She reported:

> *Supplies for craftwork were very meager but the children were eager to learn, loved to draw and march to music and do calesthenics to. . .records. There was no playground apparatus but long walks were permitted and. . .after supper (there) was often a hunt for wild flowers or for nuts and wild berries.*[39]

For handwork, she used native materials to ". . .fashion objects of interest. . . .In summer, clay from the hillsides; in fall leaves from the trees; and in winter, anything from paper dolls to hooked mats and rugs were fashioned. . ."[39] Gilbert and her patients also cultivated a garden out of the barren, wind-driven soil. The more able patients transported creek bottom soil in small cans and jars. They formed a "bucket brigade" and kept the plants alive during harsh weather. "We harvested our peanuts with much gusto, used them in candy-making and picked our flowers to adorn the shops and schoolroom."[39]

The children's cultural background was an important part of her treatment program. "We try to make much of the (various) holidays; we invent a game to use with our Indian puppets or try a health or ceremonial play or pageant to give us an excuse for 'dressing up.' "[39]

Gilbert's approach may be seen today, as therapists and assistants carry out innovative and imaginative programs in impoverished areas of the United States, and indeed, throughout the world.

Involvement of the Mind and Body.   In 1927, Ida Sands, the chief occupational therapist at Philadelphia General Hospital addressed the AOTA annual conference.[40] She stated that occupations are curative through three spheres:

Occupational therapy, through carefully selected and graded work, develops resistance: 1) spiritually, by keeping up self-respect and developing ambition and initiative; 2) mentally, by developing coordination and mental poise; and 3) physically, by developing weak muscles through adapted occupation.[40]

She defended the importance of spirituality in occupations in this way:

I have put spiritual rehabilitation first because it is often a delicate process. This form of rehabilitation is approached by the occupational therapist through understanding; . . .that subtle quality which enables a person to estimate the needs and. . .possibilities of another.[40]

The interaction of mind and body has remained a basic principle throughout our historical evolution. Beatrice Wade, a renowned clinician, educator and administrator, spoke of the treatment of the total patient in an address in 1967.[41] She stated: "This approach is unique to occupational therapy among the. . .health disciplines. . . .There has always existed a strong component concerned with the behavior of the physically ill or disabled, as well as the mentally sick; with the entirety of man and his functioning as a patient."[41] This occupational therapy concept, she continued, ". . .prevented (as has occurred in medical practice) an undesired separation of the psychiatric therapist from those who develop knowledge and skills centered in the treatment of the physically disabled."[41] Stated another way:

The major emphasis in occupational therapy is not the body as such but the individual as such. The therapist's background is strongly weighed in an understanding of personality adjustment and reactions to social situations. . .and in the patient's attitudes toward an adjustment to acute and chronic disabilities.[42]

Occupational Therapy as a Learning Process.   Throughout the formative years, occupational therapy and education

held much in common, not so much in how patients were instructed, but, in the outcomes of that instruction through changes in behavior and performance of a more complex nature. Harriet Robeson, a distinguished therapist, addressed a group of social workers in 1926 and affirmed some longstanding principles:

Many think of occupational therapy as only hand-work. It is far more than that. (It) is a program of work, play, and medicine to meet the mental, physical, and social needs of each patient. It is reeducation.[43]

The reeducation process follows the same pathway as as normal education: ". . .a gradual growth through progressive development. . . .We must teach (the patient) to creep and to creep in the right direction."[43]

Robeson also faced the challenge of crafts being central to practice: "Handicrafts are only some of the tools with which we work, not primarily with the idea that patients will earn a future livelihood. . .but because since Adam people have found expression through work with their hands; a primitive outlet, creative, educative, constructive."[43] She went on to speak about physical and emotional functions and adaptation:

Crafts may also be adapted to meet nearly all needs in mental and physical adjustments. Movements required in physical restoration of function can be found in. . .various crafts. These same techniques can produce definite results in mental cases in substituting purposeful occupation for scattered and destructive activity. . .and ideational deterioration. Furthermore, crafts can meet all degrees of scholastic background and intelligence.[43]

(See Chapter 16 for more information on the historical and contemporary use of crafts.)

Irene O'Brock, director of occupational therapy at the University of Oklahoma Hospitals in 1932, indicated that her program for children had an ". . .additional value, a deeper more intangible significance: the natural tendencies of life, play, and companionship."[44] She based her treatment program on five **lines of readiness:** 1) to construct things, 2) to communicate things, 3) to find out things, 4) to compete in things, and 5) to excel in things. The first line of readiness included a workshop with tools and materials, such as wood, metal, textiles, clay, yarn, and the like. Books and magazines were also available. The second line of readiness, to communicate things, involved ". . .stories, music, dramatizations, songs, and pictures, . . .even making musical instruments. . ."[44] The third line, to find out things, involved ". . .occupations and natural phenomena of community life, such as the building of a dog house for a pet or digging a cave for the gang to meet in. Too, gardening is of great importance in the developing of a community spirit."[44] To compete in things, the fourth line of readiness, O'Brock had a playground and gym: "Competition does much to teach good sportsmanship. We occasionally have afternoons of play. The children always help to plan these days. . .prizes are given for (those) excelling in games."[44]

Learning played an important role in what was known as *fieldwork,* treating patients who were homebound. In 1926, a therapist named Martha Emig related an experience she had with a 31-year-old homebound man, born with cerebral palsy, and living in Duluth, Minnesota.[45] He was confined to a small alcove between the kitchen and the dining room. His mother showed a great deal of concern and love, but she felt the therapist would be wasting her time, ". . .as the (mother thought the) young man was helpless and had no mind."[45] According to Emig:

During my visit I found he was mentally alert and he became interested in a few (handmade) articles I had with me, pointing to the baskets and saying "I like that." He complained that his hands were stiff, that he could hold nothing, that his mother always fed him. I had him flex and extend his fingers, which he did slowly and with difficulty, so I told him how, by using his hands, they would become stronger.[45]

In time, his skill and speed in basketry increased to such a point that the therapist was delivering additional materials almost on a daily basis. He found an outlet for his finished products and made enough money to purchase his own materials. "I helped him keep his accounts. He seldom made a mistake in calculating."[45] The patient went on to read and indulge in other studies with the family's help. Emig reported: "The home atmosphere changed; the family all are interested and they help him."[45]

Figure 1-3 shows two men engaged in activites that were typical of the times. These patients were receiving occupational therapy treatment at the Jewish Sanitorium and Hospital for Chronic Disease in Brooklyn, New York. They were painting colorful designs on wooden plates, which were sold at a bazaar, with the proceeds used to augment the hospital fund, which provided care for more than 500 disabled men, women, and children.

The Practitioner's Personal Qualities. As noted earlier, one of the 1925 principles stated that the essential qualities of the therapist and aide were at least of equal value to any instruction or procedures used in applied occupations. One of the first student papers published in *Occupational Therapy and Rehabilitation,* the official journal of the AOTA, appeared in 1930. Nelda McKee of the University of Minnesota wrote on "Ethics for the Occupational Therapist." She discussed ". . .the ideals, customs, and habits which members of the profession are. . .accumulating around the name and character

of the trained therapist."[46] Essential attributes in dealing with patients include honesty, frankness, and wisdom. She showed her insight when she stated:

A therapist should endeavor to develop a symmetrical life. We all have a physical, mental, spiritual, and social side to our make-up which needs care and cultivation. The (therapist) is under personal obligation to keep herself from growing narrow. . . .Above all, (she) must keep the quality of being "teachable." Then she will never stop developing the possibilities which she possesses.[46]

McKee ends her ethical statements with: ". . .the ideal therapist never forgets that our ambitions are all directed towards one common end. We are working for the advancement of understanding and the enlargement of human life."[46] (More information on ethics may be found in the companion volume to this text, *Practice Issues in Occupational Therapy: Intraprofessional Team Building*).

Joseph C. Doane, MD, who later became president of AOTA, gave an impromptu address to conferees at the 1928 AOTA annual meeting.[47] He distinguished between two kinds of workers, the *occupationalist* and the *therapist*:

I regret to say that the occupationalists include not a few physicians and many laymen. (They believe) that occupational therapy is a very interesting and very useful plaything which begins and stops there; they see the product, rather than the patient; they comment on the beautiful colors and difficult weaves. . . .They see nothing beyond the mere physical thing which has resulted from the activity.

Then there is the other party—the therapist. The therapist looks at yarn and raffia, not as materials to be used. . .but as the implements or tools to be employed in the handling of much more difficult material, the disposition of the persons who are ill, a most varying and a most uncertain commodity.[47]

For Doane, the critical importance is for the therapist ". . .to know what sick people do and think and why dispositions, when mixed with sickness, behave as they do—much more important than to know how to make something."[47]

WE LIVE FORWARD

Contemporary occupational theorists and visionaries, such as Mary Reilly, Phillip Shannon, Gary Kielhofner, Janice Burke, and Elizabeth Yerxa, find ample support for

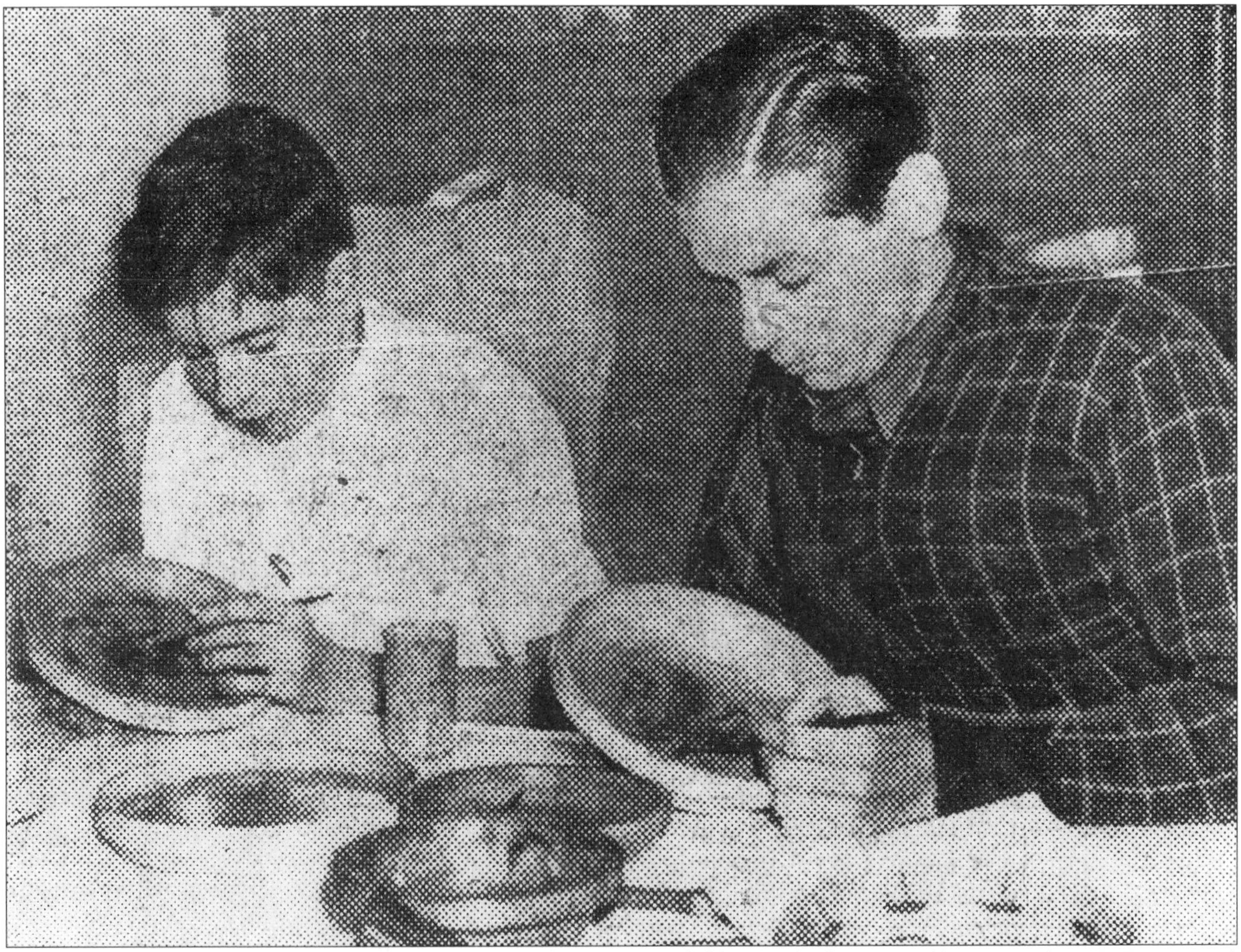

Figure 1-3. Patients in Occupational Therapy Department Jewish Sanitorium and Hospital for Chronic Diseases, Brooklyn, New York, 1937. (From personal archives. Robert K. Bing.)

their concepts in the founding, time-honored principles. In 1961, Reilly observed:

> My reexamination of our early history revealed that our profession emerged from a common belief held by a small group of people. This common belief is the hypotheses upon which our profession was founded. It was, and indeed still is, one of the truly great and even magnificent hypotheses of medicine today: That man, through the use of his hands as they are energized by mind and will, can influence the state of his own health. The splendor of its vision goes far beyond rating it as an idea conceived once in a lifetime or even once in a century. Rather, it falls in the class of one of those great beliefs which has advanced civilization.[48]

For nearly two decades, between 1958 and 1977, Reilly wrote extensively about occupational therapy principles and the profession's changing role in medicine and health care. As Madigan and Parent point out:

> She stated that the medical model is designed to prevent and reduce illness and does not address the reduction of incapacity that results from illness. It is the occupational therapist's (and assistant's) responsibility to activate residual adaptation of patients and to help deficit humans achieve life satisfaction through work and social involvement.[49]

Reilly repeatedly called for a renewed conceptualization of occupational therapy as reflected in the ideals of Dunton, Slagle and Tracy. In addition, Reilly argued that occupational therapy needed to be concerned about the difficulties people have with their occupations all along the developmental continuum, including play and work. This she called **occupational behavior,** ". . .and proposed it as the unifying concept about which occupational therapists could develop a body of theory to support practice."[49]

By 1977, much of occupational therapy practice had markedly shifted away from its foundation in the original principles. Phillip Shannon viewed with alarm what was taking place. He called it a derailment:

> *...a new hypothesis has emerged that views man not as a creative being capable of making choices and directing his own future, but as a mechanistic creature susceptible to manipulation and control via the application of techniques...is a derailment from those...values and beliefs that legitimized the practice of occupational therapy. If occupational therapy persists in this direction, what was once and still is one of the great ideas of 20th century medicine will be swept away by the tide of technique philosophy. Should this happen the ligitimacy of occupational therapy may be revoked and...its services absorbed by other health care professions.*[50]

Shannon was one of many graduate students under Reilly who advanced occupational behavior theory.

Six years later, in 1983, Kielhofner and Burke completed an exhaustive review of the early literature and were left "with a deep respect for the ideas and accomplishments of the...first generation of therapists. Both a science of occupation and the art of using occupation as a medical therapy were conceived, clearly articulated, and applied."[51] Yet, something was missing, something had been dropped out in the intervening years between the development of the principles and the time of their review:

> *A sense of confidence and enthusiasm for occupational therapy seems to have waned, and today we seem bewildered in the face of clinical problems which early occupational therapists readily embraced. Furthermore, our confusion over the identity of occupational therapy seems inexplicable compared with the unified view of early occupational therapists concerning the nature of their service.*[51]

Kielhofner and his associates proceeded with the development of what they term *a model of human occupation,* using the concepts of occupational behavior theory[52] (see Chapter 4).

The latest addition to this evolution, starting with the original principles, is called *occupational science* and is viewed by many as a foundation for occupational therapy well into the next century. Occupational science is believed to be an emerging basic science that supports occupational practice. Supporters state:

> *By identifying and articulating a scientific foundation for practice, occupational science could provide practitioners with support for what they do, justify the significance of occupational therapy to health, and differentiate occupational therapy from other disci-plines. It could provide new understanding of what it means to be chronically disabled in American society, thereby enabling occupational therapists (and assistants) to be more effective advocates for, and allies with, people who are disabled. The science of occupation could help the profession contribute new knowledge and skills to the eradication of complex problems affecting everyone in society.*[53]

OCCUPATIONAL THERAPY: POETRY OF THE COMMONPLACE

What might we carry away from this story of our profession's principles? History tells us that in turbulent times we tend to turn to structure for stability. Contrary to what many of us believe, we will not find any safety in our technology; it changes too rapidly; it is but shifting sand. Where we will find comfort and security is in the centuries-old fundamentals and principles still quite evident in today's occupational therapy practice. We will find assurance in our belief system that has emerged and will continue to develop as time moves on. Our principles and our belief that human beings can survive castastrophes of illness, disease and disabling situations and learn, perhaps for the first time, how to live life well—that is fundamental to our unique efforts.

Occupational therapy's realm consists of a carefully compounded, great vision, transforming the poetry of the commonplace into a vital sustainer and prolonger of precious life. Through the judicious use of a unique technology—human occupation—that has been grounded in research confirming the art and science, and cautiously blended with timeless values, beliefs, and principles, we will inevitably succeed where others have failed. The grand tasks of occupational therapy remain: to attend to the multiple, complex, interrelated, and critical human activities of not just living, but living well. Through the habits of attention and interest we engage the human in regaining the harmony of functions that ensure survival, in retaining those characteristics that facilitate and push balanced growth and development; and in attaining those interrelated meanings of a purposeful, fulfilled life within the context of a personal and social order.

SUMMARY

Occupational therapy's beginnings reach back more than 200 years, to the Age of Enlightenment when human beings were emerging with a new, expanded view of "why on earth they were on earth." There was a sense of economic, political, social, and religious progress. Ideas were forming about the importance of each human being, about the human ability to think and learn, about labor as the central focus of life, and about human existence being governed by a prevailing set of principles directed toward everyday living. These same ideals became significant in caring about and for the mentally ill.

In Europe, the birthplace of this new age, men and women, such as Phillippe Pinel, William Tuke, and Sir William and Lady Ellis, engaged their mental patients in a variety of occupations and amusements for a number of purposes: to restore reason; to provide feelings of security and self-worth; to allow as much freedom of choice and movement as possible, regardless of mental conditions; and to arrest delusional attention and fix it on objects that would help restore reason. From their experience, the caregivers established certain principles that were handed down to the present day. For more than 50 years, during the latter decades of the 19th century and the early 20th century, these principles all but disappeared because of social, economic, and political upheavals. They reemerged in the second decade of this century as occupational therapy.

In the United States, during the Progressive Era, a diverse collection of men and women restated and added to the inherited principles. Among these people were William Rush Dunton, Jr., a psychiatrist; Eleanor Clarke Slagle, a partially-trained social worker; Susan Tracy, a nurse; George Edward Barton, a disabled architect; and Adolph Meyer, a psychiatrist. Their contributions remain today as the cornerstone of occupational therapy principles:

1. Activity contains ingredients by which an ill or disabled individual may gain understanding of and control over one's own feelings, thoughts, and actions; habits of attention and interest; usefulness of occupation; creative expression; the process of learning by doing; skill; and concrete evidence of personal accomplishment.

2. Variations of activity provide opportunities to balance the larger rhythms of life: work, play, rest, and sleep, which must remain balanced if health is to be regained, maintained or attained.

3. Purposeful occupation involves the intricate interplay of the mind and body, which cannot be separated if the human being is to engage in activity.

4. Involvement in remedial activity has as a major purpose the acquiring or restoring of usefulness to oneself and others as a happy, productive human being.

5. The patient is the product of his or her own efforts, not the article made nor the activity accomplished.

6. One's approach to the patient is as significant to treatment and rehabilitation as is the selection and use of an activity.

7. A knowledge of the patient's needs, an appreciation of the pain that accompanies an illness or disability, a strong desire to reduce or remove it, and a gentle firmness are among the major characteristics of the provider of therapeutic occupations.

These principles remain intact, although often restated and reworded. There is considerable evidence they will remain a part of our practice through the efforts of such individuals as Mary Reilly, Phillip Shannon, Gary Kielhofner, Janice Burke, and Elizabeth Yerxa and her associates. Occupational behavior, the model of human occupation, and occupational science offer assurances that these principles will still be with us well into the next century.

Acknowledgments

The author wishes to express his profound gratitude to those people who so generously assisted in the search for materials and in the preparation of the manuscript: Lillian Hoyle Parent, OTR, FAOTA; James L. Cantwell, OTR; Gary A. Wade, OTR; Florence S. Cromwell, OTR, FAOTA; and Inci Bowman, PhD, Director, Truman Blocker History of Medicine Collection (AOTA Archives), Moody Medical Library, The University of Texas Medical Branch at Galveston.

Thanks also to the staff of the *American Journal of Occupational Therapy* for permission to use excerpts from previously published articles: "Occupational Therapy Revisited: A Paraphratic Journey," volume 35, no 6, 1981 and "Living Forward, Understanding Backwards, Part 1 and 2," volume 38, nos 6 and 7, 1984.

Related Learning Activities

1. Construct a historical timeline identifying the important events and people that shaped the profession's history.

2. Much of the impetus for the development of the profession grew out of the principles of moral treatment, yet adherence to moral treatment "died out." What implications does this have for occupational therapy today?

3. Review the summary of principles and compare and contrast them with those you see in occupational therapy literature and practice environments today. Discuss the similarities and differences.

4. If you could have spent time talking with Barton and Dunton, what would you have discussed?

5. Identify ways in which the early beliefs about habit training are reflected in occupational therapy practice today.

References

1. Neustadt RE, May ER: *Thinking in Time: The Uses of History for Decision-Makers*. New York: The Free Press, 1986, p. xxii.
2. deGrazia S: *Of Time, Work, and Leisure*. New York: Twentieth Century Fund, 1962, p. 45.
3. Pinel P: *A Treatise on Insanity in Which Are Contained The Principles of a New and More Practical Nosology of Manical Disorders*. Translated by DD Davis. London: Cadell and Davis, 1806, pp. xv-xvii.
4. Mackler B: *Phillippe Pinel: Unchainer of the Insane*. New York: Franklin Watts, 1968, p. 76.
5. Tuke W: *Description of The Retreat: An Institution Near York for Insane Persons of The Society of Friends*. London: Dawson of Pall Mall, 1813, pp. 20, 156, 180-182.
6. Hunter R, Macalpine I: *Three Hundred Years of Psychiatry: 1535-1860*. London: Oxford University Press, 1963, pp. 871-872.
7. Hass LJ: One hundred years of occupational therapy. *Arch Occup Ther* 3(2):83-100, 1924.
8. Bockhoven JS: *Moral Treatment in Community Mental Health*. New York: Springer Publishing, 1972, pp. 20-31.
9. Deutsch A: *The Mentally Ill in America: A History of Their Care and Treatment from Colonial Times*, 2nd ed. New York: Columbia University Press, 1949.
10. Bates JL: *The United States, 1898-1928: Progressivism and a Society in Transition*. New York: McGraw-Hill, 1976, pp. 18-19, 40.
11. Tracy SE: The place of invalid occupations in the general hospital. *Mod Hosp* 2 (5):386, 1914.
12. Tracy SE: Twenty-five suggested mental tests derived from invalid occupations. *Maryland Psychiatric Q* 8:15-16, 1918.
13. Tracy SE: Treatment of disease by employment at St. Elizabeth's Hospital. *Mod Hosp* 20 (2):198, 1923.
14. Tracy SE: *Studies in Invalid Occupations*. Boston: Witcomb and Barrows, 1918.
15. Barrows M: Susan B. Tracy, RN. *Maryland Psychiatric Q* 6:59, 1917.
16. Barton GE: A view of invalid occupation. *Trained Nurse and Hospital Review* 52 (6):328-330, 1914.
17. Barton GE: Occupational nursing. *Trained Nurse and Hospital Review* 54 (6):328-336, 1915.
18. Barton GE: The existing hospital system and reconstruction. *Trained Nurse and Hospital Review* 69 (4):309,320, 1922.
19. Dunton WR: The relationship of occupational therapy and physical therapy. *Arch Phys Ther* 16 (1):19, 1935.
20. Dunton WR: *Prescribing Occupational Therapy*. Springfield, Illinois, Charles C. Thomas, 1945, pp.5-6.
21. Dunton WR: The principles of occupational therapy. In *Proceedings of the National Society for the Promotion of Occupational Therapy, Second Annual Meeting*. Catonsville, Maryland, Spring Grove State Hospital Press, 1918, pp. 25-27.
22. Dunton WR: *Occupation Therapy: A Manual for Nurses*. Philadelphia, WB Saunders, 1915, pp. 25-26.
23. Barton GE: Occupational therapy. *Trained Nurse and Hospital Review* 54 (3):135-140, 1915.
24. Bing RK: Who orginated the term "occupational therapy?" Letter to the editor. *Am J Occup Ther* 41:3, 1987.
25. Slagle EC: Occupational therapy: Recent methods and advances in the United States. *Occup Ther Rehabil* 13:289, 1934.
26. Slagle EC: Training aides for mental patients. *Arch Occup Ther* 1:13-14, 1922.
27. Slagle EC, Robeson HA: *Syllabus for Training Nurses in Occupational Therapy*. Utica, New York, State Hospital Press, 1933, p. 29.
28. Slagle EC: A year's development of occupational therapy in New York state hospitals. *Ment Hosp* 22:100, 102, 1924.
29. Kidner TJ: Occupational therapy: Its development, scope, and possibilities. *Occup Ther Rehabil* 10:3, 1931.
30. Meyer A: The psychobiological point of view. In Brady JB (Ed): *Classics in American Psychiatry*. St Louis, Warren H. Green, 1975, p. 263.
31. Leif A: *The Commonsense Psychiatry of Dr. Adolph Meyer: Fifty-Two Selected Papers*. New York, McGraw-Hill, 1948, pp. vi-xi.
32. Meyer A: The philosophy of occupation therapy. *Arch Occup Ther* 1:6 1922. (Reprinted *Am J Occup Ther* 31:10, 1977).
33. Unpublished correspondence. AOTA Archives 1914-1917, Series 1. Truman Blocker History of Medicine Collection, Moody Medical Library, The University of Texas Medical Branch at Galveston.
34. Licht S: The founding and founders of the American Occupational Therapy Association. *Am J Occup Ther* 21:269-271, 1967.
35. Historical documents. AOTA Archives 1924-1970, Series 5. Truman Blocker History of Medicine Collection, Moody Medical Library, The University of Texas Medical Branch at Galveston.
36. McDaniel M: Letter to the editor. *Am J Occup Ther* 24:517, 1970.
37. Adams JD et al: An outline of lectures on occupational therapy to medical students and physicians. *Occup Ther Rehabil* 4:277-292, 1925.
38. Spackman CS: The approach to the patient in a general hospital. Unpublished paper delivered at Tri-State Institute on Occupational Therapy, Farnhurst, NJ, March 9, 1936, pp. 3-5.
39. Gilbert ME: Occupational therapy program at Chocktaw-Chickasaw Sanitorium. *Occup Ther Rehabil* 15:110-113, 1936.
40. Sands IF: When is occupation curative? *Occup Ther Rehabil* 7:117-119, 1938.
41. Wade BD: Occupational therapy: A history of its practice in the psychiatric field. Unpublished paper delivered at the AOTA 51st annual conference, October, 1967.
42. Illinois Advisory Committee on Occupational Therapy. The basic philosophy of occupational therapy. In *The University of Illinois Faculty-Alumni Newsletter of the Chicago Professional Colleges*, 6 (4):9, 1951.
43. Robeson HA: How can occupational therapists help the social service worker? *Occup Ther Rehabil* 5 (4):279-381, 1926.
44. O'Brock I: Occupational treatment for crippled children. *Occup Ther Rehabil* 11 (3):204-205, 1932.
45. Emig MR: Fieldwork: Some experiences and observations. *Occup Ther Rehabil* 5 (2):129-130, 1926.
46. McKee N: Ethics for the occupational therapist. *Occup Ther Rehabil* 9 (6):357-360, 1930.

47. Doane JC: Occupational therapy. *Occup Ther Rehabil* 8 (1):13-14, 1929.

48. Reilly M: Occupational therapy can be one of the great ideas of 20th century medicine. *Am J Occup Ther* 26:1-2, 1962.

49. Madigan MJ, Parent LH: Preface. In Kielhofner G (Ed): *A Model of Human Occupation: Theory and Practice.* Baltimore, Williams & Wilkins, 1985, pp. 25-26.

50. Shannon PD: The derailment of occupational therapy. *Am J Occup Ther* 31:233, 1977.

51. Kielhofner G, Burke JP: The evolution of knowledge and practice in occupational therapy: Past, present, and future. In Kielhofner G (Ed): *Health Through Occupation: Theory and Practice in Occupational Therapy.* Philadelphia, FA Davis, 1983.

52. Kielhofner G (Ed): *A Model of Human Occupation: Theory and Application.* Baltimore, Williams & Wilkins, 1985.

53. Yerxa EJ et al: An introduction to occupational science, a foundation for occupational therapy in the 21st century. *Occup Ther Health Care* 6(4):3, 1989.

The COTA Heritage

PROUD, PRACTICAL, STABLE, DYNAMIC

Shirley Holland Carr, MS, LOTR, FAOTA

INTRODUCTION

This chapter is a story about the birth of the certified occupational therapy assistant (COTA). The story begins in the post-World War II era with Ruth Robinson and Marion Crampton, and later Ruth Brunyate Wiemer and Mildred Schwagmeyer. With one exception, these early participants are active retirees. Colonel Robinson's thoughts were taken from the *American Occupational Therapy Association's Visual Taped History Series.*[1] Described here are 1) the circumstances that led to the creation of the COTA, 2) the roles of some individuals who were instrumental in the development of the concept, educational training, and practice of the occupational therapy assistant, and 3) COTA accomplishments.

You are carried from the "beginnings" to your own entry into our profession, with emphasis on the early years. If you discern more anecdotes than usual, consider that while you are reading contemporary history the writer was reminiscing.

USE OF PERSONNEL BEFORE 1960

Before World War II, many registered occupational therapists (OTRs) worked in psychiatric institutions. Psychiatric hospitals often had large patient populations of between 1,000 and 6,000.[2] With a shortage of therapists, occupational therapy services often were provided by a number of aides, assistants, or technicians who were supervised by one or two occupational therapists. After 1945 and influenced by military experience, increasing numbers of therapists practiced in medical and rehabilitation settings.[3,4] This added to the already severe shortage of OTRs in psychiatric settings during and after World War II.[3,4]

Supportive personnel (OT aides and technicians) working in psychiatric facilities were valuable and valued employees, having learned the "tricks of the trade" by modeling therapist behaviors or by trial and error. In contrast to the mobility of OTRs, the employment stability of aides and technicians often made them the most knowledgeable personnel about individual patient behavior and the

KEY CONCEPTS

Early use of personnel and training

Role of AOTA

Educational patterns

Rights and privileges

Developmental milestones

Roster of Honor

availability of activities and equipment in a given setting. Supportive personnel knew how to do things, but lacked goal-oriented intervention methods necessary to work without immediate supervision. This deficit motivated supervisory personnel to organize courses for occupational therapy assistants.[3,5]

EARLY TRAINING NEEDS AND SHORT COURSES

Several states and the military recognized the need for **inservice training** (on-the-job educational oppurtunities) for occupational therapy personnel and developed courses of varying lengths. As early as 1944, the US Army developed a one-month course. Crampton, employed by the state of Massachusetts, developed and conducted four- and six-week courses before approval by the American Occupational Therapy Association (AOTA). Other states with early short courses were New York, Wisconsin and Pennsylvania (for activity aides).[6]

AOTA'S ROLE IN THE DEVELOPMENT OF THE COTA

The overlapping employment and Association roles of Marion Crampton, Colonel Ruth Robinson, Mildred Schwagmeyer and Ruth Brunyate Wiemer were fortuitous to the development of the COTA. Each of these women had a long-standing interest in the use of supportive occupational therapy personnel, and all but Wiemer were members of the **Committee on Occupational Therapy Assistants.**[7] This committee was delegated responsibility for all developmental aspects of the occupational therapy assistant, including needs assessment, educational program standards, new program proposal and on-site review, and program approval.[8]

In addition, members of the Committee on Occupational Therapy Assistants reviewed applications for certification under the **grandfather clause.**[9] Of 460 applications, 336 individuals became COTAs.[10] The committee also undertook the continuing education of OTRs by preparing documents and acquiring grant funds to sponsor national workshops.[8] The focus was twofold: appropriate supervision and use of COTAs.

Schwagmeyer joined the AOTA office staff,[8] and later Wiemer became president of the AOTA from 1964 to 1967, six years after Robinson's term.[11] Those four—Robinson, Crampton, Schwagmeyer, and Wiemer—"tell it best," as they were the key players in the creation and nurturing of occupational therapy assistants.

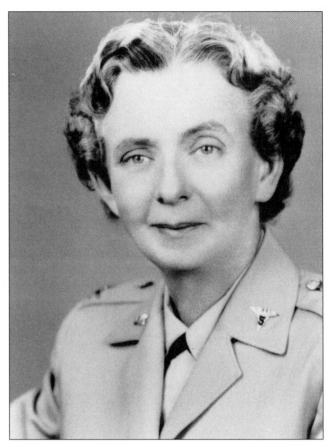

Figure 2-1. Ruth A. Robinson.

Ruth A. Robinson

Colonel Ruth A. Robinson was president of the AOTA from 1955 to 1958 (Figure 2-1). About the same time, she became Chief of the Occupational Therapy Section of the Women's (later Army) Medical Specialist Corps, and then the first Chief of the Women's (later Army) Medical Specialist Corps. Both her military and Association roles involved advocacy for the training of supportive occupational therapy personnel. She served on the Committee on Occupational Therapy Assistants from its inception, as a member, chair, and consultant.[11,12]

In an interview[1] a few years before her death in 1989, Colonel Robinson stated that she thought her greatest contribution to the occupational therapy profession was the development of the program and curriculum to train occupational therapy assistants. She also stated:

We may not realize how far advanced the occupational therapy profession was. We set a standard for other professions to follow. At first our program concentrated on the care of the psychiatric patient, just as in the early days of occupational therapy. It was frightening to some of us who felt we were not far enough advanced ourselves or secure in our own identities to be able to accept the responsibility of supervising others. We still have a long way to go. I thought the COTA ultimately would be what we thought of then as the occupational therapist, and that the COTA would be the best job in occupational therapy, leaving the OTR to do the intake work and program planning for individual patients. Recognition of the COTA through certification made me the proudest.[1]

Marion W. Crampton

Marion W. Crampton was a member of the House of Delegates, a delegate member of AOTA's Board of Management, and finally a member of the board itself (Figure 2-2). She was employed by the Massachusetts Department of Mental Health to work with the state psychiatric facilities as well as the state schools under the Division of Mental Retardation. Crampton's employment involved meeting the need for occupational therapy services in her state's institutions at a time of OTR shortages. She understood the problems and the needs of personnel with less than optimal preparation because that was her daily work. She already was involved in Massachusetts when the Committee on Occupational Therapy Assistants was formed and she was appointed chair. Crampton included "members of the loyal

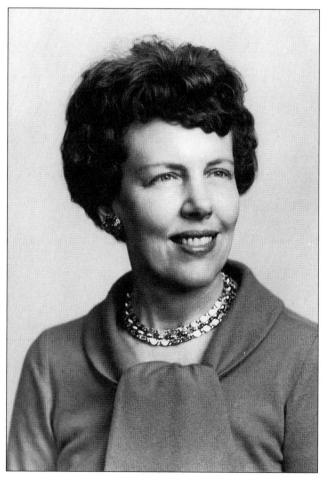

Figure 2-2. Marion W. Crampton, OTR.

opposition" as she made appointments to the committee, so all sides were heard.[6]

As noted earlier, implementation of the occupational therapy assistant program brought a deluge of applications from occupational therapy personnel seeking credentialing under the grandfather clause. She recalled, "During the two year period, applications were reviewed in a 'round robin' composed of all committee members, who worked evenings, weekends, holidays, and even vacations to process these forms."[6]

The occupational therapy assistant education program in Massachusetts was an inservice program for employed individuals with experience in occupational therapy. Crampton noted:

The first group of students thought long and hard before applying to the course, which required leaving families for a month and returning to school after many years. Exams were especially threatening, since some students had only tenth grade educations, and had school-aged children who questioned their grades.[6]

Mildred Schwagmeyer

Mildred Schwagmeyer worked in tuberculosis hospitals until recruited as assistant director of education at the AOTA national office in 1958 (Figure 2-3). Nine years later she became director of technical education, remaining in this position until 1974.[13] She became the most knowledgeable person on the subject of occupational therapy assistants at the national office and in the United States. She continued to work in occupational therapy assistant educational services through several title changes until her retirement.

In recalling those years Schwagmeyer commented:

I knew in a general way about what was going on, but not that the COTA would have a real impact on my working life. After only four months as assistant director of the education, the division became responsible for occupational therapy assistant education. I became liaison to the Committee on Occupational Therapy Assistants, which reported directly to the Board of Management. At first, occupational therapy assistants were only part of my job, but the work became increasingly time consuming, demanding, and absorbing. By the 1960's, being technical education director and working with the Committee on Occupational Therapy Assistants was a full time position.[8]

She went on to recount:

As educational programs moved from hospital-base to academic-base training, concern and discussion in-

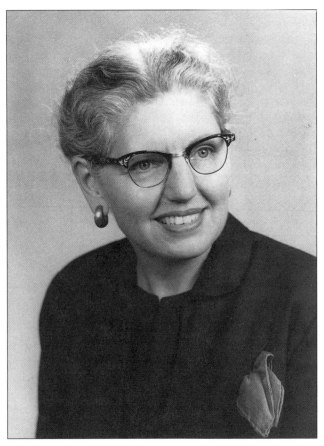

Figure 2-3. Mildred Schwagmeyer, OTR.

creased on topics such as career mobility, entry level skills, laddering, behavioral objectives, lack of appropriate textbooks and teaching aids, shortage of faculty, and over education by some programs leading to dissappointment in graduates' work experience.[8]

Five federally funded invitational workshops were held at yearly intervals between 1963 and 1968.[14] Four were attended primarily by academic and clinical faculty, and the last included an equal mix of OTRs and COTAs. Topics included role and function, COTA/OTR relationships, and supervision.[8] Excellent teaching materials came from these workshops, including a **Guide for Supervision,**[15] concepts from which are included in the 1990 document, *Supervision Guidelines for Certified Occupational Therapy Assistants.*[16] State associations were encouraged to hold meetings to disseminate information developed at the last workshop.

Schwagmeyer brought a precise use of language to her work. Among other things, she taught us that the term *certified occupational therapy assistant program* was a non sequitur. Programs are approved, but students cannot seek certification until they graduate. Even today you may sometimes hear the incorrect terminology.

After the 1964 restructuring of AOTA,[17,18] the func-

tions of the Committee on Occupational Therapy Assistants slowly were integrated into the council structure,[8] and the committee was dissolved. Seldom have so few accomplished so much.

Ruth Brunyate Wiemer

Ruth Brunyate Wiemer was employed as an occupational therapy consultant for the Maryland Department of Health and in 1964 became president of the AOTA (Figure 2-4).[11] Wiemer guided the Association through the difficult period of reorganization.[19] Of that period she said:

Communication was slow and labored, with few secretaries in the national office, or in occupational therapy departments. Flying was not common; one usually traveled by car or train. Expense accounts were unheard of, either at AOTA or on the job. Little money was available for phone, retreats, or any type of face-to-face confrontation.[20]

She continued:

Our world changed rapidly in 1965 after Medicare, with an explosion in the number of proprietary nursing homes and home health agencies. Occupa-

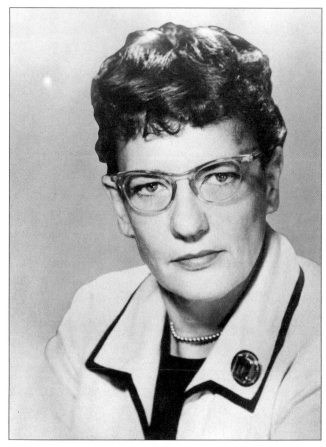

Figure 2-4. Ruth Brunyate Wiemer, OTR.

tional therapy was a small unrecognized profession without precedent for adopting such a concept (as the COTA). Nursing had supportive personnel, but were protected by licensure; we were not.[20] *For professional occupational therapists, COTAs became an added issue because of the following:*

1. *OTRs feared the unknown, especially those with no experience working with or supervising supportive personnel.*
2. *OTRs feared the AOTA was imposing the COTA on the profession.*
3. *OTRs feared giving representation to the COTA, and the consequences of COTAs voting.*
4. *Abilities of the COTA highlighted weaknesses in OTR skills such as deficits in supervisory techniques and current clinical practice, contentment in their own comfortable niche, naivety, and insufficient business acumen.*
5. *There was a lack of country-wide consensus on the appropriate role of occupational therapy, itself.*[20]

In such an environment, how then were COTAs nurtured? My belief is that the leadership came from those therapists used to hierarchical order, chain of command, and discipline, such as in the military, veterans administration, or health departments. Therapists from psychiatric settings also were familiar with working with supportive personnel.[20]

While others argued, Wiemer often seemed to be collecting her thoughts. Her responses were graceful, direct, organized, and reasoned; and they did not hide her advocacy for COTAs. She used a convincing metaphor in referring to the OTR/COTA problem: "Able seamen far outnumber captains and commodores, yet ships do not sink, and new ship forms, from sail to nuclear power, have evolved to meet man's need. So too the varied levels of our profession can be coordinated to achieve efficiency and growth."[21]

Therapists who had not stayed abreast of current clinical practice had reason to be concerned about the role of the COTA.[22] According to a 1967 "Nationally Speaking" column in the *American Journal of Occupational Therapy,* "Therapists away from current practice should be aware that what was taught fifteen years ago as functional treatment is taught to COTAs today as maintenance and supportive therapy."[23] This writer's attempt to motivate other therapists may sound harsh, but the basic premise about current practice was true.

According to Wiemer:

Change eventually came about in the profession, brought about by the advent of the COTA; these included the sharpening of the roles and functions which opened up part-time positions, increased legis-

lative efforts, and increased state licensure. A physician once asked how the occupational therapy profession had the vision to establish a subprofessional group. The profession did not; a few within it did and urged that we follow, and we did.[20]

FEELINGS OF DISTRUST

Feelings of distrust among some OTRs perodically ran high for a number of years, reigniting each time new COTA rights and privileges were initiated. The following anecdote is an example of such an emotional response in the early 1970s, when the AOTA Delegate Assembly considered **career mobility** to allow COTAs to become OTRs by fulfilling certain fieldwork requirements and passing the national certification examination for occupational therapists.[22] One evening two AOTA national office staff members spoke on the subject at a district occupational therapy meeting. Heated discussion followed the presentations as a few vocal therapists expressed concern that such legislation would directly threaten their jobs. Others disagreed, and still others sat quietly, because the hour was late and the response had become familiar. A stenotypist took notes throughout the meeting so the proceedings could be distributed to therapists statewide. Apparently to prevent such dissemination, the stenotypists tapes were "lost," but later were retrieved from a lavatory trash can. The proceedings were published,[24] the Delegate Assembly voted COTAs career mobility rights terminated in 1982,[25] and OTRs' employment was unaffected as a consequence of this or any other action pertaining to COTA rights.

"As the first COTAs practiced and practiced well at the technical level,"[20] OTRs and COTAs began building on each other's strengths, learning to identify and complement each other's skills to the betterment of the profession. As you read furthur in this and in subsequent chapters, you will see how the COTA/OTR relationship continues to mature.

OCCUPATIONAL THERAPY ASSISTANT EDUCATION

The initial short-term courses, such as those conducted under the auspices of the state hospital systems in Massachusetts, Wisconsin and New York, were inservice programs.[6] In 1961, a program in Montgomery County, Maryland, was approved in general practice to train students to practice in nursing homes.[26] The first approved program combining psychiatric and general practice was at the Duluth Vocational-Technical School in Minnesota; it also targeted student training for nursing homes.[27] Another Minnesota program at St. Mary's Junior College became the first approved two-year college program.[28] By 1966,[29] the original single-concept programs were being eliminated, and soon all students were enrolled in programs that prepared them to work in general areas of occupational therapy practice, rather than in a specialized setting.

Within the parameters set by AOTA guidelines for the number of program hours, program length remained variable depending on the academic setting, length of school day, length of fieldwork and student backgrounds. One interesting program consolidated all of the academic work into a summer. The program used the college campus and employed faculty members when the campus would otherwise be closed. All students had prior experience in occupational therapy or associated departments, or at least two years of college and experience working in a health facility. Such students had fewer professional socialization needs than typical junior college students, but received the same occupational therapy education in an eight-hour classroom day. Fieldwork was arranged when the other college students returned to campus.[30]

PRACTICE SETTINGS

As we have seen, COTAs were trained initially to work in psychiatric hospital **practice settings** and then in nursing homes and other general medical settings. Many still work in those facilities. The dispersion of COTAs into nontraditional settings came about, not because of training, but because of federal legislation.[23] Initially, Titles XVIII and XIX of P.L.89-97 (1965),[31] more commonly known as Medicare and Medicaid, opened employment in nursing homes, related facilities, and home health agencies. Other funding opened opportunities in community health and mental health centers, day care centers, and centers for the well aging. Numbers of COTAs increased at the same time some OTRs began moving from hospitals to less traditional community practice settings.[32] COTAs joined the move to community settings, sometimes in larger numbers than OTRs. Carr commented, "It may be either COTA or OTR who meanders away from traditional to new settings, but whichever goes first the other will accompany or soon follow."[24] Current employment settings for COTAs are the following:[33]

Nursing Homes and Related Facilities 20.1%
General Hospitals 18.6%
Public School Systems 14.4%
Psychiatric Facilities/Programs 8.4%
Rehabilitation Centers/Programs 8.4%

Residential Care Facilities 7.5%
Day Care Centers 4.3%
Community Mental Health Centers 3.8%
Others under 2% each 14.5%

With the passage of P.L. 94-142, The Education for All Handicapped Children Act of 1975,[34] occupational therapy personnel were recruited as a related service by public schools to assist children three through 21 years to learn skills necessary to participate in their individualized special education programs. P.L. 99-457, the Handicapped Amendments of 1986,[35] gave a direct occupational therapy role in early intervention with children from birth through two years, and COTAs and OTRs again modified their roles as they moved into schools.

As you read later in this chapter about some individual COTAs who have been singled out for honors, be aware how many have moved to nontraditional roles, some requiring OTR supervision and some not. Even in roles requiring no OTR supervision, it is observed that COTAs continue their relationships informally with their counterparts.

PRIDE IN RIGHTS AND PRIVILEGES HARD WON

The Chronology of COTA Developmental Milestones shown in Figure 2-5 chronicles hard-won rights and privileges, as well as a few not yet won. In 1980, the AOTA Executive Board formed the **COTA Task Force** to identify COTA concerns and formulate suggestions.[36,37] A year later the Task Force reported the following recommendations:[37,38]

1. Submit a resolution to the Representative Assembly to establish COTA representation. This was to include a proposal for a nationwide communication network.
2. Increase COTAs' participation on key committees and commissions and national office advisory committees.
3. Maintain a roster of COTAs qualified and interested in serving on committees at state, regional and national levels.
4. Establish "COTA Share" column in *OT Newspaper*.
5. Design COTA workshops to improve technical skills.
6. Encourage utilization of COTAs as educators in professional and technical education programs.
7. Appoint a COTA liaison in the national office.

The COTA Task Force was funded for several years[39] and then replaced by a **COTA Advisory Committee** in 1986.[40] All of the original objectives were accomplished, along with many others identified by the networking of the COTA Advisory Committee. Although a proposal to elect a COTA member-at-large in the Representative Assembly was defeated in 1982,[41] a similar measure in 1983[42] created a COTA representative with voice and vote elected by the membership. It is anticipated that when COTAs are routinely elected to the Representative Assembly from their states, such a special at-large position will be unnecessary. Two COTAs have been elected to the Representative assembly from their states, but none are currently serving.

COTAs describe the 1980s as having had two phases. In the early part, they expended their energy claiming a fair share of responsibility in the Association. Their effort paid off, and in the latter part of the decade increasing numbers of COTAs were involved in local, state and national professional activities. The maturity of the COTA group was especially obvious when the COTA Advisory Committee voluntarily withdrew the proposal to change the title of COTAs and discouraged any further action on that long-held dream because the legal and economic implications outweighed the benefits.[36]

In 1989, 21 full-time and 20 part-time COTAs were employed as faculty in technical education programs, and six full-time and 20 part-time COTAs were on faculties of professional curricula. Nine COTAs were members of state regulatory (licensure or registration) boards. Can the day be far off when COTAs are directors of educational programs?[43] Ten years ago only the visionaries among us would even have dreamed that in 1987 the American Occupational Therapy Association would change its by-laws,[44] allowing no distinction between COTAs and OTRs running for elected national office, including the office of president. Jones commented that with the labor shortage (where this chapter began), COTAs are becoming administrators, hiring OTRs as consultants and clinicians.[43]

MULTIPLYING SLOWLY

The fears of some OTRs, as outlined by Wiemer, that COTAs would become more numerous than OTRs,[20] has not yet happened. The number of COTAs has increased,[45,46] but their impact on the profession is far greater than numbers indicate. As you read the information on outstanding COTAs, compare it with the membership statistics shown in Figure 2-6 and see if you agree.

The decrease in membership from 1986 to 1988 was expected, due to a change in the method of counting after the separation of certification and membership in 1986.[45,46]

ROSTER OF HONOR

The Roster of Honor recognizes COTAs with at least five years of experience "who, with their knowledge and

expertise, have made a significant contribution to the continuing education and professional development of members of the Association, and provide an incentive to contribute to the advancement of the profession."[47] Become familiar with their names so you will recognize them when you meet them (and you will). Many of the recipients also received the **Award of Excellence,**[47] which recognizes the contributions of COTAs to the advancement of occupational therapy and provides an incentive to contribute to the development and growth of the profession.

The following recipients of these honors, which the American Occupational Therapy Association bestows on COTAs, are presented here with our pride in their accomplishments:

Sally E. Ryan of Mounds View, Minnesota, received the Roster of Honor (1979) and the Award of Excellence (1976) for "outstanding achievements and contributions in education, committee work in professional organizations at affiliate and national levels, and for identifying the needs of the COTA as a membership group."[48,49] She is a member of a professional occupational therapy curriculum faculty and is both an editor and author of textbooks for occupational therapy assistant students.

Betty Cox of Baltimore, Maryland, received the Roster of Honor (1979) and the Award of Excellence (1977) for "leadership in increasing the involvement of COTAs both in the practice arena and in the Association."[48,49] Her own business offers professional seminars in health-related subjects, both nationally and internationally. She is also president of a publishing company that produces books on occupational therapy.

Terry Brittell of New Hartford, New York, received the Roster of Honor and the Award of Excellence (1979) for "outstanding contributions to occupational therapy in the areas of practice and clinical education and for service to the profession and for services to the community."[48,49] At the same psychiatric facility where he was a traditional COTA, he was the coordinator of a stress management program for employees, and of the Mental Health Players, a community prevention program based on role playing.

Charlotte Gale Seltser of Chevy Chase, Maryland, received the Roster of Honor (1981) "in recognition of her program development for the visually handicapped."[48,49] Seltser, now retired, is employed as a volunteer at the National Eye Institute of the National Institutes of Health teaching patients appropriate independence and coping skills, and referring them to community agencies.

Toné Frank Blechert of Excelsior, Minnesota, received the Roster of Honor and the Award of Excellence (1981) "in recognition of her outstanding contributions to occupational therapy in the area of occupational therapy technical education."[48,49] As a faculty member of a junior college, she teaches mental health concepts and group dynamics to occupational therapy assistant students and coordinates

1949   AOTA Board of Management discussed a proposal to the AMA for a one-year training program for "assistants" by Guy Morrow, OTR of Ohio.[50]

1956   AOTA Board of Management approved a task force to investigate occupational therapy aides and supportive personnel.[51]

1956   AOTA Board of Management changed name of Committee on Recognition of Non-professional Personnel to Committee on Recognition of OT Aides to avoid use of term "non-professional" in all correspondence. In October of the same year, the name was changed to Committee on Recognition of Occupational Therapy Assistants.[52]

1957   AOTA Board of Management accepted the committee's plan and agreed to implement plan in October, 1958.[53]

1958   First *Essentials and Guidelines of an Approved Educational Program for Occupational Therapy Assistants* adopted.[53]

1958   Plan implemented.[53,54]

1958   Grandfather clause established.[53,54]

1959   First OT assistant education program approved at Westborough State Hospital in Massachusetts.[14]

1960   336 COTAs certified through grandfather clause.[10]

1961   First general practice program approved at Montgomery County, Maryland.[25]

1962   First COTA directory published.[14]

1963   Board of Management established COTA membership category.[55]

1965   First paper authored by a COTA published in the *American Journal of Occupational Therapy*.[56]

1966   All future educational programs must prepare occupational therapy assistant students as generalists, including both psychosocial and general practice input.[28,57]

1967   First COTA meeting held at AOTA Annual Conference.[58]

1968   Eight COTAs served on various AOTA committees.[59]

1969   Tenth anniversary of COTAs noted in Schwagmeyer paper.[60]

1970   Effort to change name of COTA to "associate" or "technician" failed in Delegate Assembly.[61]

1971   Military occupational therapy technicians eligible for certification as COTAs.[61]

1972   Fifth Annual COTA Workshop held in Baltimore on subject of COTA/OTR relationships.[14,62]

1972   First book review written by COTA published in the *American Journal of Occupational Therapy*.[63]

1973   Career mobility plan endorsed by Executive Board.[3]

1974   First COTAs take certification examination as part of career mobility plan to become OTRs.[64]

1974   COTAs get *American Journal of Occupational Therapy* as a membership benefit.[64]

1975   Award of Excellence created for COTAs.[65]

1975   COTAs became eligible to receive the Eleanor Clarke Slagle Lectureship Award and the Award of Merit.[66]

1976   First COTA elected member-at-large of the Executive Board.[67]

1977   First national certification examination administered to occupational therapy assistants.[68]

1978   Roster of Honor award established.[69]

1979   Policy adopted that the acronym "COTA" can be used only by assistants currently certified by AOTA.[70]

1980   Funding for two year (later refunded) COTA advocacy position for AOTA office.[71]

1981   COTA Task Force established.[37]

1981   Eight COTAs are faculty members of professional occupational therapy curricula.[65]

1981   Entry-level OTR and COTA role delineations adopted.[25]

1982   Career mobility plan terminated.[24]

1982   "COTA Share Column" introduced in *Occupational Therapy Newspaper*.[73]

1983   Representative Assembly agreed a COTA member-at-large elected to the assembly would have voice and vote.[42]

1985   First COTA representative and alternate to serve in the Representative Assembly elected.[74]

1987   AOTA Bylaws Revision allowed no distinction between COTA and OTR in running for or holding office, including president of the Association.[44]

1989   Twenty-one full-time and 20 part-time COTAs employed in occupational therapy assistant education programs.[43]

1989   Six full-time and twenty part-time COTAs employed in professional occupational therapy curricula.[43]

1989   Nine COTAs are members of state regulatory boards.[43]

1990   New guidelines for supervision of COTAs adopted by the Representative Assembly.[16]

1991   Treatment in Groups: A COTA Workshop was sponsored by the AOTA as the association's first continuing education program specifically for COTAs.[75]

1991   First AOTA COTA/OTR Partnership Award received by Illena Brown and Cynthia Epstein.[76]

1992   17,000 COTAs certified by AOTCB.[77]

Figure 2-5. Chronology of COTA Developmental Milestones.

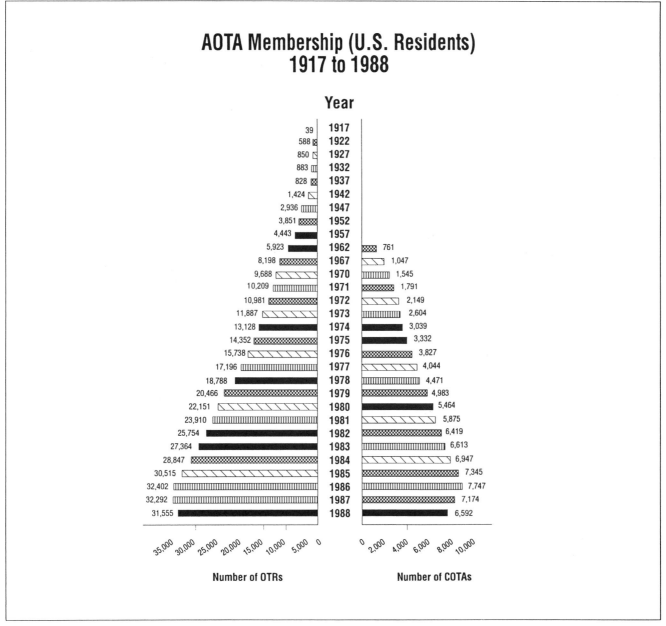

Figure 2-6. AOTA membership statistics for OTRs and COTAs.

academic advisement for all students. She is currently pursuing a master's degree in organizational leadership.

Ilenna Brown of Plainfield, New Jersey, received the Roster of Honor (1984) for "fostering pride and pursuit of excellence for COTA practitioners."[48,49] In a 550-bed nursing facility, Brown is supervising COTA and rehabilitation coordinator for programs carried on cooperatively by occupational therapy, physical therapy and rehabilitation nursing.

Barbara Larsen of Mahtomedi, Minnesota, received the Roster of Honor (1985) for "exemplary leadership and promotion of the profession."[48,49] Larson returned to school

and is now an OTR. She is the coordinator of an industrial rehabilitation clinic and is the past president of her state association.

Patty Lynn Barnett of Birmingham, Alabama, received the Roster of Honor (1986) for "dynamic leadership in the promotion of COTAs."[48,49] Barnett is a faculty member of a university occupational therapy curriculum where she teaches activity classes and coordinates clinical education for assistant students.

Margaret S. Coffey of Russiaville, Indiana, received the Roster of Honor and Award of Excellence (1986) for "excellence in role expansion, and commitment to

COTAs."[48,49] Before becoming a COTA, she completed a master's degree. She currently cares for two toddlers, coordinates a weaver's group, and recently co-authored *Activity Analysis Handbook* with two occupational therapists.[78]

Barbara Forté of Palm Springs, California, received the Roster of Honor and the Award of Excellence (1986) because "through exemplary qualities of dedication and commitment, (she) provides outstanding leadership in local, state, and national organizations. She articulates the emerging role of COTAs and serves as a role model."[48,49] Forté has broad experience in delivering community-based clinical services and is currently employed in a private mental health facility.

Robin Jones of Chicago, Illinois, received the Roster of Honor and the Award of Excellence (1987) because she "exemplifies excellence and professionalism and is recognized as a strong COTA role model by her peers. [She is] recognized as an outstanding practitioner, teacher and advocate for occupational therapy."[48,49] Jones is the director of an independent living center, and is currently enrolled in a master's degree program in public services administration. She is vice chair of her state's licensure board.

Teri Black of Madison, Wisconsin, received the Roster of Honor and Award of Excellence (1989) for "leadership modeling for COTA-OTR professional development."[48,49] She teaches in an area technical college and practices in a nursing home. Black served two terms as chair of her state's licensure board.

Sue Byers of Gresham, Oregon, received the Roster of Honor (1989) for "exemplary role modeling for COTAs and students."[48,49] As a member of the faculty of an occupational therapy assistant education program, Byers teaches in the occupational therapy assistant education program and keeps her clinical skills sharp by working in home health.

Diane S. Hawkins of Baltimore, Maryland, received the Roster of Honor (1991) in recognition of her "significant contributions in staff development and communications." Currently, Diane is a faculty consultant for the AOTA workshop "Treatment in Groups: A Workshop for COTAs" and an associate faculty member for the Sheppard and Enoch Pratt National Center for Human Development.

ELEANOR CLARKE SLAGLE AWARD

As yet, no COTA has received the Eleanor Clarke Slagle Award, the highest honor given by the American Occupational Therapy Association to any COTA or OTR. This honor may be waiting for you or one of your peers.

SUMMARY IN ALLEGORY

Picture a young fruit tree growing well, but having the potential of producing a limited amount of fruit. On advice of well-experienced practitioners, a graft of another tree is applied to increase productivity and quality of fruit. Although tramatic to the tree and to the graft bud at first, the surgery is successful. The graft takes well, and the whole tree develops and becomes stronger than before, even stronger than it could have been if left alone to grow naturally. Now after more than 30 years, the subtle difference in a part of the tree is indistinguishable, unless you are up close or know fruit trees very well.

Editor's Note
At the request of the author, the writing style has not been modified to third person, to conform with other chapters. Rather, the terms *you* and *your* have been retained where appropriate to assist in engaging the reader in the story as it unfolds.

Acknowledgments
Marion Crampton, Mildred Schwagmeyer, and Ruth Wiemer shared their early COTA stories and allowed me to use their materials; I avow my appreciation. I also thank those who helped me document memories and flesh out the intervening years. These individuals include the thirteen "ROHers," especially Patty Barnett and Sally Ryan, Robert Bing, Bonnie Brooks, Marie Moore, Dottie Renoe, Lauren Rivet, and Ira Silvergleit. Lisa Dickey has been a patient co-proofreader, and Joel G. Swetnam has generously shared his computer graphic skills in the development of the AOTA membership figure.

Related Learning Activities

1. Identify some of the barriers to acceptance of the COTA in the profession, both historically and currently.

2. Interview at least three COTAs and three OTRs and determine what the current issues are relative to supervision. What efforts are being made to resolve the issues?

3. Write a short paper discussing how COTAs will be viewed by the profession in the next decade. What challenges will assistants face? What new roles will be assumed?

4. List some of the characteristics that contribute to a positive OTR and COTA team relationship.

5. If you had the opportunity to talk to Wiemer, Schwagmeyer or Crampton, what questions would you ask? What advice would you seek?

References

1. Cox B: *American Occupational Therapy Association's Visual Taped History: Ruth A, Robinson.* Galveston, Texas, AOTA Archives, Moody Medical Library, University of Texas Medical Branch, 1977.

2. East Louisiana State Hospital: *Historical Outline.* Jackson, Louisiana, undated.

3. Hopkins H, Smith H: *Willard and Spackman's Occupational Therapy,* 5th edition. Philadelphia, JB Lippincott, 1978.

4. Willard HS, Spackman C: *Occupational Therapy.* Philadelphia, JB Lippincott, 1947.

5. Crampton M: Educational upheaval for occupational therapy assistants. *Am J Occup Ther* 21:317-320, 1967.

6. Crampton M: Presentation at 30th anniversary COTA forum. Baltimore, 1989.

7. AOTA: Annual report, committee on occupational therapy assistants. *Am J Occup Ther* 18:45-46, 1964.

8. Schwagmeyer M: Presentation at 30th anniversary COTA forum. Baltimore, 1989.

9. AOTA: Executive director's report. *Am J Occup Ther* 13:36, 1959.

10. AOTA: Board of management, midyear meeting report. *Am J Occup Ther* 14:232, 1960.

11. AOTA: Presidents of the American Occupational Therapy Association (1917-1967). *Am J Occup Ther* 21:290-298, 1967.

12. West W: In memoriam. *Am J Occup Ther* 43:481-482, 1989.

13. M. Schwagmeyer personal correspondence to S. Carr, January 4, 1990.

14. AOTA: *Development of the Certified Occupational Therapy Assistant* undated.

15. AOTA: *Guide for Supervision,* 1967.

16. AOTA: *Supervision Guidelines for the Certified Occupational Therapy Assistant.* Representative assembly minutes, 1990.

17. AOTA: Annual business meeting report. *Am J Occup Ther* 19:33, 1965.

18. AOTA: Bylaws, October 27, 1964. *Am J Occup Ther* 19:37-41, 1965.

19. Wiemer R: AOTA conference keynote address. *Am J Occup Ther* 20:9-11, 1966.

20. Wiemer R: Presentation at 30th anniversary COTA forum. Baltimore, 1989.

21. Wiemer R: Workshop Summary. Workshop on the Training of the Occupational Therapy Assistant, Detroit, Michigan, August 2, 1964.

22. AOTA: 52nd annual conference, annual business meeting. *Am J Occup Ther* 36:808-826, 1982.

23. Carr SH: A modification of role for nursing home service. *Am J Occup Ther* 21:259-262, 1971.

24. Texas Occupational Therapy Association, Southeast District: Proceedings of meeting. October 15, 1973.

25. AOTA: 1982 representative assembly report. *Am J Occup Ther* 36:808-926, 1982.

26. Caskey V: A training program for occupational therapy assistants. *Am J Occup Ther* 15:157-159, 1961.

27. Occupational Therapy Assistant Education Program brochure. Duluth Area Vocational Technical School, Duluth, Minnesota, 1964.

28. AOTA: Board of management report. *Am J Occup Ther* 19:100, 1965.

29. AOTA: Delegate assembly minutes. *Am J Occup Ther* 20:49-53, 1966.

30. Occupational Therapy Assistant Education Program Brochure. Westminister College-William Woods College, Fulton, Missouri, 1976.

31. U.S. Senate, Committe on Finance. The Social Security Act and Related Laws. December 1978 edition. Washington DC, US Government Printing Office, 1978.

32. Carr SH: Models of manpower utilization. *Am J Occup Ther* 25:259-262, 1971.

33. AOTA: 1986 Member Data Survey. *Occup Ther News* September, 1987.

34. Education for All Handicapped Children Act (Public Law 94-142), 1975, 20 U.S.C. 1401.

35. Education of the Handicapped Act Amendments of 1986 (Public Law 99-457), 20 U.S.C. 1400.

36. AOTA: 1980 Representative assembly minutes. *Am J Occup Ther* 43:844-870, 1980.

37. AOTA: COTA task force chart of concerns. *Occup Ther News* 35:8, 1981.

38. Barnett P: COTA task force report. *Occup Ther News* 35:(August) 1981.

39. AOTA: 1983 Representative assembly minutes. *Am J Occup Ther* 37:592,1983.

40. Brittell T: AOTA COTA advisory committee final report, 1986.

41. AOTA: 1982 Representative assembly minutes. *Am J Occup Ther* 36:808-926, 1982.

42. AOTA: Representative assembly minutes. *Am J Occup Ther* 37:831-840, 1983.

43. Jones R: Presentation at 30th anniversary COTA forum, Baltimore, Maryland, 1989.

44. AOTA. Bylaws revision, 1987.

45. AOTA: Member Data Survey, 1986. (Data combined with #46).

46. AOTA: Membership Data Base, 1989. (Data combined with #45).

47. AOTA: Award Nomination Form, Roster of Honor.

48. AOTA: Annual Conference Awards Ceremony Programs, 1979 to 1989.

49. Brayley CR: AOTA awardees 1977-1988. *Occup Ther News* 2(July) 1988.

50. AOTA: Education committee report. *Am J Occup Ther* 4:221, 1949.

51. AOTA: Annual reports *Am J Occup Ther* 11:41, 1957.

52. AOTA: Committee for recognition of occupational therapy assistants. *Am J Occup Ther* 12:669-675, 1958.

53. AOTA: Annual reports. *Am J Occup Ther* 12:38, 1958.

54. West W: From the treasurer. *Am J Occup Ther* 12:31, 1958.

55. AOTA: Board of management meeting. *Am J Ocup Ther* 18:34-35,45, 1964.

56. Johnson AA: Tool holder. *Am J Occup Ther* 19:214, 1965.

57. AOTA: Annual business meeting. *Am J Occup Ther* 21:95, 1967.

58. AOTA: Annual business meeting. *Am J Occup Ther* 22:99-118, 1968.

59. AOTA: Annual business meeting. *Am J Occup Ther* 23:168-169, 1969.

60. Schwagmeyer M: The COTA today. *Am J Occup Ther* 23:69-74, 1969.

61. AOTA: Delegate assembly minutes. *Am J Occup Ther* 24:438-443, 1970.

62. AOTA: 51st conference, minutes of meeting. *Am J Occup Ther* 26:95-113, 1972.

63. Knapp RL: Activity programs for senior citizens. *Am J Occup Ther* 26:224, 1972.

64. AOTA: Delegate assembly. *Am J Occup Ther* 28:549-566, 1974.

65. AOTA: Delegate assembly, *Am J Occup Ther* 29:552-564, 1975.

66. AOTA: Guidelines for AOTA recognitions. *Am J Occup Ther* 29:632-633, 1975.

67. AOTA: Annual business meeting. *Am J Occup Ther* 31:196-203, 1977.

68. AOTA: Delegate assembly. *Am J Occup Ther* 30:576-590, 1976.

69. AOTA Annual business meeting. *Am J Occup Ther* 32:671-677, 1978.

70. AOTA: Representative assembly. *Am J Occup Ther* 33:780-813, 1979.

71. AOTA 1980 representative assembly. *Am J Occup Ther* 34:844-870, 1980.

72. AOTA: Research information division, Dataline. *Occup Ther News* 36(March) 3, 1982.

73. AOTA: 1981 representative assembly. *Am J Occup Ther* 35:792-808, 1981.

74. AOTA: Newly elected officers for 1985-1986. *Occup Ther News* 39(May) 1, 1985.

75. Robertson S: COTA workshop first of its kind. *OT Week,* March 28, 1991.

76. The Association: 1991 Awards and Recognitions Recipients *Am J Occup Ther* 45:1148, 1991.

77. Gray M: Personal communication, May 1992.

78. Lamport N, Coffey M, Hersch G: *Activity Analysis Handbook* Thorofare, New Jersey, SLACK, Inc., 1989.

Section II
CORE KNOWLEDGE

Philosophical Considerations for the Practice of Occupational Therapy

Theoretical Frameworks and Approaches

Basic Concepts of Human Development

Components of Occupation and Their Relationship to Role Performance

Occupational Performance Areas

The Teaching/Learning Process

Interpersonal Communication Skills and Applied Group Dynamics

Individualization of Occupational Therapy

Building on the historical principles outlined in the beginning of the book, Section II focuses on the core concepts of the profession. These concepts are introduced through a discussion of philosophical considerations—the values and beliefs about the nature of human existence and the nature of the profession—which serve as a guide for action. These actions are further discussed in the context of theoretical frameworks and approaches frequently used as a basis for the delivery of occupational therapy services. The core elements of human development and the components of occupation that influence role performance are also presented. Another important emphasis is the occupational performance areas of activities of daily living, work and play/leisure. Following chapters address some of the people-to-people skills necessary for effective therapeutic intervention, with emphasis placed on the teaching/learning process, interpersonal communication and applied group dynamics.

The section concludes with a discussion of the important aspects of the individualization of occupational therapy, stressing such factors as environment, sociocultural considerations, change and prevention.

Consideration of the unique needs of the whole person is a prevailing theme throughout this segment. As Witherspoon stresses in regard to the profession: "[we] assist individuals in adapting to society, in assuming their occupational roles, in receiving gratification, and in reaching their full potential."

Philosophical Considerations

FOR THE PRACTICE OF OCCUPATIONAL THERAPY

Phillip D. Shannon, MA, MPA

INTRODUCTION

A vital aspect of the educational preparation of the occupational therapy assistant is an appreciation of the philosophy on which the practice of occupational therapy is based. Why is this so vital? There are at least four reasons that provide a rationale.

First, the philosophy of any profession represents the profession's views on the nature of existence. These views reflect the reasons for its own existence in responding to the needs of the population served. For example, a somewhat complex question addressed in philosophy is: "What is man?" Is man a physical being, a psychological being, a social being, or all of these? If man is perceived by a profession as a physical being only, then in responding to the needs of "man the patient" the action is quite clear: the practitioner deals only with the body, not with the mind. As incon-

ceivable as this particular belief might appear, the practices of some professions reflect a narrow perspective of man. Sometimes, as it will be discussed later, a profession does not practice what it believes.

Guided by its philosophical beliefs, a grand design evolves to specify the purposes or goals of the profession. Lacking an understanding of the philosophical basis for this grand design, the practitioner cannot be sure that the goals he or she is pursuing are worth pursuing or that the services provided are worth providing.

A second reason for understanding the philosophy of the profession is that philosophy guides action. Indeed, it is only within the context of a profession's philosophy that actions have meaning. Attending to the leisure needs of the patient, for instance, is one of the major concerns of occupational therapy, because its practitioners believe that man seeks a sense of quality to life. One aspect of a **quality**

KEY CONCEPTS

Rationale for philosophy

Metaphysical principles

Epistemological principles

Axiological principles

Philosophy of Adolph Meyer

Therapist/patient versus therapist/client relationship

life, like a satisfying work life, is a satisfying leisure life. Consequently, using arts and crafts to promote the leisure interests and skills of the patient and, therefore, the quality of life of the patient, is an action that makes sense because the action has philosophical meaning.

One of the primary reasons for studying philosophy, according to Thomas, is to clarify beliefs so that the action "which stems from those beliefs is sound and consistent."[1] Clarifying the beliefs of the profession should be regarded as a critical component of the occupational therapy assistant's education to ensure that his or her actions are sound and consistent; that is, that the occupational therapy assistant's entry-level behaviors are based on and consistent with a set of guiding philosophical beliefs.

A third rationale for understanding the philosophy of occupational therapy is the direct relationship between the growth of the profession and the ability of its practitioners to explain their "reasons for existence." In the present era of accountability, where the justification for programs and the competition for resources to support these programs is greater than in previous years, one cannot assume that those external to the profession, such as physicians, will perceive occupational therapy as an intrinsically good or essential service. Claims of goodness must be substantiated with evidence. That evidence must be supported philosophically, otherwise it will lack a context for its interpretation. For example, documented evidence that a patient's range of motion in the left elbow was increased by five degrees as a result of occupational therapy's intervention is important. What strengthens this evidence, however, are the reasons for intervening in the first place. These reasons are linked to the philosophical beliefs of the profession.

Finally, it is not sufficient for the occupational therapy assistant to be skilled in applying the techniques of the profession. On the contrary, he or she must have some appreciation, philosophical and theoretical, of the reasons why these techniques are applied. Lacking this appreciation, the occupational therapy assistant will apply these techniques without being able to communicate their value to the patient, thereby failing to motivate the patient's active involvement in treatment.

Certainly from the initial stage of patient referral to the last stage of discontinuing the patient's treatment, the philosophical beliefs of the profession must remain in the foreground. For the occupational therapy assistant, who has major responsibilities along the entire continuum of health care, these beliefs and the actions that stem from them must be understood and practiced. Indeed, this is the first duty of the occupational therapy assistant.

WHAT IS PHILOSOPHY?

To appreciate fully the philosophy of occupational therapy, one must appreciate and understand philosophy in general. Basically, philosophy is concerned with the "meaning of human life, and the significance of the world in which man finds himself."[2] Man is, by nature, a philosophical creature. Questions such as who am I?, what is my destiny?, and what do I want from life? are questions of meaning and purpose that concern all human beings. Each individual, in responding to questions such as these, develops a personalized view of oneself and the world, commonly referred to as a **"philosophy of life."** This philosophy represents a fundamental set of values, beliefs, truths and principles that guide the person's behavior from day to day and from year to year.

The philosophy of a profession also represents a set of values, beliefs, truths and principles that guides the actions of the profession's practitioners. Typically, as with individuals, the philosophy evolves over time and sometimes changes as a profession matures. Each profession, in shaping and reshaping its philosophy, has choices to make in three philosophical dimensions. These include metaphysics, epistemology and axiology.

Metaphysics

Metaphysics is concerned with questions about the ultimate nature of things, including the nature of man. With regard to the nature of man in particular, the **mind/body relationship** is of special interest to the philosopher. Are mind and body two separate entities, one superior to the other, or are mind and body a single entity representative of the "whole"—the whole person? The first position, that of mind/body separation, is the **dualistic** position. The second position, that of mind/body as one entity, is the position of **holism.**

While most (if not all) professions claim to be holistic, the truth in this claim is seen to the extent to which the actions of the profession are consistent with its beliefs. Assume, for example, that the actions of "profession X" are directed toward exercise as the means for promoting a healthy body, (ie, a healthy "physical" body). Assume also that profession X claims to be holistic, asserting a concern for the whole person. In actuality it is dualistic because the body is viewed as superior to the mind; the goal of exercise, in this case, is a healthy body, not a healthy body and a healthy mind. There is a contradiction, therefore, in what profession X believes and what it does. Its actions do not follow from its beliefs, and the claim of holism is illegitimate. When exercise is seen as promoting the health of the "whole," a more holistic approach is demonstrated.

Epistemology

The second dimension pertinent to shaping and reshaping the philosophy of a profession is the dimension of epistemology, which is concerned with questions of truth. What is truth? How do we come to know things? How do we know that we know? One way of knowing is by experience. One knows, for example, that the flame of a fire brings pleasure in terms of the warmth it provides, but also that it produces pain if it is touched by the bare hand. Usually, one only needs to experience this pain once to "know that he or she knows." Is experience the only route to truth or knowing? From a holistic perspective, there are many routes to truth and knowing. Intuition, for instance, is considered to be as truthful as experiential learning or the logic reasoned by the powers of the intellect. For the dualist, on the other hand, the subjective realities of intuition and experience cannot be accepted as truths. On the contrary, only the objective reality of rational thought can be admitted as truth; truth is logic.

Axiology

The third dimension of philosophy is axiology, which is concerned with the study of values. Two types of questions are addressed by axiology: questions of value with regard to what is desirable or beautiful in the world (aesthetics), and questions of value with regard to the standards or rules for right conduct, or **ethics.** Most people would agree that a long life is a desirable thing—something that is valued. Some people might argue that a long life without a sense of quality to one's life is a life that is not worth living. Almost everyone would maintain that it is wrong to take a life, yet, there are those who believe that "a life for a life," might be justified in some instances.

Conflicting values and standards often produce dilemmas that are difficult to resolve. If life is valued, for example, is it right or moral to disconnect the support systems maintaining the life of the person who has been certified as "brain dead?" Is it right or moral to prolong a life that may not be a life worth living? These are difficult questions of value about what is desirable or beautiful in the world and about the standards that will be applied in pursuing that which is valued.

Each profession has choices to make about what it considers beautiful and desirable in the world and the ethical principles that it will follow in achieving its goals. For medicine, the preservation of life is the first priority, and perhaps this is as it should be, for medicine. But, is this the highest priority of the other health care professions? Should it be the highest priority? A profession that claims to be holistic cannot be satisfied with saving lives. Instead, a holistic profession would maintain that a life worth saving must be a life worth living.

Given this brief glimpse of metaphysics, epistemology and axiology, each dimension can be discussed as it relates to the philosophy of occupational therapy. Specifically, four questions will be addressed:

1. The metaphysical question of "what is man?"
2. The epistemologic question of "how does man know what he knows?"
3. The aesthetic question of "what is beautiful or desirable in the world?"
4. The ethical question of "what are the rules of right conduct?"

Two approaches will be taken in responding to these questions. First, the philosophy of Adolph Meyer, who was primarily responsible for providing occupational therapy with a philosophical foundation for practice, will be examined. Second, the extent to which this philosophical base has survived the test of time will be explored.

THE EVOLUTION OF OCCUPATIONAL THERAPY

Occupational therapy evolved from the moral treatment movement that began in the early 19th century.[3] If there was a single purpose to which the champions of this movement were committed, it was to humanize and to provide more humane forms of treatment for the mentally ill incarcerated in the large asylums in this country and abroad. Marching under the banner of humanism, the leaders of this movement sought to defend and preserve the dignity of all human beings, particularly the sick and the disabled.

Among these humanists who carried the movement into the 20th century was the psychiatrist Adolph Meyer (Figure 3-1), whose paper on "The Philosophy of Occupation Therapy"[4] laid the foundation for the practice and promotion of occupational therapy. Meyer's philosophy was based on his observations of everyday living. From his beliefs about the nature of man, about life, and about a life worth living, the pioneers of the profession emerged to chart its course. Although Meyer has been quoted frequently in the literature of recent years, a more extensive discussion of his philosophy is provided here because, to date, his thoughts have not been examined within the context of metaphysics, epistemology, and axiology.

A Retrospective Glance at the Philosophy of Adolph Meyer

What is Man? Meyer's perspective of man was holistic:

Our body is not merely so many pounds of flesh and bone figuring as a machine, with an abstract mind or

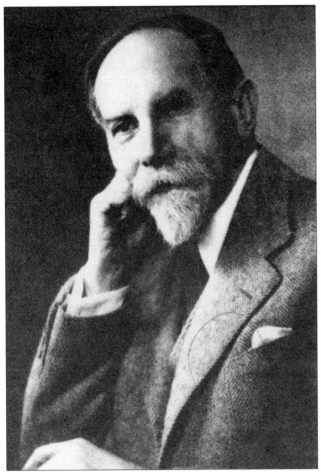

Figure 3-1. Dr. Adolph Meyer, psychiatrist and early occupational therapy proponent and philosopher (Fabian Bachrach Photo). Courtesy of the Archives of the American Psychiatric Association.

soul added to it. (Rather it is a live organism acting) in harmony with its own nature and the nature about it.[4]

For Meyer, three characteristics distinguished man from all other organisms: sense of time, capacity for imagination, and need for occupation.

A sense of time—past, present and future—was the central theme of Meyer's philosophy. He believed that a sense of time, and particularly time past, (experience) provides man with an advantage over other living organisms in terms of adapting in the present and manipulating the future. This capacity to learn from experience, when blended with the capacity for imagination or creativity, allows man to alter his environment. The squirrel, for example, is totally dependent on its environment for food and shelter during the winter months. Man, on the other hand, through experience and imagination, has been able to alter his environment to ensure survival from hunger through food preservation techniques and protection from the cold via heat-producing systems.

The need for occupation was regarded by Meyer as a distinctly human characteristic. He defined occupation as

"any form of helpful enjoyment,"[4] which clearly transcends the notion of occupation as being limited to work. On the contrary, the meaning of occupation was extended by Meyer to include all of those activities that comprise a normal day, particularly work and play. He considered occupation important to all, the sick as well as the healthy. Each individual must achieve a balance among his occupations, a balanced life of not only work and play, but also of rest and sleep.[4]

How Does Man Know That He Knows? Man learns not only by experience, but also by "**doing**": engaging mind and body in occupation. By doing, man is able to achieve. Fidler and Fidler, in reiterating this theme in the 1970s, maintained that doing is linked to becoming, to realizing one's potential.[5] Fundamental to achieving and becoming is doing. In doing, man comes to know about himself and the world. In doing, man knows that he knows.

What is Desirable or Beautiful in the World? For Meyer, man is not content simply existing in the world. Instead, man seeks a sense of quality to life that comes from the pleasure in achievement.[4] It is in engaging the total self that man comes to experience the pleasure in achievement, which Reilly, in her Eleanor Clarke Slagle lectureship, articulated so beautifully: "That man, through the use of his hands as they are energized by mind and will, can influence the state of his own health."[6] Again, it is in doing that man achieves and is able to acquire a sense of quality in his life.

What are the Rules of Right Conduct? Meyer, in outlining the guiding principles for the practice of occupational therapy, maintained that the occupation worker should provide **opportunities**, not **prescriptions**.[4] Prescriptions tend to constrain the development of one's potential, whereas opportunities nourish it. To apply prescriptions is to treat the patient as an object; to offer opportunities is to regard the patient as a person. Inherent in this principle of right conduct is a belief in the type of relationship that the occupation worker should maintain with the patient—a helping relationship, a caring relationship, a relationship where patients are indeed treated as persons and not as objects.

To summarize, Meyer's perspective of man was holistic. He emphasized doing as the primary route to truth and to achieving a sense of quality in one's life. Prerequisite to doing, however, is opportunity. Lacking the opportunity to do, man, like the squirrel, cannot control his own destiny. On the contrary, man becomes the squirrel, controlled and manipulated by his environment.

The Test of Time

Has the philosophy of Adolph Meyer, which provided the direction for the practice and promotion of occupational therapy, survived the test of time; or has the profession, as it matured, changed its direction, based on a different set of values, beliefs, truths, and principles? The answer is reflected in the report to the American Occupational Therapy Association on the Project to Identify the Philosophical Base of Occupational Therapy, which was submitted to the Executive Board of the AOTA in 1983.[7] This report does not represent "an official position" of the AOTA with regard to the philosophy of occupational therapy, but it is the documentation of a six and one-half-year project designed to trace the philosophical beliefs of the profession historically and to interpret those beliefs within the context of more modern times. In reviewing the degree to which the beliefs of Adolph Meyer have withstood the test of time, the four philosophical questions addressed earlier are once again discussed in the following sections.

What is Man? The belief in holism has persisted in the profession.[7] Indeed, one of the unique aspects of occupational therapy is its integrating function, where mind and body are activated to promote the patient's total involvement in the treatment process. To lose sight of this function is to lose sight of one of the major contributions of occupational therapy—attending to the "whole person."

One might speculate that it is the profession's commitment to holism that has attracted people to occupational therapy rather than to some of the other health professions that appear less holistic. Even in occupational therapy, however, the concept of holism, although universally professed, is not uniformly applied in practice. Action is not always consistent with belief. When practice takes the form of dealing only with the mind, only with the body, or worse yet, with only parts of the body, the commitment to holism has been compromised; and there is a contradiction between what one believes and what one does.

For example, hand rehabilitation has become a highly specialized area of practice. Unquestionably, there is a significant contribution to be made to health care in this area. However, when some of the practitioners in rehabilitation begin to refer to themselves as "hand therapists" versus "occupational therapists," there is an implicit shift away from holism. The belief in holism may remain, but the explicit actions that follow are sometimes not holistic. Only when hand rehabilitation focuses on the whole person does it retain its holistic function.

Another contradiction between belief and action is in mental health practice. Probably one of the first signs indicating the shift away from holism in mental health is when the practitioner uses the title "psychiatric occupational therapist" or "psychiatric occupational therapy assistant." "Psychiatric occupational therapy" personnel tend to focus only on the mind of the patient to the exclusion of the patient's body. Furthermore, when the practitioner's actions are directed primarily toward the unconscious mind, as in providing activities for the sublimation of innate drives,

attention is not even focused on the whole mind, much less the mind and body. Again the belief in holism may be contradicted by the practitioner's actions.

Surely these examples are not characteristic of most practitioners in mental health; nor is "hand therapy" necessarily limited to the treatment of the hand. However, when the broad concerns of occupational therapy are narrowed, the patient is somehow cheated in the process.

Also surviving the test of time is the belief in Meyer's distinguishing characteristics of man. Indeed, in responding to the needs of "man the patient," occupational therapy has placed a high priority on time as a continuum in the life of a patient, designing programs of treatment within the context of the patient's past, present and future. In implementing these programs, the patient's capacity for imagination or creativity is challenged in the interest of serving the need for occupation.

Occupation, as defined in the report from the AOTA Project to Identify the Philosophical Base of Occupational Therapy, is "goal-directed behavior aimed at the development of play, work and life skills for optimal time management."[7] If, as Reilly proposed, man's need for occupation is "that vital need of man served by occupational therapy,"[6] then to reduce the concept of occupation to the level of exercising bodily parts with weights and pulleys, or to the level of occupying the patient's mind with activities that bear little or no relationship to the nature of his or her occupation, is to deny this vital need. In addition, another unique aspect of the profession is somehow lost in the transformation of belief into action.

In contrast, by drawing on the patient's past experiences in work and play and in exploring the patient's values, capacities, and interests, the therapist should provide experiences that will serve the patient's need for occupation. In addition, in tapping the creative potential of the patient in areas such as problem solving and decision making, the therapist can expand the patient's capacities for altering the environment, thereby, expanding the potential for adapting in the present and for controlling his or her own destiny into the future.

How Does Man Know That He Knows? From the beginning, occupational therapy has believed in the active versus the passive involvement of the patient in treatment, that is, in doing. As Meyer believed, however, doing is but one way of knowing. There are multiple routes to truth—experience, thinking, feeling and doing—which the modern-day practitioner also accepts as reality.[7] One knows, for example, what happiness means because it has been experienced and because it can be felt. Happiness cannot be measured, but this does not make it any less real.

Among the many ways of knowing, doing is emphasized in the profession as the means for acquiring the skills for daily living and knowing one's capabilities in the present and one's potential for the future. Here again, the opportunities for doing must be framed within the context of the whole person. Consider, for example, the active engagement of the patient in sensory-integration activities. One of the major reasons for involving a patient in this type of activity is that the ability to receive and process sensory information is one way of knowing. For example, one knows that it is cold, and, therefore, that the body should be protected with warm clothing because one is able to feel cold, process this input, and take the appropriate steps to protect oneself.

Lacking the ability to process sensory information, the person is denied an important, if not critical, source of information. In this case, doing, in the form of involving the individual in sensory-integration activities, is an important step in the process of knowing. On the other hand, if the patient benefits from involvement in occupational therapy are limited to those derived by applying the techniques of sensory-integration, then occupational therapy has not served its holistic function; nor has it served the patient's need for occupation.

The practitioner takes a step away from this belief in doing when the action of "having the patient do" is replaced with the action of "doing to the patient." Another unique aspect of occupational therapy is obscured when the patient is denied the opportunity for doing.

What is Desirable or Beautiful in the World? To subsist, according to Meyer, is not enough for man. Man seeks something beyond subsistence or survival: the "good life," a life of quality. In maintaining this position over the years, occupational therapy has focused its attention in two directions, minimizing the deficits and maximizing the strengths of the patient.[7] Attending to one without attending to the other is incomplete and insufficient if the goals go beyond mere survival.

Traditionally, occupational therapy has minimized its contribution to the survival aspects of care and maximized its role in promoting a life of quality for its patients. Perhaps this is as it should be, perhaps not. Perhaps it is a matter of interpretation, that is, how one defines survival in terms of whether or not this position is legitimate. Consider, for example, the patient who has not learned the techniques of wheelchair mobility. This individual will not survive, at least not as a self-sufficient being. Consider also the patient who cannot dress him- or herself and is unable to organize time to meet the demands of daily living. This patient will not survive with any degree of autonomy or self-respect. Furthermore, as Shannon stated, "bodies and minds that are not active will atrophy from disuse, they will die. Also, people who lack quality in their lives sometimes engage in self-destructive behaviors, such as alcoholism, that lead to deterioration and death."[8] Does occupational therapy contribute to the preservation of life? Surely, as these examples suggest, occupational therapy contributes to the survival of the patient directly, if survival is interpreted to mean the ability to care for self, and indirectly, by adding a sense of quality to the lives of those served by the profession.

Reilly stated that "the first duty of an organism is to be alive; the second duty is to grow and be productive."[6] If survival is the first priority of the organism, then perhaps the position of the profession can be strengthened by developing an argument for the practice and promotion of occupational therapy that includes a commitment to the survival of the patient, as well as to the quality of his or her life.[8] In developing this argument, it must be made clear that the first priority of the profession is to teach the patient skills that will ensure survival. The second priority is to guide the patient toward the realization of his or her potential and social worth as a member of society, as evidenced, according to Heard, by the ability to perform an **occupational role**.[9] Indeed, it is for these reasons that man engages in occupation; it is also for these reasons that occupational therapy exists.

Occupational therapy has expressed its commitment to the second priority, but its actions are often directed to the first.[7,8] As Heard maintained, it is in addressing the second priority, and particularly the social worth of the patient, that occupational therapy has been most negligent.[9] Yet, in attending to the social worth of the patient, the profession is making a major contribution to a more healthy society. Certainly, in making this contribution, as Yerxa argued that it must,[10] the profession's value is increased and its survival guaranteed.

What are the Rules of Right Conduct? Meyer's principle of providing opportunities, not prescriptions, for patients has been one of the distinguishing characteristics of the profession. In applying the rule of non-prescription, the patient becomes an active partner in treatment. Why is this important?

First, the skills and habits necessary for the performance of occupational roles cannot be administered to the patient, but must be acquired by the patient. Second, prescriptions tend to foster pawnlike behaviors (externally controlled), whereas opportunities encourage origin-like behaviors (internally controlled), as defined by Burke.[11] In applying prescriptions, the patient is treated as a pawn, externally controlled by those responsible for his or her care; in offering opportunities, the patient is treated as origin, drawing upon the strengths within him- or herself to assume control for his or her own life. If taking charge of one's own life is important and assuming control for one's own destiny is valued, providing opportunities and not prescriptions is a necessary first step.

In offering opportunities for patients to take charge of their own lives, two major ethical principles guide the actions of the practitioner. The first of these is the principle *nonmaleficence,* which states that not only should one do no

Table 3-1
Summary of Philosophical Beliefs, Principles and Contradictory Practices

Philosophical Beliefs	Principles for Practice	Beliefs/Principles Compromised
Metaphysical Position		
The belief in holism, in mind and body as one entity	Attending to the whole person	Attending only to the mind or only to the body or parts of the body
The belief in the uniqueness of or in man's distinctly human qualities, which include an appreciation of time, past, present and future	Designing intervention programs within the context of the patient's past, present and future	Attending to the present needs of the patient without considering the patient's past experiences and goals for the future
The capacity for imagination	Challenging the patient's capacity for imagination or creativity	Providing prescriptions versus opportunities
The need for occupation	Promoting a balanced life of work, play, rest and sleep	Placing an emphasis on the treatment of pathology to the extent that the acquisition of skills that will support occupational role is minimized or ignored
Epistemologic Position		
The belief that there is not just one, but many routes to knowing or learning	Valuing experience, thinking and feeling in the process of doing en route to knowing or learning	Treating the patient as a passive versus active participant during the process of intervention
Axiologic Position— The Aesthetic Component		
The belief that man seeks a life beyond subsistence, a life of quality	The first principle: teaching survival skills by minimizing deficits and maximizing strengths	Teaching survival skills without attending to the patient's potential beyond survival and to the patient's social worth
	The second principle: providing opportunities for achievement, for the realization of one's potential and one's social worth	
Axiologic Position— The Ethical Component		
The humanistic belief that patients should be treated as persons, not objects	Protecting the patient from harm; promoting good	Neglecting the patient's safety or security needs and/or failing to protect the patient's rights as a patient and as a human being
	Demonstrating kindness and caring	Promoting a therapist-client versus therapist-patient relationship
	Providing opportunities versus prescriptions	Applying remedies that discourage individual initiative

harm, but also that one should promote the good. The second is the principle of *beneficence,* or the rule that one should show kindness and caring.[12] Perhaps no profession can lay greater claim to applying these principles than occupational therapy. The principle of showing kindness and caring, however, raises the issue of patient versus client.

Which is more legitimate: a therapist-client relationship or a therapist-patient relationship?

In a therapist-client relationship, the client is perceived as an object, an "it," because only one aspect of the client becomes the focus of attention. The therapist-client relationship is similar to that of a used car salesperson who has only one goal: to sell the client a used car regardless of whether the client can afford gasoline to operate the car, or whether the client has the financial resources to insure and maintain it.

In a therapist-patient relationship the patient is perceived not as an object, but as a person. Patients expect that their total well-being will be improved when seeking health care. Reilly argues that there is a special bond in the therapist-patient relationship, similar to the bonding relationship of teacher-student, that is not present in a therapist-client relationship. Like teacher-student, the therapist-patient relationship is reciprocal, one involving mutual loyalties, obligations and caring.[13]

Over the years occupational therapy has prided itself on the fact that it cares. In caring about its patients, the profession has demonstrated that it is holistic and humanistic. If a different type of caring evolves, as implied by the use of the term "client," then any future claim of being a holistic, humanistic enterprise will have to be denied.

SUMMARY

The philosophical beliefs guiding the contemporary practice of occupational therapy can be traced to Adolph Meyer, whose philosophy of *occupation therapy* was framed within the context of metaphysics, epistemology and axiology. Meyer's philosophy was both holistic and humanistic. As it persists in the present to guide the actions of the occupational therapy practitioner, so will it persist in the future to provide direction for the profession as it continues to mature.

The philosophical beliefs identified in this chapter and the principles for practice that evolved from these philosophical beliefs are summarized in Table 3-1, which also contains descriptions of situations when these beliefs and principles are compromised. The COTA owes allegiance to these beliefs and principles when responding to the needs of those served by the profession.

Editor's Note

In the context of this chapter, the term "man," in the philosophical sense, refers to the generic term "mankind," which is considered standard and gender inclusive.

Related Learning Activities

1. The author cited several ways in which occupational therapy practitioners fail to retain a holistic approach to

rehabilitation. Outline how occupational therapy personnel in a physical dysfunction setting and in a psychosocial dysfunction setting would proceed with evaluation and treatment applying a holistic approach.

2. Reilly, Heard and Yerxa were cited regarding whether the profession of occupational therapy should be concerned with survival or with quality of life. What are the pros and cons of each position? What are the implications of each course of action?

3. Make a list of your basic beliefs about occupational therapy. Compare and discuss your list with a classmate or peer.

4. List at least four reasons why it is important for COTAs to be able to communicate the philosophy on which the profession of occupational therapy is based.

5. Discuss the following questions with a peer: According to Meyer, what three characteristics distinguish man from all other organisms? What are the implications for occupational therapy practice?

References

1. Thomas CE: *Sport in a Philosophic Context*. Philadelphia, Lea and Febiger, 1983, p. 19.
2. Randall JH, Buchler J: *Philosophy: An Introduction*. New York, Barnes and Noble, Inc., 1960, p. 5.
3. Bockhoven JS: Legacy of moral treatment 1800's to 1910. *Am J Occup Ther* 25:223-225, 1971.
4. Meyer A: The philosophy of occupation therapy. *Am J Occup Ther* 31:639-642, 1977.
5. Fidler GS, Fidler JW: Doing and becoming: Purposeful action and self-actualization. *Am J Occup Ther* 32:305-310, 1978.
6. Reilly M: Occupational therapy can be one of the great ideas of 20th century medicine. *Am J Occup Ther* 16:1-9, 1962.
7. Shannon PD: Report on the AOTA Project to Identify the Philosophical Base of Occupational Therapy. January, 1983. Condensed under the title: *Toward a Philosophy of Occupational Therapy*. August, 1983.
8. Shannon PD: From another perspective: An overview of the issue on the roles of occupational therapists in continuity of care. *Occup Ther Health Care* 2:3-11, 1985.
9. Heard C: Occupational role acquisition: A perspective on the chronically disabled. *Am J Occup Ther* 31:243-247, 1977.
10. Yerxa E: The philosophical base of occupational therapy. In *Occupational Therapy: 2001 AD*. Rockville, Maryland, American Occupational Therapy Association, 1979, pp. 26-30.
11. Burke JP: A clinical perspective on motivation: Pawn versus origin. *Am J Occup Ther* 31:254-258, 1977.
12. Beauchamp TL, Childress JF: *Principles of Biomedical Ethics*. New York, Oxford University Press, 1983, pp. 106-107, 148.
13. Reilly M: The importance of the patient versus client issue for occupational therapy. *Am J Occup Ther* 6:404-406, 1984.

Theoretical Frameworks and Approaches

M. Jeanne Madigan, EdD, OTR, FAOTA
Sally E. Ryan, COTA, ROH

INTRODUCTION

Confusion about the terminology related to theory has been reflected in the occupational therapy literature. Terms that have been used by occupational therapy personnel include *theory, paradigm, model of practice, frame of reference, and conceptual framework.* These terms have been used very specifically by some to differentiate levels of theory development, whereas others have used the terms loosely and interchangeably.

This chapter emphasizes the term *theoretical frameworks,* which is defined as the interrelated set of ideas that provide a way to conceptualize the fundamental principles and applications inherent in the practice of occupational therapy. The reader should note that some theoretical frameworks are more fully developed than others.

In addition, some are much more general, allowing application in many areas of practice with a variety of patients, whereas others are more appropriate to specific populations and conditions. The chapter is organized based on this fact with the more general theoretical frameworks presented in the beginning. With this understanding, the purposes of this chapter are twofold: to indicate why the consideration of theoretical frameworks is important and to introduce the occupational therapy assistant student and practitioner to a variety of theoretical frameworks proposed and used by members of the profession.

Parham[1] has pointed out that theory is critically important for occupational therapy to be recognized as a profession and valued as a unique and necessary service to patients. She indicated that theory provides reasons

---

KEY CONCEPTS

Occupational behavior	Mosey's four frameworks
Model of human occupation	Sensory integration
Adaptive responses	Spatiotemporal adaptation
Facilitating growth and development	Neuromotor approaches
Doing and becoming: purposeful action	Cognitive disabilities model

for making decisions and taking actions in regard to patients. Theory is also the key to systematic research and increased development of a knowledge base.

When one engages in theory-based practice, one selects certain things to consider when evaluating patients and determining goals and the methods to accomplish those goals.

Parham[1] has stated that theory helps us "set the problem" (by identifying the appropriate problem to solve) and "solve the problem" (by applying the appropriate procedures for intervention). Sands[2] indicated that *setting the problem* is the responsibility of the occupational therapist, but that the COTA collaborates with the OTR in *solving the problem*. This approach indicates that both must have some knowledge of the theoretical foundations for practice, although at different levels of understanding.

This chapter focuses on some of the more well-known and used theoretical frameworks proposed by occupational therapists. Basic information is provided to acquaint the reader with primary principles, concepts and applications. The reference and bibliographic listings should be used for more in-depth study.

OCCUPATIONAL BEHAVIOR

In her Eleanor Clarke Slagle address, Mary Reilly concluded "that man, through the use of his hands, as they are energized by mind and will, can influence the state of his own health."[3] This hypothesis was formulated from her examination of the heritage of our founders. She returned to the principles of moral treatment and the concepts of health-restoring properties of occupation; habit training; and a balance of work, play, rest, and sleep, proposed by Adolph Meyer, Eleanor Clarke Slagle, Louis Haas, Susan B. Tracy, George Barton, and other founders of the profession (see Chapter 1).

Using these basic ideas and borrowing related concepts from many other disciplines, she built her framework, which emphasizes the critical importance of occupation to the well-being of the individual—that each person has a need to master his or her environment, to alter and improve it. She stated that the goal of occupational therapy is "to encourage active, open encounter with the tasks which would reasonably belong to (one's) role in life"[3] and the occupational therapy clinic is a "laboratory setting for human productivity."[3] According to this framework, occupational therapy practice is based on the assumption that "the mind and will of man are occupied through central nervous system action and that man can and should be involved consciously in problem solving and creative activity."[3] Reilly defined the developmental continuum of play and work as occupational behavior. She proposed that this definition should be the

unifying concept around which occupational therapists could build a body of knowledge to support practice in all areas of the profession and to guide education and research.

Using a psychiatric occupational therapy clinic as a proving ground for her ideas, Reilly examined **life roles** relative to community adaptation and to identify various skills that would support these roles. She then built a milieu to encourage competency, arouse curiosity, and develop appropriate skills and habits. Patients' daily living was to be balanced among work, play and rest at appropriate times and with opportunities for decision making. Occupation, therefore, would become the integrating factor for improving patient behavior.[4]

During the 1960s and the 1970s, Reilly and her students at the University of Southern California researched, discussed and refined the various concepts that became the occupational behavior body of knowledge. Since reduction of disease does not necessarily lead to improved function and increased engagement in activity, the purpose of occupational therapy was "to prevent and reduce the incapacities resulting from illness" and to "activate the residual adaptation forces within the patient."[5] Occupational therapy's focus was the patients' achievement and the ability to carry on the daily activities required by their social roles. It was proposed that the achievement drive generates interests, abilities, skills and habits of competition and cooperation. The environment for this was engagement in play and work (occupational behavior). Play was seen as both preparatory and facility to work, oftentimes offering support to a work pattern through the application of adaptive skills learned through play activities.

Temporal adaptation was also considered to be an important element. How one occupies time and the appropriate balance of activities within specific and general time frames was considered a sign of one's ability to adapt.[6] According to Reilly, organization of time and behavior to carry out one's roles was necessary and involved a complex process that follows a ranked system (in ascending order), which moves from *rules* to *skills* to *roles*.[7]

Evaluation was viewed as identifying role-function problems. Treatment planning and implementation were aimed at role reconstitution so that individuals could go about their activities of daily life having achieved the necessary competence and deriving a level of satisfaction as they fulfilled their occupational roles.[5]

MODEL OF HUMAN OCCUPATION

As students of Reilly, Gary Kielhofner and Janice Burke were involved in identifying concepts and adding to the theoretical foundation of the occupational behavior framework. They developed a theoretical framework based in part on occupational behavior framework. Since then, Kielhofner has enlisted the aid of many students and associates in developing the model of human occupation and in further defining and refining the basic concepts.

Kielhofner and Burke organized the concepts of occupation into a **general systems** theoretical framework. They conceptualized humans as an open system composed of input, throughput, output and feedback.[8] Thus there is a dynamic interaction between the parts of the system and with the environment. The parts are defined as follows:[8]

- *Input* describes information received from the environment.
- *Throughput* refers to one's internal organizational processes.
- *Output* is defined as the mental, physical and social aspects of occupation.
- *Feedback* means information received regarding consequences of actions taken, which guides future behavior.

This system is self-transforming; that is, output and feedback provide input and, in turn, throughput modifies output. Society makes demands of the system in the form of norms and role requirements. The internal part of the system (throughput) is composed of the three following subsystems:[8]

- **Volition** guides individual choices and is influenced by values, goals and interests. It refers to motivation and the resulting actions. If the will to act is not present, action will not occur.
- **Habituation** refers to the individual's habits and internalized roles. It helps to maintain activity and action and is characterized by activities that tend to be routine.
- **Performance** means actions produced through skill acquisition. It is seen through the individual's performance and operates on rules and procedures for using skills.

The interaction of these three subsystems is critical for determining the composition of the systems output; higher subsystems control the lower ones and the lower subsystems constrain the higher ones.[8]

Three levels of motivation in the volitional subsystem govern change in other subsystems:[8]

- *Exploration* promotes generation of skills.
- *Competency* helps organize habits.
- *Achievement* influences the acquisition of competent role behavior.

"Occupation is the purposeful use of time by humans to fulfill their own internal urges toward exploring and mastering their environment that at the same time fulfills the requirements of a social group to which they belong and personal needs for self-maintenance."[9] It is a lifelong series of experiences and a changing balance of play and work. The occupational therapy clinic should provide a hierarchical set of challenges that corresponds to the exploration,

competency and achievement hierarchy of motivation.[9]

The goal of therapy is to achieve a balance among the subsystems, which is necessary for fulfilling both internal satisfaction and external demands. Changes in the system must begin with the lowest level of the subsystem (exploration) and the lowest level of behavior (skills). Occupational therapy creates an environment that presents demands for performance and elicits enactment of responses that can result in positive feedback. Challenges should then be increased to elicit a sense of competency.[10] Therapy is a process in which the system experiences the organizing involvement in planned occupations.[11]

Kielhofner views the occupation of human beings as a dominant activity, which is the result of evolutionary development. It is reflected in the individual's need for both productive and enjoyable behavior.[12] Roann Barris has also contributed to the development of this model, particularly in relation to the environmental aspects. Figure 4-1 illustrates the model of human occupation.

ADAPTIVE RESPONSES

Lorna Jean King believes that occupational therapy needs a unifying theory that ensures cohesiveness between the different areas in which occupational therapy personnel practice, especially in this time of specialization. The theory should also distinguish occupational therapy from other disciplines. In her Eleanor Clarke Slagle lecture in 1978, King said that she was struck by A. Jean Ayre's phrase "eliciting an adaptive response." After reviewing the literature, she concluded that adaptation was the common thread which ran throughout the history of occupational therapy.

She outlined the following four characteristics of the adaptive response:[13]

1. It requires active participation (the person must act rather than being acted on by another).
2. It must be evoked by the demands of the environment.
3. It is usually most efficiently organized subcortically (conscious attention directed to objects or tasks rather than specific movements).
4. It is self-reinforcing (each success acts as a motivation for greater effort or a more complex challenge).

Occupational therapy personnel must know principles and milestones of **human development** and which adaptive response is needed so that they can provide the proper environment and stimuli for a given action. The stimuli must also be given at an opportune time when a successful response is most likely to occur. King[13] states that occupational therapy consists of structuring the surroundings, materials, and especially the demands of the environment in

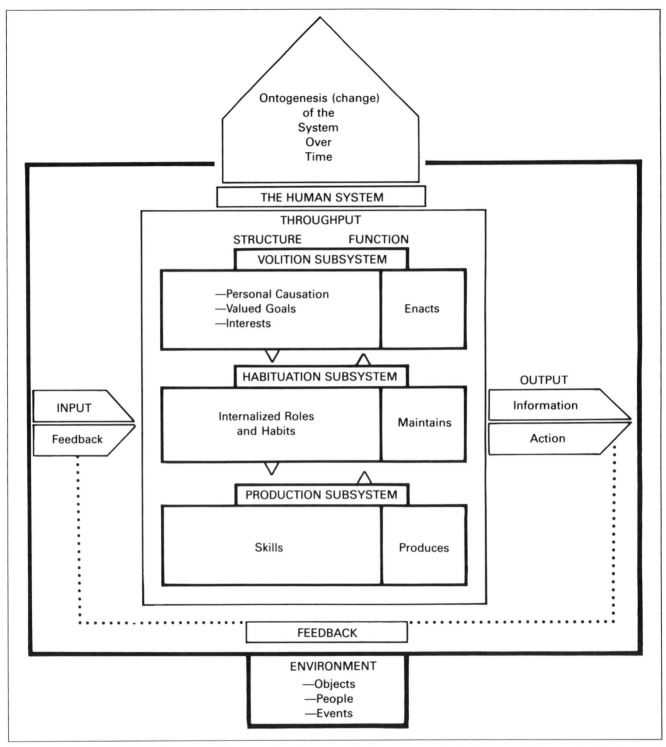

Figure 4-1. Model of human occupation. From Kielhofner G and Burke JP: A model of human occupation. Part I: Conceptual framework and content. *Am J Occup Ther* 34:572-581, 1980. Used with permission.

such a way as to call forth a specific adaptive response.

Kleinman and Bulkley,[14] in attempting to apply King's theoretical framework in 1982, presented an adaptation continuum, consisting of the following basic categories:

1. Homeostatic reactions
2. Adaptive responses
3. Adaptive skills
4. Adaptive patterns

They pointed out that the first relates to the capacity to perform, the second and third relate to performance, and the fourth relates to the constellations of performance over time. They also stated that the major function of all health disciplines is to foster adaptation. However, the second and third levels of the continuum are more appropriately the responsibility of occupational therapy because the focus is an integrated response to the whole person.[14]

FACILITATING GROWTH AND DEVELOPMENT

The facilitating growth and development framework was presented by Lela Llorens in her 1969 Eleanor Clarke Slagle address. The following premises were cited as a basis for her theory:[15]

1. Human development occurs horizontally in the areas of neurophysiologic, physical, psychological, and psychodynamic growth and in the development of social language, daily living, and sociocultural skills.
2. Humans develop longitudinally in the preceding areas in a continuous process as they age.
3. Mastery of skills, abilities, and relationships in each of these areas is necessary for satisfactory coping behavior and satisfactory relationships.
4. This mastery usually occurs naturally through the experience with the environments of home, school and community.
5. When physical or psychological trauma interrupts this growth and development process, a gap in development occurs, resulting in a disparity between expected behaviors and skills necessary to the adaptation process.
6. Through the skilled application of activities and relationships, occupational therapy can provide growth and development links to assist in closing this gap by increasing skills, abilities and relationships.

Using the work of many other theorists, Llorens constructed a matrix detailing selected development expectations, facilitating activities and adaptive skills. She pointed out that the occupational therapist is the enculturation agent who must understand the needs of the individual (determining function and dysfunction). The therapist then chooses activities and relationships to attain the following goals:[15]

1. Ameliorate (improve) or modify dysfunction.
2. Enhance remaining function.
3. Facilitate growth consistent with the individual's developmental stage.

She stressed that, while emphasis may be put on facilitating growth in a specific area of dysfunction, simultaneous attention should be given to all other areas of development so that an integrating experience will take place. The occupational therapist must determine the level at which the individual is functioning in the various aspects along the developmental continuum and program activities accordingly. It is necessary to meet the individual's needs at the present level of development and to monitor progress so that treatment can move to a higher level. If all areas of development are not considered, it is unlikely that there will be much success in restoring *integrated* function.[15]

In 1984, Llorens indicated that functional adaptation is the goal of occupational therapy. This adaptation depends on the dynamic interaction between the individual and the environment. She differentiated between three levels of environment as follows:[16]

1. First level—the individual (interior environmental factors are biologic, psychophysiologic, and sociologic
2. Second level—family, spouse, and partner interactions
3. Third level—community relationships

Through research that she and her students have carried out, Llorens concluded that occupational therapy objectives are concerned first with the patient as an environment that needs to gain or regain integrity to function adaptively within the sociocultural and person-made environments.[16]

DOING AND BECOMING— PURPOSEFUL ACTION

Gail Fidler and her husband Jay, a psychiatrist, first introduced a framework for occupational therapy as a communication process. This framework was concerned with action and its use in communicating feelings and thoughts as well as nonverbal communication. The occupational therapy experience was structured according to the following factors:[17]

1. The action itself
2. Objects used in the **action process** and ones that result from the action process
3. Interpersonal relationships that influence the action and, in turn, are influenced by it

They concluded that activity and objects function as catalytic agents or stimuli eliciting intrapsychic and interpersonal responses.[17]

Fourteen years later the Fidlers introduced a framework that modified these ideas somewhat and became known as "doing and becoming—purposeful action." They concluded that we realize our being in doing; what is potential becomes actual.[18] Their work was based on the belief that doing is a sense of performing, producing or causing; it is purposeful in contrast to random and is directed toward the following:[18]

1. Intrapersonal—testing a skill
2. Interpersonal—relationships
3. Nonhuman—creating an end product.

Through action and feedback, individuals know their potentials and limitations of self and the environment and achieve a sense of competence and worth. Becoming occurs when actions are transformed into behavior that satisfies individual needs and contributes to society. Activity must match maturation, developmental needs, and skill readiness and be recognized by the group as relevent to values and needs.[18] This framework has been used primarily in mental health.

MOSEY—FOUR FRAMEWORKS

Anne Cronin Mosey has long been a contributor to enunciating the parameters of occupational therapy and its theoretical frameworks. Four of her contributions, spanning more than 20 years, are presented here. It is interesting to identify various concepts and to note their evolution and relative emphasis over time.

Recapitulation of Ontogenesis

In 1968, Mosey developed a theoretical framework for the practice of occupational therapy called *recapitulation of ontogenesis*. This model was influenced by Mosey's clinical work with Gail Fidler.[19] The term reflects the biologic concept that there is a "repetition of evolutionary stages of a species during embryonic development of an individual organism."[19] She stated that an individual is able to move from a state of dysfunction to a state of function through participation in activities similar to those object interactions believed to be responsible for the development of an adapting human organism. She outlined the following seven adaptive skills:[20]

1. Perceptual-motor
2. Cognitive
3. Drive-object
4. Dyadic interaction
5. Primary group interaction
6. Self-identity
7. Sexual identity

Each of these adaptive skills was further divided into hierarchical components, so that one must learn a lower-level component before learning a higher-level one. She also said that these components are interdependent; one must learn some components in one skill before being able to learn certain components in another skill. She concluded that a state of function was the intergrated learning of those adaptive skills components needed for successful participation in the social roles expected of the individual in the usual environmental setting.[20] Learning occurs through involvement in activities that allow the individual to progress sequentially through those stages of development that previously were never completely mastered. She stressed the importance for occupational therapy personnel to analyze activities, first according to **skill components** and then according to their environmental elements. Initial, immediate goals are related to learning the most elementary skill components, whereas long-term goals are the patient's successful participation in expected social roles.[20]

Activities Therapy

The activities therapy framework, developed by Anne Mosey and introduced in 1973, is based on the assumption that many individuals who are unable to learn to function in the community have mental health problems.[21] These problems occur due to basic skill deficits, such as failure in planning and carrying out activities of daily living, and inability to express feelings in a socially acceptable way, among others.[22]

Activities therapy takes place in the present in a therapeutic community; both one to one and groups are used in treatment. It is immediate and action-oriented, with the treatment focusing on the patient's future needs and the knowledge and skills necessary to meet these needs.[19] Individual values are also considered in planning the treatment activities, which emphasize learning by doing.[22] Examples include how to plan meals, shop and prepare nutritious food, or read a bus schedule and take a bus to and from a specified location. This model is used primarily in adult mental health.

Biopsychosocial Model

In 1974, Mosey proposed the biopsychosocial model for the profession of occupational therapy as an alternative to the medical model and the health model. She stated that it directs attention to body, mind and environment of the individual.[23] The major assumption of this model is that humans have a right to a meaningful and productive existence—not only to be free from disease, but to participate in the life of the community. It is oriented toward the delineation of the learning needs of the person and the teaching/learning process (see Chapter 8). Initial evaluation is the assessment and delineation of the individual's learning needs. Next is the specification of what knowledge, skills and attitudes should be the focus of the treatment program (learning sequence and priorities). The selection and organization of learning experiences are a statement of the teaching plan. Occupational therapy personnel should follow the principles of teaching and learning, which include the following:[23]

1. Beginning where the learner is and proceeding at a rate that is comfortable for the learner

2. Involving the learner as an active participant
3. Facilitating learning through frequent repetition and practice
4. Moving from simple to complex

This model is oriented to the client-in-the-community and views occupational therapists, assistants, and the individual receiving services working together to solve problems of living. It focuses on humans as a biologic entity, a thinking and feeling person, and a member of the community[23] (see Chapter 6 for related information).

Domains of Concern and Tools

In 1981, Mosey outlined what she considered to be a model for the practice of occupational therapy. She identified the following domains of concern: performance components (sensory integration, neuromuscular function, cognitive function, psychological function, and social interaction) within the context of age, occupational performance, and an individual's environment.[24] She also stated that the legitimate tools of occupational therapy are the nonhuman environment, conscious use of self, the teaching-learning process, purposeful activities, activity groups, and activity analysis and synthesis.[24]

SENSORY INTEGRATION

The sensory integration approach to occupational therapy intervention was introduced by A. Jean Ayres in the 1960s and resulted from her various and extensive research projects, which were an integral part of her clinical practice. It was based on her earlier work with perceptual motor deficits.[21,25] Sensory integration may be defined as the ability to develop and coordinate sensory information, motor response, and sensory feedback.[26]

Deficits were originally found through the administration of the *Southern California Sensory Integration Tests,* which included visual, kinesthetic, tactile and motor areas. The tests were revised and extended in the 1980s and renamed the *Sensory Integration and Praxis Tests.* As with the original battery, it measures sensory integration processes that provide a foundation for learning and behavior. Test scores are viewed as a "total picture" rather then individually.[27] They provide information about how the human brain receives and processes sensory messages and organizes a response to the sensory information.[21]

Sensory integration treatment procedures focus on "control of sensory input that proceeds according to a developmental sequence and requires an adaptive response."[19] Activities and appropriate therapeutic equipment are selected to obtain the desired sensory input and response. For example, treatment might include rubbing the skin with terry cloth to provide tactile stimulation or having a child lie prone on a scooterboard and move about in a specific way to provide vestibular stimulation.[21] This approach has been widely used with children. Other applications have been proposed, eg, King, with adult schizophrenics, and Lewis,[28] with elderly patients.

SPATIOTEMPORAL ADAPTATION

Spatiotemporal adaptation is a model developed by Elnora Gilfoyle and Ann Grady based on the human development milestones and learning sequence of Gesell and Piaget, respectively, as well as biopsychosocial elements and the Bobath approach.[21] The model focuses on adaptation to space and timing of movements to build postural and movement strategies, which are adapted to achieve purposeful behaviors such as creeping, crawling and walking. The behaviors are a foundation for development of skills and the performance of purposeful activities.[21] Gilfoyle and Grady view the behaviors in a spiraling continuum in which adaptation begins before birth. When considering the present status of a child, past behaviors are called up to improve the present situation and enhance future skill acquisition and adaptation. Figure 4-2 illustrates the sequence of the model and the relationship of sensory input, motor output and sensory feedback. The following are brief definitions of the terms used in the continuum to achieve spatiotemporal adaptation:[29]

1. **Assimilation**—the ability to absorb, to make information a part of one's thinking
2. **Accommodation**—the ability to modify or adjust in response to the environment
3. **Association**—the ability to relate factors from the past to experiences in the present
4. **Differentiation**—the ability to determine what differences exist between objects and events

To provide further illustration, the following scenario describes a little boy who is just beginning to crawl. The child learns that reciprocal movement of the arms and legs will move him forward a given distance. He also learns that he can crawl that distance at a fast or slow rate. This information is assimilated and recalled the next time the child has an opportunity to crawl. The child is crawling on another occasion and becomes distracted. He crawls too close to the wall and hits his head. The child then crawls away from the wall thus accommodating to this environmental barrier. He continues crawling about the room and touches a lamp cord. The mother responds by lightly tapping the child's hand and saying "no." He touches the cord again and the mother responds in the same way (association). Eventually the child learns to differentiate what he can touch and what should not be touched.

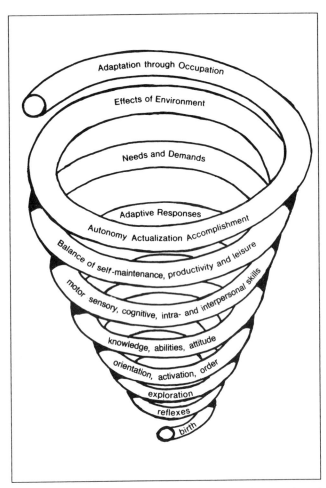

Figure 4-2. Spatiotemporal adaptation model. From Gilfoyle, Grady, and Moore: *Children Adapt*. Thorofare, New Jersey, Slack Inc., 1981.

NEUROMOTOR APPROACH

Neuromotor approaches are a group of treatment strategies based on a reflex (peripheral) model and/or a hierarchical (central) model of motor control. In the reflex model, sensory input controls motor output. Another way of stating this is that sensation is essential for movement to occur. Various sensory stimuli, such as vibration, tapping and quick stretch, are used to elicit more normal motor output. In the hierarchical model of motor control, motor programs in the brain control movement. To enhance motor performance, normal movement patterns are practiced repeatedly to develop motor programs that are thought to underlie all movement patterns. All of the neuromotor approaches emphasize that the nervous system controls movement, and view other systems within the body and the environment as subservient. These approaches also emphasize the importance of the normal developmental sequence in treatment. Proponents believe that the changes seen during development are a result of the maturation of the nervous system.

The Rood Approach

Margaret Rood was a physical and occupational therapist who developed her neurophysiologic approach to treatment while working with patients having cerebral palsy and hemiplegia.[21,30] Her treatment centered on the principles that sensory stimulation can assist in developing normal muscle tone and motor response, and that stimulation of reflex responses is the first step in motor control development.[31]

Sensory stimulation is a central focus to effect the desired motor response. Treatment includes relaxation techniques, such as slow stroking of the spinal column, slow side-to-side rolling, and neutral warmth, which entails wrapping the patient or a part of the patient in a blanket. Sensory stimulation may be provided by using a vibrator or brush or through rubbing the belly of a muscle to facilitate or make the desired response easier.[32]

Rood was a strong advocate of purposeful activity and promoted the use of her techniques in conjunction with such woodworking tasks as sanding a bread board. Through engagement in an activity, the patient's attention is focused on the task at hand and achievement of that task rather than the correct motor response.[32]

Proprioceptive Neuromuscular Facilitation

The proprioceptive neuromuscular approach (PNF) was developed by the physiatrist Herman Kabat. It was later expanded by Margaret Knott and Dorothy Voss, both physical therapists. PNF is used with patients with cerebral palsy as well as those with spinal cord injuries, orthopedic problems and other disabilities affecting the neuromuscular system. The basic thrust of this approach is stimulation of the proprioceptors. **Proprioceptors** are located in the muscles, tendons, and joints, which, through movement, make the patient aware of position, balance and equilibrium changes. Mass movement patterns are developed first through activities such as washing a floor in a creeping position or finger painting on the floor on "all fours." Making a macramé project is an example of how fine motor coordination might be used. Diagonal patterns of motion are stressed to facilitate the appropriate motor responses. The patient's active participation in the process is emphasized.[33]

Neurodevelopmental Approach

The late Karel Bobath, a neuropsychiatrist, and Berta Bobath, a physical therapist, developed the neurodevelopmental approach to treatment (NDT) while they were practicing in London. This approach, used with cerebral palsy and hemiplegia patients primarily, is based on the following concepts:[31]

1. Patterns of movement are learned and refined to enable the individual to develop skills.
2. Abnormal patterns of posture, balance and movement occur when the brain has been damaged.

3. Abnormal patterns interfere with the individual's ability to carry out normal activities of daily living.

Basic treatment centers on the inhibition or restraint of abnormal reflex patterns through handling and sensory stimulation. The goal is to help the patient produce the desired normal movement pattern. For example, the therapist might place a child on top of a large, inflated ball and roll the ball from side to side. The desired response is that the child will extend his or her hands and arms to maintain balance and as a protection against falling off the ball.[31] As this activity is repeated, changes will occur in muscle tone that promote normal movement.[32]

Movement Therapy

The movement therapy approach to treatment was developed in the 1950s by a physical therapist, Signe Brunnstrom, as a method for treating patients with hemiplegia. Based on the principles of neurodevelopment, she defined specific states of recovery of the hand, arm and leg. She also developed related techniques to establish patterns of motion or **synergies**.[31] Some of these techniques include tapping the belly of a muscle, applying pressure on a tendon, and quickly stroking a muscle.

Primitive reflexes, present in the early stages of normal development, often reappear in a patient who has had a cerebral vascular accident. These reflexes are facilitated in occupational therapy through activities that offer resistance (eg, weaving and woodworking) to promote the functional return of movement patterns. Such activities allow a neurologic impulse to spread to other muscles in a group. Visual and verbal clues are also a very important part of the total treatment process.[31,34] Brunnstrom noted that the movement therapy patterns that deal primarily with the lower extremities should be dealt with by a physical therapist.[31]

COGNITIVE DISABILITIES MODEL

In the early 1980s, Claudia Allen proposed a theory to guide occupational therapy practice. She indicated that identification of functional units of the brain would help specify elements that could assist in uniting our profession.[35] She constructed a matrix of six levels of cognitive function, which indicates the complexity of sensorimotor association formed during the process of performing a task:[36]

1. Automatic actions
2. Postural actions
3. Manual actions
4. Goal-oriented actions
5. Exploratory actions
6. Planned actions

She defined a *cognitive disability* as a series of functional units of behavior that cut across diagnostic categories and interfere with task behavior. According to her findings, cognitive disability is a restriction in sensorimotor actions originating in the physical or chemical structures of the brain. These changes produce observable and measurable limitations in routine task behavior. These dysfunctions restrict performance of social roles, limit ability to function in carrying out activities of daily living, and signal that disease exists.[36]

Allen devised a method of measuring the degree of social dysfunction and constructed another matrix, identifying levels of cognitive disability that corresponded to the the the six levels of cognitive ability and disability. These range, in ascending order, from level 1, severe impairment, to level 6, no impairment. At each cognitive level, specific motor actions and associated sensory cues are provided. For example, the following characteristics would be exhibited by a level 4 patient:[37]

1. Spontaneous motor actions are goal-directed
2. Can copy or reproduce a task from an example, such as chopping vegetables or sanding wood
3. Responds to visual sensory cues, ignoring what is not in immediate view

A third matrix, task analysis for cognitive disability, indicates the type and amount of assistance required to complete the task and specifies the kinds of directions a care giver needs to provide for each of the six cognitive levels.[35]

Allen pointed out that other disciplines frequently focus on verbal behavior and that occupational therapists who emulated them did little to help patients or the profession. Now, more neuroscientists are recognizing the importance of voluntary motor actions as a way to clarify the brain-behavior association. Occupational therapy personnel are unique in their approach, however, because of what we can do with motor action by applying task analysis.

According to Allen *task analysis* refers to the examination of each step that is followed in a typical procedure to achieve a goal. Occupational therapists and assistants use task analysis to modify the task procedure so that patients can achieve greater independence. The task analysis is a guideline for selecting and designing activities that correspond to the patient's level of ability (see Chapter 17). The structure of an activity is modified by using elements of the physical environment as substitutes for deficient patterns of thought.[35]

Allen also points out that occupational therapy treatment objectives differ according to the medical condition of the patient (unstable, acute versus stable, chronic). These objectives can be directed toward treatment (changing the condition) or compensation (modifying the task to offset deficits). In the case of cognitive deficit, the therapist or assistant can do little to improve the deficit. By reporting changes in the patient's behavior, however, occupational therapy personnel as well as other team members can identify what kinds of therapy would be most appropriate and report on the effectiveness of drugs and other forms of treatment. Another extremely important use of this framework is the ability to identify when a patient should be discharged and to plan the appropriate community support and placement.[35,36]

Originally used with psychiatric patients, this framework is also effective across other diagnostic categories and can be used whenever cognitive limitations are involved, such as stroke, head injury, dementia and mental retardation. This model focuses on measurement and management rather than improvement as goals of occupational therapy treatment. Allen emphasizes, however, the importance of providing activities that require increasingly complex abilities as the patient's cognitive functioning changes. Occupational therapy personnel can also provide tasks that a person can do successfully during acute illness or recovery by changing a task to place it within the patient's range of ability. In addition, Allen points out that the cognitive disabilities model can provide a mechanism to objectively assess occupational therapy services. She believes that we must achieve greater specificity about objectives and methods to increase the ability to facilitate independence through activity.[35]

FUTURE CONSIDERATIONS

The profession has not yet identified or adopted a singular theoretical framework or group of frameworks.[38,39] The debate continues as to the relative advantages and disadvantages of taking such a position. Some advocates of endorsing one comprehensive framework point to the need to achieve a greater degree of professional unity and to guide important research. Others feel that this is a narrow approach, emphasizing that multiple theoretical perspectives are more appropriate for the multifaceted practice of occupational therapy.[39] Although some practitioners indeed believe that it is advantageous to use more than one theory, Parham[1] cautions therapists to be sure that the theories they combine are compatible (based on similar assumptions and values).

It is unlikely that this issue will be resolved in the near future. As both the profession and society continue to grow and change, some frameworks and approaches will be discarded, others will be combined, and new ones will emerge. Certain common denominators, however, will survive the test of time: historically significant guiding principles, philosophical values and beliefs, ethics, and core concepts of *occupation*. These elements will continue to be in the forefront and provide a strong influence in further defining the theoretical foundations and guiding the profession in its research and continued development of its knowledge base.

SUMMARY

Definitions and basic concepts relative to some of the theoretical frameworks and approaches proposed by occupational therapists and others have been presented. The importance of using theoretical frameworks is stressed as a means of helping practitioners "set the problem" and "solve the problem," as well as being a key to systematic research and the continued building of a knowledge base specific for occupational therapy. Examples are provided that are general and have application to all areas of practice, such as occupational behavior and the model of human occupation, whereas others deal with specific clinical settings, such as psychiatry and pediatrics. Theoretical approaches related to the application of definitive techniques, such as sensory integration, proprioceptive neuromuscular facilitation, and cognitive disabilities, are also addressed. Reference is often made to human development and occupation as a base for many of these theories. Nevertheless, the profession has yet not adopted a singular theoretical framework or group of frameworks. This is currently evidenced by the pioneering work being done by the faculty and students at the University of Southern California in developing an emergency science of occupation (see Chapter Six).

Acknowledgment

Appreciation is extended to Virgil Mathiowetz, PhD, OTR, for his provision of content related to neuromotor approaches.

Related Learning Activities

1. Select any two of the more general theoretical frameworks and compare and contrast them in terms of basic values and beliefs, variety and age of patients, specific treatment techniques, and any additional pertinent factors. Use references and bibliographic material as needed. Organizing the material into a chart may be helpful.

2. Write a list of the theoretical frameworks and approaches you have personally observed being carried out in practice. Compare the list with at least two peers and determine which frameworks and approaches seem to be used most often in your area.

3. Develop a list of at least 20 different treatment activities for a variety of different patients with varying diagnoses. Adapt these activities to at least two different theoretical frameworks and approaches. Demonstrate some of these modifications to peers.

4. Stage a debate with your peers focusing on whether the profession should adopt a single theoretical framework as a foundation for practice. Provide a rationale for the stand taken.

5. Which of the many theoretical frameworks and approaches discussed in this chapter could be combined? What would be gained? What would be lost?

References

1. Parham D: Toward professionalism: The reflective therapist. *Am J Occup Ther* 41:555-561, 1987.
2. Sands M: Applying theory to practice: A response from technical education. In: *Occupational Therapy Education: Target 2000.* Rockville, Maryland, American Occupational Therapy Association, 1986, pp. 125-126.
3. Reilly M: Occupational therapy can be one of the great ideas of 20th century medicine. *Am J Occup Ther* 16:1-9, 1962.
4. Reilly M: A psychiatric occupational therapy program as a teaching model. *Am J Occup Ther* 20:61-67,1966.
5. Reilly M: The educational process. *Am J Occup Ther* 23:299-307, 1969.
6. Shannon P: Occupational behavior frame of reference. In Hopkins HL, Smith HD (Eds): *Willard and Spackman's Occupational Therapy* 7th edition. Philadelphia, JB Lippincott, 1988.
7. Reilly M: Defining a cobweb, an explanation of play. In Reilly M (Ed): *Play as Exploratory Learning.* Beverly Hills, California, Sage Publications, 1974.
8. Kielhofner G, Burke JP: A model of human occupation. Part 1: Conceptual framework and content. *Am J Occup Ther* 34:572-581, 1980.
9. Kielhofner G: A model of human occupation, Part 2: Ontogenesis from the perspective of temporal adaptation. *Am J Occup Ther* 34:657-663, 1980.
10. Kielhofner G: A model of human occupation, Part 3: Benign and vicious cycles. *Am J Occup Ther* 34:731-737, 1980.
11. Kielhofner G, Burke JP, Igi CH: A model of human occupation, Part 4: Assessment and intervention. *Am J Occup Ther* 34:777-788, 1980.
12. Kielhofner G: Occupation. In Hopkins HL, Smith HS (Eds): *Willard and Spackman's Occupational Therapy* 6th edition. Philadelphia, JB Lippincott, 1983, p. 31.
13. King LJ: Toward a science of adaptive responses. *Am J Occup Ther* 32:429-437, 1978.
14. Kleinman BL, Bulkley BL: Some implications of a science of adaptive responses. *Am J Occup Ther* 36:15-19, 1982.
15. Llorens LA: Facilitating growth and development: The promise of occupational therapy. *Am J Occup Ther* 24:93-101, 1970.
16. Llorens LA: Changing balance: Environment and individual. *Am J Occup Ther* 38:29-34, 1984.
17. Fidler GS, Fidler JW: *Occupational Therapy: A Communication Process in Psychiatry.* New York, McMillan, 1964.
18. Fidler GS, Fidler JW: Doing and becoming: Purposeful action and self-actualization. *Am J Occup Ther* 32:305-310, 1978.
19. Miller BRJ et al: *Six Perspectives on Theory for the Practice of Occupational Therapy.* Rockville, Maryland, Aspen, 1988.
20. Mosey AC: Recapitulation of ontogenesis: A theory for practice of occupational therapy. *Am J Occup Ther* 22:426-438, 1968.
21. Reed KL: *Models of Practice in Occupational Therapy.* Baltimore, Williams & Wilkins, 1984.
22. Mosey AC: *Activities Therapy.* New York, Raven Press, 1973.
23. Mosey AC: An alternative: The biopsychosocial model. *Am J Occup Ther* 28:137-140, 1974.
24. Mosey AC: *Occupational Therapy: Configuration of a Profession.* New York, Raven Press, 1981.
25. Ayers AJ: The development of perceptual motor abilities: A theoretical basis for treatment of dysfunction. *Am J Occup Ther* 17:221-225, 1963.
26. *Uniform Terminology for Reporting Occupational Therapy Services.* Rockville, Maryland, American Occupational Therapy Association, 1979.
27. Vezie MB: Sensory integration: A foundation for learning. *Acad Ther* 10:348, 1975.
28. Lewis SC: *The Mature Years.* Thorofare, New Jersey, Slack Inc., 1979, p. 93.
29. Gilfoyle EM, Grady AP, Moore, JC: *Children Adapt.* Thorofare, New Jersey, Slack Inc., 1981.
30. Cromwell FS: In memoriam. *Am J Occup Ther* 39:54, 1985.
31. Trombly CA, Scott AD: *Occupational Therapy for Physical Dysfunction.* Baltimore, Williams & Wilkins, 1977, pp. 70, 78, 87, 91, 98.
32. Huss AJ: Overview of sensorimotor approaches. In Hopkins HL, Smith HD (Eds): *Willard and Spackman's Occupational Therapy,* 6th edition. Philadelphia, JB Lippincott, 1983, pp. 116-117.
33. Voss DE: Proprioceptive neuromuscular facilitation: Application of patterns and techniques in occupational therapy. *Am J Occup Ther* 13:193, 1959.
34. Huss AJ: Sensory motor treatment approaches. In Willard H, Spackman C (Eds): *Occupational Therapy* 4th edition. Philadelphia, JB Lippincott, 1971, pp. 379-380.
35. Allen CK: Independence through activity: The practice of occuptional therapy (psychiatry). *Am J Occup Ther* 36:731-739, 1982.
36. Allen CK, Allen RE: Cognitive disabilities: Measuring the social consequences of mental disorders. *J Clin Psychiatry* 48:185-190, 1987.
37. Early MB: *Mental Health Concepts and Techniques for the Occupational Therapy Assistant.* New York, Raven Press, 1987, pp. 47-53.
38. Hopkins HL: Current basis for theory and philosophy of occupational therapy. In Hopkins HL, Smith HD (Eds): *Willard and Spackman's Occupational Therapy,* 6th edition. Philadelphia, JB Lippincott, 1983, p. 28.
39. Punwar AJ: *Occupational Therapy Principles and Practice.* Baltimore, Williams & Wilkins, 1988, p. 221.

Basic Concepts of Human Development

Sister Genevieve Cummings, CSJ, MA, OTR, FAOTA

INTRODUCTION

Human development is the essential basis for all occupational therapy practice. Although the subject of human development is vast and cannot be covered completely in this discussion, the elements most applicable to the practice of occupational therapy are addressed here: motor, cognitive and psychosocial development. Language development, although important, is not considered.

Basic theorists who will be discussed are Arnold Gesell, Jean Piaget, Erik Erikson, Robert Havighurst, and Abraham Maslow. There are, of course, many others who could be included and have contributed greatly to the field of human development. This chapter should be regarded as a summary and as a review of material studied in detail in courses in human growth and development.

MOTOR DEVELOPMENT

Many investigators have contributed to the body of knowledge about motor development. Among the most important is Arnold Gesell. Gesell studied and developed his theories first at Yale University and eventually at the Gesell Institute of Child Development. His important work is in the area of infant and child development.

Motor development occurs in a relatively unvaried sequence; however, the timing of each step in the sequence may be highly varied. Some of the principles that guide motor development are the **cephalocaudal development** and **proximal-distal development** (ie, development proceeds from the head to the lower extremities [tail] and from the parts close to the midline to the extremities, respectively). Control of the head occurs before

---

KEY CONCEPTS

Gesell's principles of motor development

Piaget's principles of cognitive development

Erikson's stages of psychosocial development

Havighurst's developmental life tasks

Maslow's hierarchy of needs

Relationship to disability

control of the limbs; control of the trunk and shoulder occurs before the hand.[1] The principle of **reciprocal interweaving** has been defined as well. This term refers to the fact that immature behavior and more mature behavior alternate in a constantly spiraling manner until, eventually, the mature behavior is firmly established. Therefore, development does not occur in a straight-line manner, but by this interweaving or circling pattern. Through careful studies, Gesell determined milestones of development that the infant should accomplish at particular times. The major milestones are shown in Table 5-1.[1-3]

Most children follow this sequence, although sometimes the sequence is altered or a stage is omitted. The actual time spent becoming stable in these tasks varies greatly. Reciprocal interveaving may be of short or long duration, or it may not be apparent to observers of the development. There is also a distinction between the time when the child is capable of performing these tasks, given optimal conditions, and when the tasks appear spontaneously. How strongly the parents desire to have a child perform the particular task seems to influence the development; children who are encouraged and given many opportunities to practice or perform may master a task sooner than those not having that encouragement. Motor development depends highly on both reflex and sensory development.

Reflex Development

A **reflex** is a constant response to a given stimulus. Reflexes generally precede voluntary movement control and later are integrated with motor function. Reflex action is observed as early as the seventh week in utero. By the 14th week in utero, the fetus reacts to stimulation with multiple motor responses.[4] Primitive reflexes, present at birth, involve the entire body and limbs. Rooting, sucking, incurvatum, crossed extension, withdrawal, Moro's reflex, primary righting, primary walking, and grasp are the major reflexes present at birth[4-5] (see Appendix A). A discussion of these reflexes and their development is beyond the scope of this chapter.

Sensory Development

At birth, the sensation of touch is highly developed and serves as the main source of sensory information for the neonate. All of the somatosensory **perceptions,** such as pain, temperature and touch, are present.

Visual perception is also present at birth, but is probably limited to light/dark perception and vague visual images. Fixing on an object for a brief time occurs at approximately one month, with more stable fixation occurring at three to four months. The visual system continues to develop for about ten years. Hearing appears to become acute a few days after birth. Smell and taste are present at birth and well developed by the second and third months[4] (see Appendix A).

Table 5-1 Milestones in Gross Motor Development and Postural Control	
Accomplishment	**Age in Months**
Lift head to 45° when prone	2
Lift chest off floor when prone	3
Sit up when supported	4
Sit by self	7
Crawl	8
Pull self up on furniture	9
Creep	10
Walk when led	11
Stand alone	14
Walk alone, straddle-toddle (feet far apart, full sole step)	15
Toddle (longer steps, narrower width, lower step height)	18
Run	21

Reach and Early Manipulation

Reaching in the supine position using small incipient movements occurs between eight and 12 weeks of age. Spontaneous regard of objects occurs at about 16 weeks, accompanied by greatly increased arm activity. Bilateral approach movements begin around 20 weeks, and at 24 weeks bilateral grasp of the object occurs. Beyond 28 weeks, the activity becomes more and more unilateral.

In the sitting position only passive and brief regard for reaching occurs from 12 to 16 weeks. At 20 weeks, the child makes movements that are likely to cause contact with the object. At 24 weeks, the child grasps the object and can **manipulate** it somewhat. A 28-week-old child can move an object such as a rattle from hand to hand and manipulate it in a variety of ways. By 18 months, the toddler reaches for near objects easily and automatically, but reaches for distant ones more awkwardly. This reaching for distant objects gradually becomes smoother and more coordinated by five years of age.

Grasp and Release

Grasp occurs as a reflex prenatally. There are two aspects to this reflex action: finger closure and gripping. Light pressure or stroking on the palm elicits closure; stretching the finger tendons elicits gripping. The closure aspect of the reflex disappears from 16 to 24 weeks after birth; the gripping aspect weakens and then disappears from 12 to 24 weeks.

Voluntary grasping, in contrast to reflex grasping, follows a relatively precise pattern. Initially, the ulnar side of the hand is used in a raking manner. Objects are palmed rather then handled precisely by the fingers. At 18 months the hand is open until it contacts the object; the thumb is in opposition.[2,3]

At 24 weeks, squeeze grasp is normally achieved. By 28 weeks, hand grasp is accomplished, and a palm grasp usually is performed by 32 weeks. At 52 weeks, the baby shows improved ability to use a four-finger grasp. Other milestones, which may be termed predrawing, include the ability to hold a crayon or object of similar size at 12 months, to "scribble" at 18 months, and to follow a horizontal line with a crayon at 30 months.

When the infant is eight weeks, a swiping movement is used to reach an object, but contact is not made; at three months, swiping results in some contact. By four months, the child is using a palmar grasp (ie, all fingers and the palm are in contact with the object). At six months, a mitten pattern of grasp appears whereby all of the fingers are together and the thumb is in opposition. At the baby reaches the age of seven months, the fingers, particularly the middle finger, are used as a rake to get an object into the palm with the thumb in opposition. At eight months, there is a beginning palmar prehension-thumb, index and middle fingers in opposition to each other. By one year, the child can use a more advanced palmar or fingertip prehension.[6]

Releasing is a more difficult motor activity than grasping. At nine months, the child begins to release objects voluntarily. At this age, the child will drop things spontaneously or will release an object when an adult takes it. At approximately 11 to 12 months, the child will release things on request.[7] Table 5-2 presents a list of grasp, release and manipulation milestones.[1]

COGNITIVE DEVELOPMENT

Jean Piaget is primarily responsible for the theory of cognitive development. Born in Switzerland in 1896, he did his early work in biology, but he eventually became interested in normal child development, particularly in the cognitive area. He used a clinical method of careful observation of children, beginning with his own, to study and analyze behavior and thinking. He did not use control groups, random sampling, or other research techniques of that type; but instead studied children in their natural environment doing their normal activities. He later developed a series of tasks to be presented to children as a basis of observation and analysis. Piaget died in 1983.[6,8-10]

Piaget's theory of intellectual development includes the concepts of organization and adaptation. **Organization** refers to a person's tendency to develop a coherent system, ie, to systematize. Adaptation is the tendency to adjust to the environment. As new knowledge is attained, it must be brought into balance with previous experience. This balance is called **equilibration**.[6,8]

Organization and adaptation are two tendencies within each person. Experiences are changed into knowledge through two complementary processes: assimilation and accommodation. Assimilation is a process by which an experience is incorporated into existing knowledge; in accommodation what is known is adjusted to the environment.

Knowledge is gained when experiences are organized, systemized, and related to previous experiences. This knowledge is adjusted according to the outside environment, the reality of things around the individual. A dynamic balance is being sought between what is known and what is objectively present. "Accommodation and assimilation, which are two complementary aspects of adaptation, are

Table 5-2
Milestones on Grasp, Release and Manipulation

Accomplishment	Age
Hands fisted	4 weeks
Hands open; scratches and clutches	16 weeks
Grasps cube in palm; rakes at pellet	28 weeks
Crude release	40 weeks
Prehends pellet with neat pincer grasp	52 weeks
Builds tower of 3 cubes; turns 2-3 pages at once	18 months
Builds tower of 6 cubes; turns pages singly	24 months
Builds tower of 10 cubes; holds crayon adult-fashion	36 months
Traces with lines	48 months

perpetually in action, are trying to maintain an equilibrium which is perpetually disrupted."[11]

Piaget described four stages of cognitive development: *sensory-motor* period, *preoperational* period, the *concrete-operational* period, and the *formal-operations* period (Table 5-3). The order of acquiring the skills in each period is constant, but the timing is not. Piaget emphasized the integrative aspect of stages, ie, structures of each stage become an integral part of the next stage. Each stage includes a period of preparation and a level of completion.[12]

Table 5-3
Piaget's Four Major Stages
of Cognitive Development

Stage	Name	Age
I	Sensorimotor	Birth to 2 years
II	Preoperational	2 to 7 years
III	Concrete Operations	7 to 11 years
IV	Formal Operations	12 to 15 years

Sensory-Motor Period

The sensory-motor period extends from birth until the appearance of language, or about two years of age. It is a period that begins with reflex activity, particularly sucking, eye movements and the palmar reflex. Through the use of reflexes, the baby brings information in and begins the process of assimilation. The child reacts to objects through reflex activity and gradually develops habits of response. These habits become organized as the baby learns to perceive and identify objects. The child learns to relate actions to objects and to see objects as something outside self. As children move through this stage, they learn the names of objects but do not name them because this is a preverbal stage. A child will search for objects that are not visible, try out different means of securing objects, and experiment with different properties of objects. At this point, the child begins to relate the means (actions) to the end (achieving what he or she wants).

Preoperational Period

The preoperational period is the time from approximately two to seven years of age. An operation is defined as a mental action that can be reversed; Preoperational refers to the period in which the child is unable to reverse mental actions. The child's reasoning is from the particular to the particular.[11] Generalization is not possible, and neither inductive nor deductive reasoning is present. The child is not

able to distinguish between reality and fantasy. One strong characteristic of this period is animistic thinking. The child regards inanimate objects as living and gives feelings and thoughts to them. The child is able to be aware of past and future, as well as present, but of short durations in each direction. Concepts of time are limited but present.

Concrete-Operational Period

The concrete-operational period occurs between about seven and 11 years. In this stage the child is able to use logic in thinking and is able to reverse mental actions. The child can analyze, understand part and whole relationships, combine or separate things mentally, put things in order, and multiply and divide. This stage is concrete because the mental processes are limited to those that are present and deal with the concrete. The child is not able to generalize. Abstract thinking begins to occur at the end of this period.

Formal-Operational Period

Toward the end of elementary school age and into the high school age, the young person develops the ability to reason hypothetically. The person in the formal-operational period is able to think about thinking. He or she is able to think abstractly; objects need not be present. Logical thinking and the ability to reason with syllogisms (a form of reasoning involving three propositions) are present. Theories can be developed and understood.

The development of the abilities in this stage lead to adult thinking patterns. Experience has shown that many adults do not think with adult thinking patterns, but may use concrete-operational patterns. It is also apparent, that the development of cognition is closely related to sensorimotor development. Lack of normal sensorimotor development will limit the child's ability to experiment with and explore cognitive skills. When a disability or condition interferes with the active exploration of the environment, it is necessary to make such exploration central in treatment.

PSYCHOSOCIAL DEVELOPMENT

Erik Erikson contributed greatly to the development of theories of psychosocial development and provided a framework for looking at development throughout the life span. He is usually classified as a neo-Freudian. He defined "eight ages of man," first described in his book *Childhood and Society* (Table 5-4). For each of the eight ages he identified a pair of alternative attitudes toward life, the self and other people. The person must resolve each of the issues identified as the alternatives. **Ego strength** develops from this process at each age, and these strengths continue throughout life; this development is cumulative.[13,14]

Table 5-4
Erikson's Eight Stages of Psychosocial Development

Stage	Name	Age
I	Basic Trust versus Mistrust	Birth to 18 months
II	Autonomy versus Shame and Doubt	18 months to 3 years
III	Initiative versus Guilt	3 to 5 years
IV	Industry versus Inferiority	5 to 11 years
V	Identity versus Role Confusion	12 to 17 years
VI	Intimacy versus Isolation	Young Adulthood
VII	Generativity versus Stagnation	Maturity
VIII	Ego Integrity versus Despair	Old Age

First Stage: Trust Versus Mistrust

Erikson's first stage centers on the polarity between trust and mistrust. This stage occurs during infancy when there is complete dependence on others who provide care. How this care is given determines the basic outlook of the infant. If the quality of the care is good and loving, then the infant develops a sense of expecting the good. If the child's needs are not fulfilled in a caring manner, a sense of expecting the worst develops. Trust, then, is the result of the relationship between feeling comfort and having that feeling relate to the world. This does not mean that mistrust does not occur or is not appropriate in some situations. Part of the balance is the recognition of when to trust and when not to trust.

The appropriate resolution of trust-mistrust leads to hope. Hope refers to an expectancy that needs will be met. As growth and development proceed, a basic attitude of hope means that the person expects the good and will have an optimistic approach to all aspects of life. If mistrust is emphasized, the person lacks this expectancy, is pessimistic, and usually looks at the dark side of any situation. This stage corresponds to Freud's oral stage of development.

Erikson points out that it is not the quality of food and basic care that influences this feeling of trust, but the quality of the relationship between the provider, usually the mother, and the infant. The mother-child relationship is crucial.[13]

Second Stage: Autonomy Versus Shame and Doubt

The second stage, autonomy versus shame and doubt, is the beginning of independent action by the child. As the child begins to move independently by standing and walking, develops control over bodily functions, and clearly distinguishes self from others, he or she begins to establish control over self and the environment. How the parents react to these efforts at independence and how much control they feel they must exert determines the balance between auton-

omy and shame. Again, this is a dynamic balance, not a matter of all or none.

Resolution of this stage results in will or free choice, the ability to choose to behave in a certain way because it is the best way to behave under the circumstances. A person who successfully resolves this conflict will be able to accept law and act independently within it as an adult.[13,14]

Third Stage: Initiative Versus Guilt

The third stage focuses on the balance between initiative and guilt. At this stage, the child is highly active, is able to use language effectively, and is learning to control the environment. The balance needed is between having confidence to try new activities and fearing the consequences of behavior. Questions of what others will think, how they will react to behavior, and what will happen as the result of the behavior are factors. This balance may result in a person who is confident to strike out on new things, to explore possibilities, and to work for goals; or a person who is fearful, feels guilty about doing or not doing, and is overly concerned about what will happen as a result of behavior. The resolution of this stage is purpose, the ability to establish goals and act to reach them.

Play, particularly the use of toys, is of great importance in the development and the resolution of this stage. The child uses this method to try new behaviors to learn of the reactions of others. Toys and play can help to develop initiative and confidence at this stage.

Fourth Stage: Industry Versus Inferiority

As the child reaches school age, which in most societies is approximately five years of age, the world becomes a wider arena. Play becomes the child's work. Tasks take on a greater degree of importance; how the child relates to these tasks determines the balance within this stage. Industry versus inferiority is the focus of this fourth stage. If the child succeeds and gains confidence from the tasks attempted, the ability to take on new tasks and the feeling of being able to achieve whatever is desired is fostered. If the child feels a failure in comparison with other children, a sense of inferiority results. This feeling can interfere with the ability to experiment and enjoy new activities. The use of tools, generally the same tools used by adults, is an important task at this stage.

The resulting quality of the dynamic balance in this stage is competence, described by Erikson as the ability to use dexterity and intelligence in the completion of tasks, which implies a sense of satisfaction in the completion. This developmental stage spans the elementary school ages of approximately five to 13 years of age.

Fifth Stage: Identity Versus Role Confusion

The fifth stage is that of identity versus role confusion and is the stage of adolescence. Erikson describes this stage as that in which youths are concerned with how they appear in the eyes of others in comparison to how they appear to themselves.[13] It is a time of great physiologic change. It is also a time of solidifying the skills developed in earlier stages and focusing these on the adult world of work. Knowing who they are and how they will relate to the world is an essential task. Peer relationships are highly important. Casual observation of adolescents confirms that being a part of a group, experimenting with all aspects of behavior, being different from those of any other age, and at the same time seeking acceptance are characteristics of this time.

Role confusion is the other end of this dynamic balance. It is characterized by an individual's inability to identify with the adult world of work and define his or her role in the environment. Much of the behavior of adolescence is an attempt to avoid this role confusion and to seek out and establish the appropriate boundaries.

The quality that develops in the successful fulfillment of this stage is fidelity. This is the ability to maintain loyalties in spite of differences. This loyalty is the result of strong peer identification.

Sixth Stage: Intimacy Versus Isolation

Young adulthood, the early twenties, focuses on the development of the capacity for intimacy. Erikson defines intimacy as "the capacity to commit oneself to concrete affiliations and partnerships and to develop the ethical strength to abide by such commitments, even though they may call for significant sacrifices and compromises."[14] Sexual relations are an important part of achieving this intimacy. The achievement of unity with another person and the development of a new identity that includes that person within it is the purpose and the result of a sexual relationship. Previous sexual relationships may have had the different purpose of establishing and solidifying self-identity.[14] The opposite pole is isolation: avoiding contacts that might lead to intimacy.[13]

Love is the result of the successful resolution of this stage. Although marriage is often the societal expression of this stage, marriage itself does not necessitate true intimacy.

Seventh Stage: Generativity Versus Stagnation

Generativity refers to the concern for the establishment and the guidance of the next generation. It does not necessarily include the bearing and rearing of children, although this is a common way for this stage to be expressed, but centers on a concern that what is important to human beings and society be passed on to the next generation. Erikson indicates that productivity and creativity are facets of this stage, but cannot replace generativity itself.[13] Older, more mature persons need to be able to share and to give. Generativity implies giving without expecting return. Care (concern for what has been generated) is the quality that emerges from the resolution of this stage.

The opposite pole of generativity is stagnation. Without sharing or giving, the person becomes preoccupied with self, without concern for growth or change. Erikson likens stagnation to having self as a child or pet. People may turn in on themselves and lavish the love and care they would give their children or pets on themselves.

Eighth Stage: Ego Integrity Versus Despair

Ego integrity includes an acceptance of self, of nature, and of one's life. It means that the person recognizes the value of the particular life led and does not grieve over what might have been. Such a person has inner satisfaction and is not compelled to try desperately to "live life to the fullest" or to make up for lost time. No time is regarded as "lost."

The opposite pole is despair, in which the person fears death with a feeling of unfulfillment: "There's so much left to do and no time to do it." This is characterized by an agonizing concern and penetrating dissatisfaction.

The quality of the resolution of this stage is wisdom. A person who is wise has knowledge of what is true and has the necessary judgment to act on what is right. This is a culmination of all the qualities described. As indicated, these qualities are cumulative, each being incorporated into the next, and surviving in the subsequent stage. Thus, a fully developed person has a sense of hope, determines options by free choice, establishes purpose, is competent, is faithful to self and to others, is capable of loving and caring, and is able to know and act on the truth.

Erikson made a major contribution to the field of development by the exploration of psychosocial development throughout the life span. He has pointed out that each of these stages presents a crisis or critical choice. This does not mean that it is catastrophic, but rather what emerges is particular to the stage. The way in which each polarity is resolved serves as the basis for the development in the next stage.

DEVELOPMENTAL LIFE TASKS

Robert Havighurst is credited with the concept of developmental life tasks. His book, *Developmental Tasks and Education,* is the primary source of information on this concept.[15] This approach is based on the idea that living and growing involve learning. Both inner and outer forces influence the development of life tasks. For instance, a child does not have the life task of walking until the physical condition and nervous system development allow for it. These are inner forces. The fact that the child is expected, encouraged, and helped to walk at a certain age is an outer force. In addition, some forces come from personal motives and values. These three types of forces combine to create the need to accomplish tasks.

Developmental life tasks must be accomplished by each person for successful living. It is also necessary to learn tasks at the most appropriate time. It is useless to try to teach a developmental task before the time when the combined physical, psychological, and personal forces are present to make the task appropriate.

Havighurst divides development into six age periods and discusses six to ten developmental tasks for each period (Table 5-5). He emphasizes that this is an arbitrary presentation of the tasks and that additional tasks may occur within each period. Each set of developmental tasks needs to be accomplished for adequate development and to form the basis for development in the next period.

Infancy and Early Childhood

Havighurst lists nine developmental life tasks of this period, in which the age range is from birth to about six years of age. He indicates that many of these tasks could be broken down into a number of separate tasks. However, the principal tasks are as follows:

1. Learning to walk
2. Learning to take solid foods
3. Learning to talk
4. Learning to control the elimination of bodily wastes
5. Learning sex differences and sexual modesty
6. Achieving physiologic stability (the only one of these tasks that appears to be purely biologic)
7. Forming simple concepts of social and physical reality
8. Learning to relate oneself emotionally to parents, siblings and others
9. Learning to distinguish right from wrong and developing a conscience

Middle Childhood

Middle childhood extends from about six to 12 years of age and is equivalent to Erikson's school age (industry versus inferiority). Havighurst points out that there are three "great outward pushes" on the child during this period: into

Table 5-5 Havighurst's Developmental Stages		
Stage	**Name**	**Age**
I	Infancy and Early Childhood	Birth to 6-7 years
II	Middle Childhood	6 to 12 years
III	Adolescence	12 to 18 years
IV	Early Adulthood	19 to 30 years
V	Middle Age	30 to 60 years
VI	Later Maturity	Over 60 years

the peer group, into games and work requiring neuromuscular skills, and into adult concepts and communication. Nine developmental life tasks relate to these three outward thrusts:

1. Learning physical skills necessary for ordinary games (throwing, catching, handling simple tools)
2. Building wholesome attitudes toward oneself a growing organism (habits of self-care, cleanliness, ability to enjoy using the body, wholesome attitudes toward sex, etc.)
3. Learning to get along with peers
4. Learning an appropriate masculine or feminine social role (the cultural basis of this is the most important, since there appears to be no basis for sexual differences in motor skills, and since role expectations are changing)
5. Developing fundamental skills in reading, writing and calculating
6. Developing concepts necessary for everyday living ("The task is to acquire a store of concepts sufficient for thinking effectively about ordinary occupational, civic, and social matters"[15])
7. Developing conscience, morality and a scale of values (the latter develops slowly during this period)
8. Achieving personal independence (developing the authority to make choices for oneself)
9. Developing attitudes toward social groups and institutions (religious and economic groups)

Adolescence

Adolescence extends from 12 to 18 years of age. The principal developmental life tasks during this period, according to Havighurst, are as follows:

1. Achieving new and more mature relationships with peers of both sexes (The goal is to "become an adult among adults"; working with others and leading without dominating are the most crucial part of the adolescent's life.)

2. Achieving a masculine or feminine social role (a changing phenomenon in our society—It is now more difficult to define the appropriate and acceptable sex role, or to be certain that there is one, then it was when Havighurst considered these tasks.)

3. Accepting one's physique and using the body effectively (Physiologic maturity affects the chronologic age at which this becomes an important task.)

4. Achieving emotional independence of parents and other adults (The important task is the development of affection and respect for parents and older adults without dependence on them.)

5. Achieving assurance of economic independence (feeling able to make a living—Today most adolescents begin some type of work early in this period, but are not financially independent until later.)

6. Selecting and preparing for an occupation

7. Preparing for marriage and family life (There is a great deal of variation in how adolescents view marriage and their own desire for it.)

8. Developing intellectual skills and concepts necessary for civic competence (Direct or vicarious experiences in government, economics, politics and psychology are the bases for the development of concepts necessary for civic competence.)

9. Desiring and achieving socially responsible behavior (Older adolescents often develop altruism and want to be able to "make a difference" in society.)

10. Acquiring a set of values and an ethical system to guide behavior (Solidifying present values, developing new ones, and becoming aware of values held are aspects of this task.)

Early Adulthood

This period extends from 18 to 30 years of age. For most individuals, a great many things happen during this time. It is usually the period in which marriage takes place, children are born, full-time career-oriented employment is begun, and independent living arrangement is achieved. Havighurst feels that this is a time when the person is most able to learn, but that it also is a time when there is little effort to teach.[15] The eight developmental tasks are as follows:

1. Selecting a mate (the most interesting and disturbing of the tasks, it is usually considered almost totally the responsibility of the persons involved.)

2. Learning to live with a marriage partner (success is built on successful fulfillment of the previous life tasks.)

3. Starting a family (both mother and father assume new roles and adapt psychologically to the changes that this brings.)

4. Rearing children (meeting the physical and emotional needs of the child, adapting to new circumstances, and taking on responsibilities for another person.)

5. Managing a home physically (furnishing, repairing, decorating, cleaning, and providing an atmosphere conducive to living), psychologically (providing an environment that allows those living in the place to feel comfortable and to be themselves), and socially (providing for relationships between the persons who reside there). Havighurst indicated that much of this was the responsibility of women, although men also contributed.[15]

6. Getting started in an occupation (Havighurst first related this task to men, and noted that this is so important that a young person may delay fulfilling other tasks, such as choosing a partner, until this task has been accomplished.)

7. Taking on civic responsibility (This task is less important early in the period; young adults begin to see the advantages of belonging to and influencing organizations of all kinds once the other tasks have become more solidified.)

8. Finding a congenial social group (The group of friends from adolescence is often psychologically and geographically distanced, so new friendships must be established.)

Middle Age

From about 30 to 55 years of age the individual is exceedingly active in fulfilling what are perceived as life goals. It is a time of great productivity. The life tasks of those who are married and have a family have a different focus from tasks of those who have not married. For family members, the tasks will be reciprocal as individuals react to each other.[15] Havighurst lists seven developmental tasks for this period:

1. Achieving civic and social responsibility by taking part in organizations and taking on responsibilities in effecting change (Middle age is the period in which most people are able to make their best contributions in this area—they have the greatest interest, the most energy to give, and the most available time.)

2. Establishing and maintaining an economic standard of living (This is the most important task of the period for many people, with social and even psychological needs sacrificed for econmic necessity.)

3. Assisting teen-aged children to become responsible and happy adults (being a good role model—The middle-aged parent has the task of facilitating the adolescent in maturing and becoming independent.)

4. Developing adult leisure-time activities (This task results from the increase in leisure time and changes in the kinds of leisure activities that appeal to the person.)

5. Relating oneself to one's spouse as a person (Husbands and wives relate to each other in different ways as parenting becomes less demanding and securing economic stability is of less concern.)

6. Accepting and adjusting to the physiologic changes of middle-age (The gradual aging that went unnoticed earlier is replaced by more dramatic changes that can no longer be ignored, particularly the stress of female menopause.)

7. Adjusting to aging parents (Taking on the care of parents and working out new psychological relationships, which reflect the way developmental tasks were handled early in life, the socioeconomic realities, the ages and physical and mental conditions of both parents and adult children, and a host of other factors.)

Later Maturity

This later time of life is still a period of learning. Many new circumstances require adaptation by the older person. Usually retirement from the occupation that has sustained the person for decades will occur. Marked economic changes often occur during this period, as well as major changes in interpersonal relationships. The life tasks are many. Havighurst lists the following six:

1. Adjusting to decreasing physical strength and health (The rate of decrease is different for each person, but all must adjust to a loss of vigor and independence in action, and many older persons have health problems affecting the cardiovascular system, the nervous system, and the joints.)

2. Adjusting to retirement and reduced income (Work is often intimately related to self-worth, although some people look forward immensely to retirement.)

3. Adjusting to death of a spouse (This task is probably the most difficult life task faced by individuals, often including a change of living arrangements, learning to do things that the spouse always did, dealing with loneliness, and handling changes in financial stability.)

4. Establishing an explicit affiliation with one's age group (This task includes receiving social security payments, moving to a retirement village, requesting a senior citizen discount, joining a senior citizen group, etc.)

5. Meeting social and civic responsibilities (as the population ages, it becomes increasingly important for older people to maintain their interest and concern with the political and social climate.)

6. Establishing satisfactory living arrangements (This task includes preferably making housing decisions themselves, keeping the physical condition of one's home in satisfactory repair and cleanliness, moving into smaller quarters while remaining independent, living with relatives, becoming acclimated to some form of congregate living, or accepting skilled nursing care.)

Havighurst's life tasks were originally published in 1948. Society has changed in many ways since then, but most of the life tasks remain valid for most people. One of the areas to which he did not refer is adjustment to divorce by both the couples and children.

Havighurst's work has formed an important basis for occupational therapy. When completion of the life tasks is disrupted by illness or disability, an essential role of therapy is to provide the opportunities for those life tasks to be accomplished.

PSYCHOSOCIAL NEEDS

Another approach to the consideration of human development was formulated by Abraham Maslow. Maslow described a hierarchy of needs, which must be fulfilled to achieve full development as a human being. Maslow feared the misapplication of his theories and emphasized the flexibility of this hierarchy and the importance of other motivating factors.[16]

Maslow's theory centers on the idea that the individual has basic needs, which are never completely satisfied, but which approach satisfaction to varying degrees. These needs are in a hierarchy: Usually the most basic must be partially met before the next set emerges. This progression is in many ways cyclical: One always moves back to more basic needs and then further up the hierarchy before coming back to the basics. There are five sets of needs: physiologic, safety, belongingness and love, esteem, and self-actualization; and two sets of needs that are integrated throughout the hierarchy, cognitive and aesthetic (Figure 5-1).[16]

Physiologic Needs

The physiologic needs are the basic drives to attain what is necessary to maintain homeostasis in the body. The needs related to homeostasis usually are food and water to supply nutrients to the body. There are other basic physiologic needs, however, that do not appear to relate closely to homeostasis, such as the need for sexual activity, sleep and activity.[16] These needs must be met to some extent before other needs emerge. Maslow points out that if these needs are seriously unmet, no other needs exist; a person who is starving is unable to appreciate any other needs. Gratification of the basic physiologic needs will lead to the emergence of the next level of needs (safety), whereas deprivation of these needs will lead to an all-encompassing concern for their fulfillment.

Safety Needs

Safety needs include the need for security, protection, structure, law and similar components that create a feeling of safety. Maslow indicates that this need can be seen more clearly in infants and young children, but that the needs are also important in the adult. All people appear to have a need

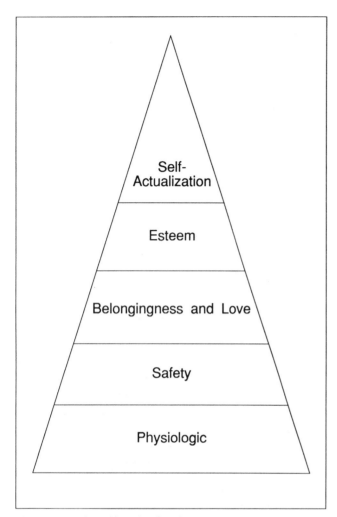

Figure 5-1. Maslow's hierarchy of needs.

for routine, predictability, and protection from danger. The infant reacts strongly to any threat to security; adults have learned to be more controlling of reactions.

The need for adequate housing is a prominent safety need that is often lacking in society. Many elderly people feel that they are in danger whenever they leave their own homes. People also seek to give themselves structure and routine, both of which meet safety needs.

Belongingness and Love Needs

The needs to experience love and affection, to have deep relationships with people, to have friends, and to feel a secure place in one's family or group are some of the aspects of this level of Maslow's hierarchy. When physiologic and safety needs are met, these needs for belongingness become prominent.

Maslow points out that mobility in our society creates problems in relation to these needs. Adjusting to new neighborhoods, making new friends, leaving old friends, establishing new roots, and relating to a totally new set of

persons cause upheaval in the fulfillment of these needs. Developing loyalties to country, city, neighborhood, employer, and family are ways in which this need is demonstrated. Persons who are alienated do not feel a sense of belonging; their needs on this level are thwarted. The great interest in tracing family history may well be a response to the difficulties people in our mobile society are experiencing and a strong expression of the need to belong.

The more severe psychological disorders may be traced to the person's lack of fulfillment of these needs.[16] One of the major problems of aging is the gradual loss of relationships with spouse and friends, and consequent isolation.

Esteem Needs

These needs are divided by Maslow into those related to the concept of self (feelings of adequacy, sense of competency, self-esteem and self-respect) and those related to other people's estimation of the person. Reputation, status, attention and recognition are some of the elements of these needs that come from outside the person and may or may not be correlated with the person's own perceptions. A person with an excellent reputation and high status and recognition may still feel inadequate and incompetent. Maslow also includes the need for independence and freedom in this category.

Cognitive Needs

Maslow discussed the needs to know and understand as cognitive needs that were integrated with the basic hierarchy of needs. He saw these as related to both the need for safety and the need for self-actualization. Curiosity, the desire to seek out answers, and the need to give meaning to events, circumstances and life itself are some of the aspects of cognitive needs. Active searching for explanations for what is observed or perceived is an on-going expression of this need. Cognitive needs are present in infancy and early childhood, and persist throughout life.

Aesthetic Needs

The need for beauty, for what is aesthetically pleasing, is a motivating factor for at least some persons. Maslow believed that healthy children universally demonstrate this need. As with the cognitive needs, he proposed that these needs are integrated into the basic hierarchy of needs, rather than being a step in the hierarchy.

Need for Self-Actualization

Self-actualization is the highest level of need. It is the desire to be fulfilled and to be all that one is capable of being. This need includes the ability to carry out most capably what one is most fitted for. Many people search for a number of years yet never find their real place in the world. For these needs to emerge, it is usually necessary for the physiologic, safety, belongingness and love, and esteem needs to be at least partially filled.

Although these five levels of needs are described as a hierarchy, there is a great deal of flexibility. For some people, the need for self-actualization is so strong that it overrides hunger or the need for status. Maslow also points out that one's values may change the relative importance of the levels of need. The framework of the hierarchy, however, is valid for most people.

CONCLUSION

It is essential that all occupational therapy personnel be knowledgeable in the areas of human development. Development occurs over the entire life span. There are a number of areas of development (motor, social, speech and language, psychological, cognitive, and sensory) but a person should be thought of as a whole person. It is necessary to think of the patient as *person* and to consider all of the areas of development at the particular stage of that individual. To facilitate the correlation of some of the developmental data from birth to adolescence, Mary K. Cowan, MA, OTR, FAOTA has developed a useful chart, which is shown in Appendix A.

Disability, whether physical, psychological, or both, affects development at all ages. Understanding the appropriate aspects of development will help to direct the formation of occupational therapy treatment goals and assist in the selection of suitable treatment approaches and media.

SUMMARY

Basic concepts of human development have been presented. These include motor development from birth through five years of age, primarily as described by Gesell and associates; cognitive development as studied by Piaget; psychosocial development throughout the life span according to Erikson; the developmental tasks first discussed by Havighurst; and the basic needs hierarchy of Maslow.

Related Learning Activities

1. Start a collection of children's drawings that represent the acquisition of fine motor skills at various stages of development.

2. Observe a group of children six to 12 years of age who are playing in a school yard during a recess period. Describe the play activities taking place and identify specific physical and social skills observed.

3. Chaperone an adolescent party at which both young men and women are guests. Compare and contrast behaviors seen with the work of two developmental theorists.

4. Develop a short, ten-item questionnaire that focuses on the life tasks defined by Havighurst. Use the questionnaire as a guide for interviewing a young adult, a middle aged person, and an elderly person, each of whom has a physical or mental disability.

5. Discuss the results of the questionnaire information from item four with peers. Were any additional life tasks identified? Did sociocultural background, economic status, educational level, or disability have an influence on the achievement of any life tasks?

References

1. Knoblock H, Pasamanick B (Eds): *Gesell and Amatruda's Developmental Diagnosis.* Hagerstown, Maryland, Harper & Row, 1974.
2. Gesell A: *The First Five Years of Life.* New York, Harper and Row, 1940.
3. Ames L et al: *The Gesell Institute's Child from One to Six.* New York, Harper & Row, 1979.
4. Noback CR, Demarest RJ: *The Human Nervous System,* 3rd edition. Lisbon, McGraw-Hill, 1981.
5. Fiorentino MR: *Normal and Adnormal Development.* Springfield, Illinois, Charles C. Thomas, 1972.
6. Biehler RF: *Child Development.* Boston, Houghton Mifflin, 1976.
7. Barclay LK: *Infant Development.* New York, Holt, Rhinehart & Winston, 1985.
8. Ginsberg H, Opper S: *Piaget's Theory of Intellectual Development.* Englewood Cliffs, New Jersey, Prentice Hall, 1969.
9. Flavell JH: *The Developmental Psychology of Jean Piaget.* Princeton, New Jersey, D. Von Nostrand, 1963.
10. Rosen H: *Pathway to Piaget.* Cherry Hill, New Jersey, Postgraduate International, 1977.
11. Wursten H: *Jean Piaget and His Work.* Unpublished paper presented at the American Occupational Therapy Conference, Los Angeles, 1972.
12. Gruber H, Coneche JJ: *The Essential Piaget.* New York, Basic Books, 1977.
13. Erikson EH: *Childhood and Society.* New York, WW Norton, 1963.
14. Stevens R: *Erik Erikson.* New York, St. Martin's Press, 1983.
15. Havighurst RJ: *Developmental Life Tasks and Education.* New York, David McKay Company, 1952.
16. Maslow AH: *Motivation and Personality.* New York, Harper & Row, 1970.

Chapter 6

Components of Occupation
AND THEIR RELATIONSHIP TO ROLE PERFORMANCE

Ben Atchison, MEd, OTR, FAOTA

The same stream of life that runs through my veins night and day, runs through the world and dances in rhythmic measure.

—**Rabindranath Tagore**

INTRODUCTION

One concept that drives the practice of occupational therapy is the idea of occupation. Both the student and practitioner must understand the importance of occupation and its impact on biological, psychological, and sociocultural mechanisms. Putting that understanding into action to enhance role performance is the essence of the profession and appropriate intervention.

This chapter reviews the concept of *occupation* and describes three components that are vital to successful occupation. A review of the literature related to the impact of occupation on these three mechanisms is presented. Illustrations of the connection among these components, or their integration, are presented through brief case studies, which provide examples of how role performance is influenced. Elements of the teaching/learning process are also addressed.

THE MEANING OF OCCUPATION

In the development of a profession like occupational therapy, it is vital to define and articulate the unique aspects of the field. As occupational therapy personnel examine the basic philosophical beliefs of practice as described in Chapter 3, a return to the profession's early roots is evident. In this vein, as early as 1917, the founders of the National Society for the Promotion of Occupational Therapy established these objectives (see Chapter 1):[1]

1. The advancement of occupations as a therapeutic measure
2. The study of the **effects of occupation** (outcome of purposeful, meaningful activity) on the human being
3. The dissemination of scientific knowledge on this subject

ESSENTIAL VOCABULARY

Effects of occupation

Occupational science

Human activity

Choice of occupation

Biopsychosocial

Integrative school

Immunity

Culturally sensitive

Teaching/learning process

Disruption

KEY CONCEPTS

Meaning of occupation

Biologic components

Psychologic components

Sociocultural components

Relationship of components to role performance

Based on these founding ideas, a movement is currently underway to establish an academic discipline called **occupational science,** which is clearly rooted in these early principles set forth by the founders of the occupational therapy profession.[2] To understand the rationale for developing such a discipline, one needs to look at the concept of occupation and, in doing so, appreciate the complexity of its components as well as its relevance as a field of study that will ultimately increase the knowledge base of the profession.

Occupation refers to **human activity** and includes those basic needs for survival, as well as those activities we choose to pursue to live a productive, full life. The term *to occupy* does not connote passivity; rather, it conveys action, employment and anticipation.[3] Occupation includes the full repertoire of our daily activities, which are self-directed, purposeful, and socially acceptable.[4] Our **choice of occupation** comes from our cultural exposure, individual values and interests, and special abilities. It is a choice that is individualized and complex. Occupation is of symbolic importance to humans.[5] What a person does to occupy time has significance in social, cultural and spiritual contexts.[6] According to Reed,[7] occupation is dynamic and occurs through the influence of biologic, psychologic and sociocultural environments.

The occupational therapy assistant will have the opportunity to affect the occupational well-being of patients through intervention in the areas of self-maintenance (activities of daily living), work, play and leisure, and rest. Each recipient of occupational therapy treatment must be given the opportunity to teach the assistant what those areas mean in his or her life before effective therapeutic intervention can take place.

COMPONENTS OF OCCUPATION

Occupation can be seen as an end product of the human systems that interact to enable one to function. The interaction of these systems is of interest to many health practitioners, including occupational therapy personnel. These systems, including biologic, psychologic and sociocultural, are concepts on which rehabilitation is founded.[8] The impact of these systems, individually and in an integrated form, has been put forth as one model of intervention in occupational therapy practice. According to Reed, "The **biopsychosocial** model is designed to weigh the relative contributions of social and psychologic, as well as biologic factors, in determining the degree of health and illness and dysfunction."[7] The occupational therapy process of analyzing individuals through a systems approach provides understanding that a change in any subsystem may affect the whole human system.[7] The person is not to be viewed in

terms of a diseased organ or traumatized limb, but as a total organism with psychologic, social and biologic factors all being equal. If one considers the impact of amputation, it is not difficult to think beyond the obvious biologic changes. One must also appreciate the impact on the individual's psychologic and social functioning. Consideration is critical in therapeutic assessment and appropriate intervention. However, it is not easy to quantify the degree of impairment in all three areas, which is a limitation of this model.[7] For example, observation of biologic and physiologic changes after amputation of a limb are quantifiable, whereas psychological recovery, which may involve a change in values, interests, self-esteem, and emotions, is not as easily measured (Figure 6-1).

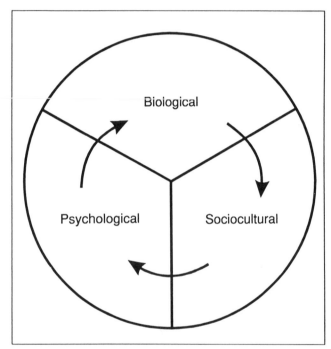

Figure 6-1. Relationship of subsystems.

Among several schools of thought in psychiatry is the **integrative school,** also known as the biopsychosocial school. Tiffany[8] points out that this approach is based on the idea that psychologic behaviors are determined by the complexity of physical, emotional, social and cultural processes that are interrelated. The theoretical frameworks that address the broad areas of knowledge that compose this school of thought include occupational behavior and those based on human development[9] (see Chapter 5).

Mosey[10] described the advantages of viewing the biopsychosocial model as a frame of reference for occupational therapy. She stresses that the first advantage is that our information about an individual is composed of information about the body, mind and environment. An appreciation of the relevance of this information strongly parallels the holistic approach to intervention, which is generic to occupational therapy philosophy. The second advantage is that this model addresses teaching/learning theory, which is a practical aspect of occupational therapy. The following sections detail information on these points, beginning with the first advantage.

Biologic Component

Biologic components include those internal systems that the individual must have to function, ie, the anatomic and physiologic components of the body. Disease and illness have an impact on these functions, as in the case of a cerebral vascular accident. The therapeutic intervention strategy for such a condition, which requires increasing musculoskeletal function (among others), includes engagement in activities to gain greater range of motion, muscle strength, and coordination. This approach has its basis in knowledge of the biologic component.

There are numerous reports in the scientific literature about the relationship of engagement in activity and biologic health. Bortz[11] presents a review of biologic changes that take place with aging. These changes are similar to those that take place as a result of enforced physical inactivity. The physiologic changes that take place at the cellular level and across total organs suggest that changes take place by disuse and not just from the aging process.[11] Specific studies related to the impact of exercise and activity on **immunity** are more prevalent. Simon[12] summarizes ten studies indicating that athletes, because of their habitual engagement in activity, have special defenses against illness. His studies focus on the effects of exercise on various "host-defense" factors, indicating that an active body has decreased potential for infection.

The study by Valliant[13] on the effect of exercise on older adults concluded that those who were actively involved experienced a significant reduction in depression and body fat concentration, leading to improved biologic health. Siscovick et al.[14] present information that outlines the benefits of physical activity on specific diseases. Many other studies clearly support the notion that humans who are actively engaged in physical activity have a healthier biologic profile. A number of these studies, including those specifically noted, present evidence of actual cellular changes as a result of physical activity. It is important for the occupational therapy assistant to be aware of these research findings because they provide needed justification for the inclusion of activity in a patient's overall health care management program.

Psychologic Component

The psychologic component is based on developmental, learning and behavioral theories. The occupational therapist's and assistant's knowledge of activity design and implementation is based on these theories as well. The certified occupational therapy assistant should review the literature for a basic understanding of these theories to appreciate their relevance in the intervention process. When planning activity, occupational therapy personnel consider the psychologic components of occupational performance, which include role acquisition, development and clarification of values and interests, initiating and terminating activity, and development of self-concept.

There is support for the relationship between engagement in activity and enhanced psychologic behavior. Soenstrom and Morgan[15] present a detailed analysis of self-esteem theory and provide an empirically based (experiential) rationale for self-esteem enhancement through engagement in activity. Valliant[13] also reports increased cognitive performance among older adults as a result of participation in an exercise program on a regular basis. Cook[16] describes the "alternatives approach" to drug abuse prevention based on the concept that individuals provided with healthful, non-chemical ways of gaining rewards and pleasures will be less likely to engage in drug or alcohol abuse. He presents a series of guidelines for the selection and development of activities from a "biopsychological" model of alternatives.

Sociocultural Component

The sociocultural component of this model addresses issues of individual values, roles and social patterns that must be a focus in effective intervention. The social skills related to occupational performance include social conduct, conversational skills, and self-expression. Although patients are expected to function within general social norms, it is critical that each of these skills be addressed in the context of the individual's cultural background. For intervention to be truly effective, the variation among patients with respect to ethnic values, interests, requirements, needs and roles must be considered. The social dynamics of one group will be unique from others and intervention must be sensitive to this fact.

Boyle[17] addresses these points in an excellent article on the multiple issues related to rehabilitation of individuals with physical performance deficits. She recommends that the profession of occupational therapy become more **culturally sensitive** (ie, aware of others' traditions, customs and beliefs) to meet the needs of the varied groups of patients who receive services. Recruitment of a more heterogenous group of therapists and assistants is one important way to address this issue. Further, she suggests that occupational therapy educational programs require certain courses that lead to a better understanding of and interaction with various cultural groups, including requirement of foreign language courses (see Chapter 10).

The Teaching/Learning Process

The second advantage of the model is that it focuses on the **teaching/learning process**.[10] This process emphasizes team effort in rehabilitation—the team being the therapist or the assistant and the patient. One guiding principle of occupational therapy intervention emphasizes "doing with" rather than "doing to." This model presents less emphasis on "treating" and more on "teaching." The therapist or assistant begins where the patient is and proceeds at a rate appropriate to the individual's ability. The teaching/learning process takes into account the learner's biologic, psychologic and sociocultural capacities and requirements (see Chapter 8).

ILLUSTRATIONS OF THE BIOPSYCHOSOCIAL CONNECTION

The occupational therapy assistant who views intervention from a biopsychosocial point of view will have an appreciation of the impact of dysfunction on role performance. It is important to remember that each system, if dysfunctional, can precipitate breakdown of function in the others. Illustrations of this point follow in brief case examples.

Case Study 6-1

Joe. Joe has a serious respiratory disease. He needs to be supported by a mobile oxygen unit, which causes a great deal of emotional discomfort. Because of this disease, he has great difficulty breathing during any activity, is often nauseated, and has a poor appetite. Since he is unable to perform many activities, he is deconditioned, which leads to fatigue and further discomfort. He is afraid that he is going to continue to get worse. His previously active social life is no longer as full. Joe spends a great deal of time alone, worrying about his health. When he worries, he feels his need to take in more oxygen as his respiration and demands for oxygen increase.

Joe's case illustrates the impact of biologic dysfunction on social and psychologic components and the disruptive cycle that can occur among the components. His biologic disease leads to disruption of his mental health, which creates a breakdown in socialization. This in turn continues to contribute to his biologic dysfunction. The cycle continues.

Case Study 6-2

Katherine. Katherine has been diagnosed with rheumatoid arthritis. The course of her condition has been stable for about five years. She has been able to maintain a high level of function, in spite of the disabling hand condition typified by this disease. Recently, she learned that her father was diagnosed as having pancreatic cancer and would not likely survive beyond one year. She has suffered considerable grief over this news and has noted increased swelling and pain, and decreased motion in all her joints. She also is experiencing increased inflammation. Her appetite is decreasing, she feels very fatigued, and she is not sure she can continue to work every day, as she has done in past years. Her anxiety grows over the impending loss of her father, as well as her potential loss of function.

Katherine's case presents an example of someone who is suffering exacerbations of a dormant condition due to psychosocial stressors. The biologic manifestations are real, but precipitated by emotional stress.

Case Study 6-3

Tom. Tom sustained a head injury as a result of a swimming accident two years ago. He had rather intensive rehabilitation, including residency for six months at a community reentry program for head-injured individuals. His discharge from the program and subsequent return to his home has been difficult. The rehabilitation team at the community reentry program has made great efforts to assist Tom in developing functional skills to allow a transition to independent living. Yet, after a short time at home, Tom is lonely, depressed, and unable to cope independently. He also drinks heavily, a behavior that led to the accident causing his injury. Tom's premorbid lifestyle, a critical factor in the overall success of his rehabilitation program, was not addressed. He is again at risk.

RELATIONSHIP TO ROLE PERFORMANCE

The ability of an individual to achieve success in role performance is a result of biopsychosocial competence. **Disruption** of any of these three components will result in dysfunctional patterns of role performance. The term "disruption" refers to a forced interruption in a person's life. It is the degree of disruption that the occupational therapy assistant should question. That is, some individuals will be unaffected by biopsychosocial stressors that cause total breakdown in others. This difference is due to adaptation and, as demonstrated by the case studies, occurs within the limits of the individual. Thus, it is important to provide opportunities that allow for adaptation and manipulation of the environment. This goal might be accomplished in a clinical setting initially and then gradually approached in "real world" situations. The process of adaptation must be approached through engagement in occupation. Through occupational therapy intervention, the patient can learn problem-solving methods that will assist in occupational performance and effective adaptation.[18] To illustrate this idea, application of the process will be applied to the cases described earlier.

Joe

Because of the severity of his respiratory disease, Joe will have considerable difficulty in performing all of his previous occupations. He requires mechanical adaptations and adaptive devices to allow for energy conservation, so that he may be able to achieve independently self-care tasks. Allowing him to dress himself, through work simplification techniques, will result in his feeling more capable and less regressive. Feeling less exhausted due to simple environmental adaptations will allow Joe to resume some aspects of his role as a husband. Although alteration of the biologic deficit is not possible, adaptation of his environmemt will lead to enhanced competence in some activities leading to improved psychologic health and resulting in less stress on an already taxed biologic system.

Katherine

Katherine is clearly suffering biologic symptoms as a result of psychologic stressors. Allowing her to work through her grief by expressing her feelings of loss, fear and anxiety will provide the "nourishment" needed to replenish her physical strength. Symptoms as noted will decrease along with her opportunity to express her grief.

Tom

Tom's case represents a critical problem in rehabilitation. To provide proper treatment for Tom, the rehabilitation team must better understand his background, particularly his social history. An understanding of his lifestyle and experiences that place him at high risk for disability is needed if rehabilitation is to be effective. Boyle[17] speaks to this issue when she points out that a single impulsive act, such as drinking and driving, "may cause a person to cross the threshold for disability, that point at which a physiologic or psychologic effect begins to be produced."[17] Boyle recounts the story of John Callahan, a successful cartoonist with quadraplegia. His disability was the result of an automobile accident, caused by driving while intoxicated. It wasn't until six years after his injury that he realized that the true source of his disability was not his physical limitations, but the fact that he was an alcoholic.[17]

IMPLICATIONS FOR OCCUPATIONAL THERAPY

Taking a holistic view of the individual, with consideration as to how the biologic, psychologic and sociocultural components impact on occupation and role perfomance, is critically important for all members of the profession if we are to be successful in our intervention efforts. When specializing in areas such as neurodevelopmental therapy or hand therapy, it is important to continue to view the whole person, not just the immediate problem.

SUMMARY

The concept of occupation was reviewed, together with the three important components: biologic, psychologic and sociocultural. All must be considered to have a holistic approach to therapeutic intervention. Case studies were presented to illustrate the interrelationship of the components and their impact on role performance and the health of the individual. Scientific evidence was introduced that clearly demonstrates that changes at the cellular level, as well as changes in psychological behavior, occur as a result of engagement in occupation. Biologic conditions are often exacerbated by sociocultural conditions, which must be addressed as a part of a therapeutic intervention program. The importance of the teaching/learning process was also emphasized.

Editor's Note

This chapter builds on the content found in the preceding chapters. To gain maximal appreciation for the information presented here, the reader should have a good understanding of historical, philosophical, theoretical and developmental principles of the profession. The author's discussion of the components of occupation in relation to role performance provides the necessary background for the student to proceed to the study of the remaining chapters, particularly those on occupational performance areas.

Acknowledgment

The author and the editor wish to thank Sr. Genevieve Cummings, CSJ, MA, OTR, FAOTA for her content and editorial suggestions.

Related Learning Activities

1. Define the term *occupation* in your own words.

2. Discuss your primary occupations and roles with a peer. Identify similarities and differences.

3. Interview a child, a teenager, an adult and an elderly person, all of whom have a physical or psychosocial disability. Determine in what ways, if any, their disability changed their primary roles and occupations.

4. What were some of the specific biologic, psychological, and social factors that had an influence on the patients interviewed in item 3?

5. Review the case study about Katherine. List potential treatment activities that could be used as a part of an occupational therapy program.

References

1. Dunton WR: The principles of occupational therapy. *Proceedings of the National Society for the Promotion of Occupational Therapy: Second Annual Meeting.* Catonsville, Maryland, Spring Grove State Hospital, 1918.

2. Yerxa E et al: An introduction to occupational science, a foundation for the occupational therapy in the 21st century. *Occup Ther Health Care* 6:1-17, 1989.

3. Englehardt HT: Defining occupational therapy: The meaning of therapy and the virtues of occupation. *Am J Occup Ther* 31:666-672, 1977.

4. University of Southern California, Department of Occupational Therapy: A proposal for a new doctor of philosophy degree in occupational science. Unpublished manuscript, 1987.

5. Campbell J: *The Power of Myth.* New York, Doubleday, 1988.

6. Fraser JT: *Time, the Familiar Stranger.* Amherst, Massachusetts, University of Massachusetts Press, 1987.

7. Reed KL, Sanderson S: *Concepts of Occupational Therapy.* Baltimore, Williams & Wilkins, 1983.

8. Tiffany E: Psychiatry and mental health. In Hopkins HD, Smith HL (Eds): *Willard and Spackman's Occupational Therapy,* 5th edition. Philadelphia, JB Lippincott, 1978.

9. Adams JE, Lindemann E: Coping with long-term disability. In Coelho GV, Hamburg DA, Adams JE (Eds): *Coping and Adaptation.* New York, Basic Books, 1974.

10. Mosey AC: An alternative: The biopsychosocial model. *Am J Occup Ther* 28:137-140, 1974.

11. Bortz WM: Disuse and aging. *J Am Med Assoc* 248:1203-1208, 1980.

12. Simon HB: The immunology of exercise. A brief review. *J Am Med Assoc* 252:2735-2738, 1894.

13. Valliant PM: Exercise and its effects on cognition and physiology in older adults. *Percept Mot Skills* 61:1031-1038, 1985.

14. Siscovick DS, LaPorte RE, Newman JM: The disease specific benefits and risks of physical activity and exercise. *Public Health Rep* 100:180-188, 1985.

15. Soenstrom RJ, Morgan WP: Exercise and self-esteem: Rationale and model. *Medicine and Science in Sports and Exercise* 21:329-337, 1989.

16. Cook R: The alternatives approach revisited: A biopsychological model and guidelines for application. *Int J Addict* 20:1399-1419, 1985.

17. Boyle M: The changing face of the rehabilitation population: A challenge for therapists. *Am J Occup Ther* 44:941-945, 1990.

18. Ryan SE: Theoretical frameworks and approaches. In Ryan SE (Ed): *The Certified Occupational Therapy Assistant: Roles and Responsibilities.* Thorofare, New Jersey, Slack Inc., 1986.

Occupational Performance Areas

Doris Y. Witherspoon, MS, OTR

INTRODUCTION

Occupational performance areas are those things accomplished each day that sustain and enhance life. Everyday life presents few problems to individuals who have "good" physical and emotional health. Occupational therapy personnel work with patients with health problems brought about by causes such as birth defects, injury or illness. These impairments can affect a person's ability to meet needs and fulfill desired roles and life goals.[1] Early occupational therapy practice was founded on the idea that activity promotes mental and physical well-being and that, conversely, absence of activity leads to deterioration or loss of mental and physical function.[2]

Occupational therapy assumes that daily activities play a central part in everyone's life. This assumption grew out of knowledge and concern that people must be able to perform certain tasks at prescribed levels of competence.[3] These activities have been identified as occupation.

The three major **categories of occupation** are referred to collectively as occupational performance areas and include activities of daily living (ADLs), work activities, and play or leisure activities. Healthful living and self-esteem depend on the balance established among these three types of occupational performance. Individuals who fail to develop balanced living routines or whose routines have been disrupted may learn to regain their occupations through participation in occupational therapy.[3]

The individual's view of an activity varies considerably. In one situation a task may be considered work, but in another setting it may be a leisurely activity. For example, a woman does house cleaning in clients' homes and considers her tasks gainful employment. When she cleans her own home in preparation for guests, however, the same activity could be described as leisurely.

KEY CONCEPTS

Occupational therapy process

Activities of daily living: physical and psychological components

Play classifications

Contributions of play to development

Purposes, functions, and goals of leisure

Recreation

Significance of work

Relationship of work to physical and psychosocial elements

Where does work fit into the daily living routine? Because of cultural dictates, ADLs, also referred to as self-care, are a precursor to work; and work, a precursor to leisure. American culture, for the most part, dictates that one's grooming and hygiene be completed before going to the work place. It is also generally accepted that leisure is a reward activity for one's hard work. In addition, many of the functional abilities acquired through work activities and training are used in everyday leisure activities. The interrelationship of the primary components of occupational performance areas is shown in Figure 7-1.

The relationship among ADLs, work and leisure changes markedly as individuals progress from infancy to adulthood. Consequently, the daily living routines of infants and adults are very dissimilar.[4] One's **cultural environment** (ie, human and non-human elements that relate to traditions, customs and beliefs) and related social status help in defining the balance among activities. Routine activity for blue collar workers will differ substantially from the regular activity of executives and homemakers.

A lack of balance in healthful activity can cause withdrawal, depression, or deterioration in the individual's capacity to meet daily needs. Occupational therapy assists in developing, redeveloping, or maintaining necessary activity skills for occupational performance, which lead to productive and satisfying lifestyles. **Skill acquisition** allows the impaired individual to return to independent, wholesome living in the community.[3]

Everyone needs balanced activity to adapt to societal living. An important goal of occupational therapy is to correct deficiencies that interfere with the exercise of independence by teaching ADLs, work, and play and leisure activity skills.

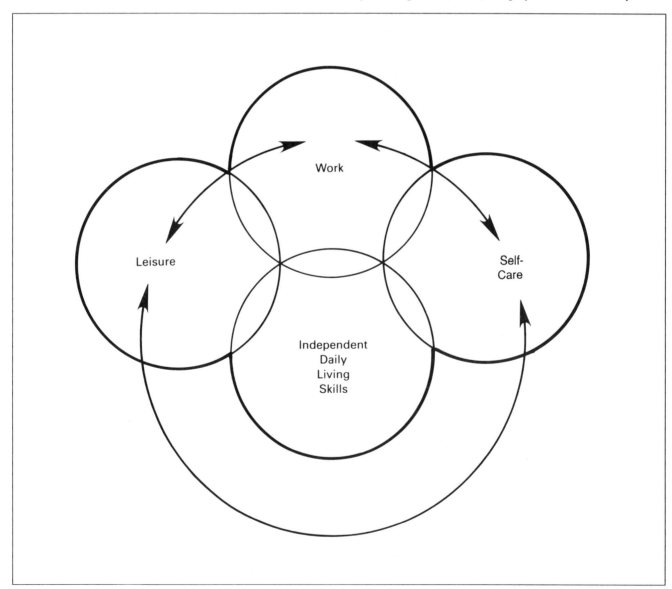

Figure 7-1. The interrelationship of primary components of occupational performance areas.

THE OCCUPATIONAL THERAPY PROCESS

The essential focus of the occupational therapy evaluation is on the occupational skills and roles of the patient in relation to occupational performance responsibilities. Occupational therapy personnel study these skill levels, roles, and responsibilities and determine how the patient's normal patterns of dealing with them have changed. Both the family and the patient are involved in determining the specific discrepancies between past and present activities and the level of performance, and discovering what level of function is necessary and acceptable to the patient in the personal environment and social/cultural setting. An objective assessment of the patient's needs and potential is essential for the registered occupational therapist and the certified occupational therapy assistant to plan and implement a treatment program that will allow the patient to gain or regain as many functional abilities as possible. ADLs are a primary focus of the occupational therapy process.

Occupational therapy assistants must understand and appreciate the importance of occupational performance activities to provide the most effective therapeutic intervention strategies in meeting the patient's needs. They can assist patients in determining their present status and the additional skills and attitudes they may need to acquire to achieve their goals.[5]

ACTIVITIES OF DAILY LIVING

While play/leisure and work activities are equally important skills, ADLs (self-care) are presented first because they are prerequisite to work and play/leisure, and are paramount to independent survival.[6]

An individual is expected to perform routine tasks such as dressing, feeding, and grooming before he or she is considered well adapted to community life.[7] Occupational therapy personnel are responsible for assessing the patient's basic potential and teaching primary skills in ADLs. Such assessments are based on mental and chronological age, and the goals for children and adults differ greatly. Moreover, the methods for teaching these two groups vary considerably.

Self-help and daily living skills training is critical in dealing with attitudes that patients may have formed about their conditions. If they receive adequate instruction and support, routine life may be less burdensome, and self-care skill may be a motivating force for pursuing work and leisure activities.[7] The specific activities are categorized as follows:[8]

1. Grooming
2. Oral hygiene
3. Bathing
4. Toilet hygiene
5. Dressing
6. Feeding and eating
7. Medication routine
8. Socialization
9. Functional communication
10. Functional mobility
11. Sexual expression

Skills are developed in three essential ways. First is the ability to perform tasks independently. Second, assistive devices may be developed to aid the physically impaired in accomplishing such tasks. Finally, other persons within an individual's environment may be trained to assist the patient in the performance of certain tasks. Many disabled persons learn to achieve daily living skills through a combination of these three methods.

Evaluating Physical Daily Living Skills

The first step in any rehabilitation plan is to evaluate the patient's abilities and dysfunctions. Figure 7-2 provides an example of a form that may be followed to evaluate daily living skills. A variety of other **evaluation tools** are available and are used to determine performance definitions.

Independence is the focus of ADLs; therefore, the certified occupational therapy assistant (COTA), working under the supervision of the registered occupational therapist (OTR), must observe and analyze each action. It is not enough merely to identify skills that the patient is unable to perform. How the patient performs the task is equally important, as this determines the level and quality of the skill performance in carrying out selected tasks. The patient may be able to complete some tasks independently, but the evaluator needs to study the "how" very closely and answer the following questions:

1. How long did it take to perform the activity?
2. Did the activity take twice as long as it would for a person of average ability?
3. Did the patient complain of fatigue and need frequent rest periods?
4. Was the patient, despite working steadily, still unable to complete the task because movements were too slow?
5. Which motions are functional, and how do they function?
6. When did the patient first require assistance, and what kind of assistance was needed?

Although terminology often varies, COTAs may report patient needs in terms of the following observations:

- *Stand-By Assistance (SBA):* The patient completes the activity independently, but may lack confidence. The patient may require verbal or physical assistance in completing the activity.
- *Minimal Physical Assistance (Min PA):* The patient requires physical assistance to complete the activity.
- *Moderate Physical Assistance (Mod PA):* The patient requires physical assistance to continue and complete the activity.

Name _____ Age _____

Address _____

Diagnosis _____ Occupation _____

GROOMING	Date	Needs Equipment	Needs Assistance	Needs Minimal Assistance	Needs No Assistance
Comb/brush hair					
Wash hair					
Set hair					
Shave					
Apply make-up					
Trim nails					
File nails					
Manage feminine hygiene					
Brush teeth					
Manage toothpaste or powder					
BATHING					
Shower					
Turn on/off faucet					
Bathe					
Dry self					
DRESSING					
Over shirts					
Button shirt/blouse					
Ties					
Jacket/coats					
Hats/gloves					
Zipping					
Putting on shoes					
Tying shoes					
Lace shoes					
Putting on socks/hose					
Pants					
Skirts/slacks					
Dress					
Secure clothes from drawer					
Hang up clothing					
COMMUNCATION					
Read book or magazine					
Write/type					
Speaks coherently					
Comprehends spoken words					
TRANSPORTATION					
Bus					
Drive					
Walk					

Figure 7-2. Daily living skills evaluation. Used with permission of Wayne County Community College, Occupational Therapy Assistant program.

Name _____ Age _____

Address _____

Diagnosis _____ Occupation _____

COOKING	Date	Needs Equipment	Needs Assistance	Needs Minimal Assistance	Needs No Assistance
Peel					
Measure basic ingredients					
Mix					
Follow simple directions					
Follow complex directions					
Prepare cold meal					
Prepare hot meal					
Convenience foods					
Boxed					
Frozen					
Canned					
CLEAN-UP					
Wipe counters					
Sweep floors					
Scour sink					
Wash pots/pans					
Dishes/silver, glasses					
Put away supplies					
Dishes, bowls, spoons					
Find supplies (memory)					
Dusting					
Mop floor					
Make bed					
Change bed					
Wash clothes					
Vacuum					
Clean tub					
Clean toilet					
Windows					
TIME MANAGEMENT					
Planning day					
Planning meals					
Coordinating schedules					
Manage watch					
MONEY MANAGEMENT					
Making change					
Checks					
Paying bills					

Figure 7-2. Continued.

Name _____				Age _____	
Address _____					
Diagnosis _____		Occupation _____			
EATING	Date	Needs Equipment	Needs Assistance	Needs Minimal Assistance	Needs No Assistance
Eat with fingers					
Pick up utensils					
Use fork/spoon					
Cut food					
Spread butter on bread					
Use salt and pepper					
Drink from glass/cup					
Open milk container					
Pour from container					
Stir liquid					
Open screw-top bottles					
MOBILITY					
Sit balanced on edge of bed					
Get in/out of bed					
Turn over in bed					
Sit in straight chair					
Rise from straight chair					
Open doors					
Stand unsupported					
Walk					
Walk carrying objects					
Pick up objects from floor					
Independent transfers					
MISCELLANEOUS					
Manage keys					
Manage glasses					
Operate radio or TV					

Figure 7-2. Continued.

- *Maximal Physical Assistance (Max PA):* The patient requires physical assistance to initiate, continue, and complete the activity.
- *Mechanical Assistance:* The patient completes the activity independently with the use of an assistive or adaptive aid.

During the evaluation it is important for the COTA to remember to actually observe the patient in the performance of each task. This gives the assistant an opportunity to monitor the patient rather than to rely on the patient's descriptive statements about how the activity was or will be performed. Such a procedure also provides a more accurate assessment of how the patient will function in the performance of ADLs when he or she no longer is receiving direct care.

The COTA, in collaboration with the OTR, determines the underlying reason or reasons for lack of independence in ADLs, such as muscle weakness, lack of coordination, poor balance, or visual perceptual deficits. Short-term goals should focus on improving functional impairment, whereas long-term goals should emphasize independence of function in the activities.

Case Study 7-1

The patient is unable to dress himself. He lacks trunk balance and has limited shoulder range of motion. Short-term goals would center on improving balance, thus freeing the upper extremities for functional activities, while allowing trunk range and "righting" and increasing range of motion at the shoulder joints. This will allow more reaching and extending movements. The result will be improved physical function, thus allowing the patient to focus on the long-term goal of achieving greater independence by improving skills in ADLs where deficits exist.

Adaptations in Physical Daily Living Skills—Definition and Purpose

The physical ADLs have been enumerated in the early part of this chapter. They may be defined as those daily activities necessary for fulfilling basic needs, such as personal hygiene and grooming, dressing, feeding and eating, use of medications, socialization, functional communication and mobility, and sexual expression. In every aspect of life—play, leisure or work—daily living needs act as both prerequisites and corequisites to accomplishing everyday routines.

The COTA, under the supervision of the OTR, evaluates patient's abilities to perform daily living activities and identifies deficiencies and strengths. The COTA may assist the OTR in the establishment of goals for the treatment plan and the methods that will be used to accomplish these goals through acceptable levels of activity. Patients and their families are informed about the occupational therapy treatment plans and are encouraged to participate in the rehabilitation/habilitation process. A variety of methods are used to teach skills, including verbal instruction, demonstration, and visual or verbal cues.[9] More information on specific teaching techniques may be found in Chapter 8.

The need for independence in daily living skills is often more acute for the physically disabled population. The need to eat, dress, work, recreate, and manipulate the environment generally does not diminish for the individual, although he or she is limited in physical abilities. The person with a disability learns to perform necessary daily living tasks by adapting the surrounding environment through manipulation of those elements within his or her control. This manipulation may take many forms, including:

1. Assistive aids
2. Adaptive equipment
3. Energy conservation techniques
4. Work simplification skills
5. Effective time management
6. Positioning
7. Designs to eliminate barriers
8. Vocational modifications

These techniques entail using the environment in creative ways to fulfill tasks that are easy for the physically able.

Beyond environmental concerns, a patient's functional impairments, such as spasticity and rigidity, may contribute to an inability to perform daily living tasks. These functional impairments are attributable to various pathol-

ogic diseases and disorders. The combination of functional impairment and environmental barriers cause a need for change in the patient's daily routine through adaptation. They compel the patient to rethink or relearn otherwise simple activities commensurate with the changes in abilities.

Spasticity may result in the following:
1. Joint motion limitation
2. Muscle weakness/paralysis
3. Motor ataxia/sensory ataxia
4. Lack of trunk control/balance
5. Athetoid/tremorous movements
6. Impaired cognition
7. Concentration/attention span

Rigidity may cause the following:
1. Contractures/deformities
2. Decreased physical tolerance/endurance
3. Sensory impairment
4. Impaired visual perception
5. Impaired coordination
6. Motor/sensory/kinetic apraxia

Assessing the Need for Assistive/Adaptive Equipment

Assistive/adaptive equipment is often the key to independence for the person who is disabled. Not only can it assist in improving the quality of life for the patient, but it can often help to restore the patient's sense of dignity and self-esteem through newly found independence.

Several important factors should be considered before recommending, constructing, or ordering adaptive aids for patients. Cost, design and maintenance are three of the primary considerations (see Chapter 15).

Cost. The following questions must be answered: Is the recommended item covered as reimbursable in the patient's insurance plan? If so, what percentage of the cost will be covered? If not, what is the maximum amount the patient can afford? Is it less expensive and more feasible for the occupational therapist or assistant to construct the item than to purchase it?

Design. The following questions must be answered: Will the recommended item serve more than one purpose? How durable is the item (especially if it will be used frequently)? Is it attractive as well as functional? Is the item easy to use or wear, or is it too cumbersome? Is the patient embarrassed about using the device? (If so, it may not accomplish the intended purpose.)

Maintenance. The following questions must be answered: If the item requires repair or replacement, can a local vendor fulfill this need? Can the patient make minor repairs or adjustments? Can the device be cleaned easily?

Adaptations in Treatment Implementation

Many assistive devices are available to help the patient with various functional impairments, such as muscle weakness, paralysis, joint limitation, or poor grasp. Although too numerous to list in detail, the more common items are illustrated in Figures 7-3 and 7-4.

Grooming and Hygiene. Grooming and hygiene include the skills of bathing, oral hygiene, toileting, hair and nail care, shaving, application of cosmetics, and other health needs.[8,10] When the patient is unable to perform tasks without assistance, an assessment for the potential use of the adaptive equipment should be made. The following aids are commonly used to improve independence in grooming and hygiene: long-handled bath brush, hair brush, scrub sponge, hand mirror and shaver, built up handle on toothbrush and comb, tube squeezer, electric razor holder, deodorant/shaving cream dispenser handle, suction denture brush, toilet tissue dispenser holder, raised toilet seat, toilet and bath safety rails, bath seat/chair lift, tub chair, hand-held shower nozzle, and rubber tub mat.

Dressing. The skill of dressing includes the ability to choose clothing that is seasonal and occasion-appropriate, remove it from a storage area, and don it in a sequential fashion, including use of special fasteners and adjustments.[8] Dressing instruction usually begins with dressing the disabled side first and undressing it last.[10] Clothes that are loose-fitting and open are recommended for easy wear. Some of the common adaptive equipment used for dressing tasks include long-handled shoe horns, sock aids, dressing sticks and reachers; stabilizing botton hooks, Velcro or clip shoe fasteners and elastic laces, one-handed belts, zippers and trouser pulls, and Velcro fasteners, elastic waistbands, and suspenders.

Feeding and Eating. Feeding includes the skills of setting up food, use of appropriate utensils and dishes, the ability to bring food or a beverage to the mouth, chewing, sucking, swallowing, and coughing to avoid choking.[8,10] The patient must be alert; proper body positioning is critical. It may be necessary to instruct the patient in sucking, chewing and swallowing. Some of the more common types of adapted equipment used to increase functional use of feeding utensils include long-handled, lightweight, or swivel spoons; forks with built up handles or triangular finger grips; plastic handle mugs with pedestal cups and other modified drinking utensils; splints with palmar clips; straw holders; scoop dishes; plate/food guards; suction plates; rubber mats; weighted utensils; rocker knives; ball bearing and offset suspension feeders; and universal cuffs and splints.

Medication Routine. Medication routine may be defined as the ability to obtain medication, open and close containers, and take the prescribed amount at the specified time.[8] Adaptive devices may include enlarged, easy-to-open containers or a divided container with medications placed in specific compartments with time noted when they should be taken.

Socialization. Socialization is defined as one's skill in interacting appropriately in contextual and cultural ways.[8] Adaptive equipment may include proper positioning devices to allow greater comfort and ease in social situations and slings that are made of fabric to match or complement clothing, thus improving self-image. In addition, a number of the adaptations listed under functional communication, such as the telephone, assist in promoting greater socialization in some cases.

Functional Mobility. Mobility includes the ability to move physically from one position or place to another. Such movement includes bed mobility; transfers to and from bed, chair, toilet, tub, and automobile; wheelchair mobility; ambulation; and driving.[8,10] Some of the common adaptive equipment used to facilitate mobility includes manual and electric wheelchairs, motorized scooters, mechanical and hydraulic lifts, trapeze bars, walkers (which may or may not have bag attachments), canes and cane seats, crutches, transfer boards, elevated chair and toilet seats, and modified vans, cars, and public transportation vehicles.

Functional Communication. Communication includes the ability to receive and transmit information verbally or nonverbally. Adaptive devices used to enhance communication skills include telephones, talking books, tape recorders, computers with printers and Braille writers, typewriters, radios, television, prism glasses, page turners, clip boards, and mouth sticks.[10]

Sexual Expression. Sexual expression has been defined as the ability to "recognize, communicate, and perform desired sexual activities."[8] Adaptive equipment such as pillows may be used to enhance function and increase comfort.

Related Adaptations. A large variety of adaptive devices are available to assist with performing work tasks. They will be discussed briefly here in relation to the specific areas of general object manipulation and cooking.

Object manipulation includes the skill and performance of handling large and small objects such as calculators, keys, money, light switches, doorknobs and packages. To assist the patient in manipulating common objects, positioning splints and other types of adaptive equipment are useful. These devices include tweezers, mouthstick holders/wands,

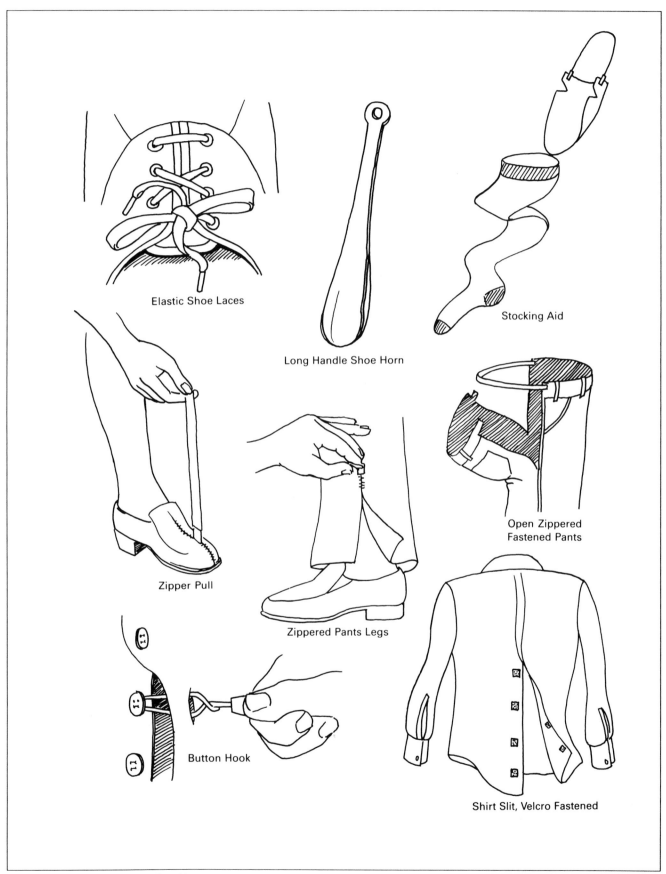

Elastic Shoe Laces

Long Handle Shoe Horn

Stocking Aid

Zipper Pull

Zippered Pants Legs

Open Zippered Fastened Pants

Button Hook

Shirt Slit, Velcro Fastened

Figure 7-3. Adaptive/assistive dressing aids.

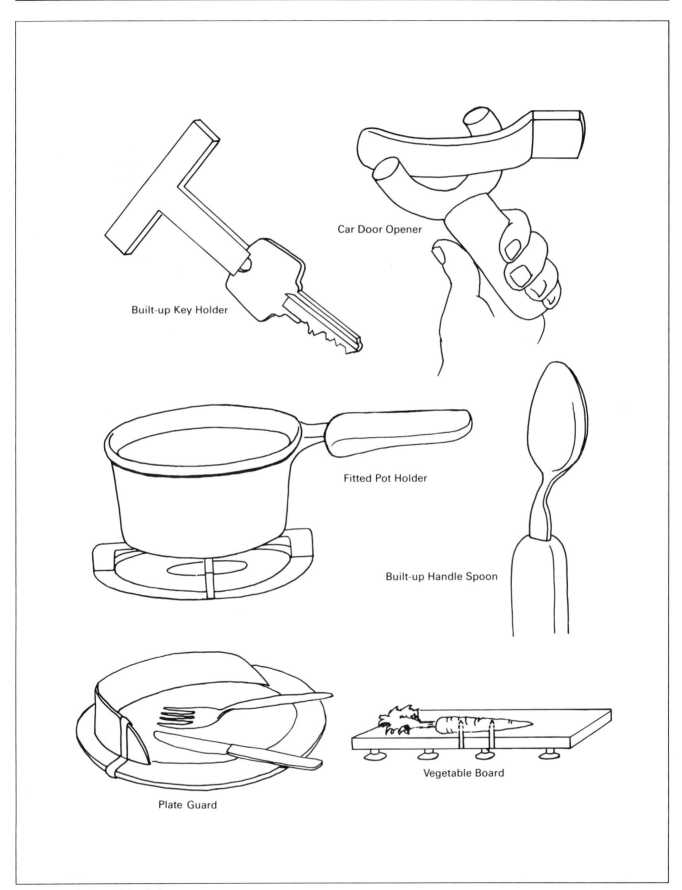

Figure 7-4. Adaptive/assistive devices.

light switch extensions/levers, key holders, and door knob extenders and turners.

Physical cooking skills range from simple peeling skills to preparing entire meals. Some of the common types of cooking adaptations are built up handles on utensils, plate guards, rubber mats, fitted potholders, and vegetable boards (see Figure 7-4).

Psychological/Emotional Daily Living Skills

Although this section focuses on the patient with psychosocial/emotional problems, these problems may also be seen in a patient with a physical disability. Conversely, the patient with psychiatric problems, owing to medication for example, may experience difficulty with gross motor, fine motor, and coordination skills.

ADLs for psychiatry are also centered around self-concept, self-identity, and coping with life situations in family, organizational and community involvement. Unlike patients with physical disabilities, individuals with psychiatric conditions have the motor ability to perform the tasks in most cases, but emotional conflicts may reduce the desire or motivation to carry them out. Patients may not attend to personal hygiene and grooming without assistance or verbal prompting from others. Occupational therapy provides a structured setting in which to learn how to take charge of their lives and be responsible for personal actions. Through therapy, the patient is guided in decision-making activities with the assurance that behaviors exhibited can be acceptable. With the contemporary emphasis on community mental health, the COTA is an important team member responsible for contributing to program planning and carrying out day-to-day activities.

The occupational therapy program in psychiatry provides service to the individual whose ability to meet psychosocial needs is impaired. This inability may be demonstrated through socialization, personal self-care, and play. For example, an individual may become disorganized or preoccupied, resulting in an inability to perform some task. The person may be very demanding and hostile, resulting in upsetting relationships with family and peers. The person may withdraw, become fearful, and reject communication.

Treatment begins with a psychosocial evaluation to assess the individual's self-concept, orientation to reality, and ability to communicate with others and to perform life tasks. Determining the patient's level of motivation, maturity, socialization, interpersonal relationships, and ability to cope with frustration and conflicts is another important part of the evaluation. Evaluation tools, techniques and methods used by occupational therapy personnel are the following:

1. Observation
2. Interest checklist
3. Anecdotal notes
4. Cumulative records
5. Rating scales
6. Self-report forms
7. Sociometric devices
8. Psychological tests
9. Standardized tests
10. Interviews
11. History taking

Patients who are referred to occupational therapy in psychiatry may have problems with occupational performance areas for a number of reasons, such as depression, which leaves them with little energy to cope with routine activities. The patient who is out of touch with reality may be unable to cook and eat because of fear that the food is poisoned.

Teaching task skills to patients can be very challenging and offers the therapist and the assistant opportunities for creativity. The most common areas of treatment addressed by the COTA practicing in psychiatry are grooming and hygiene, cooking, time management, socialization and organizational skills. Helping patients learn or relearn skills in these areas can increase their awareness and self-esteem.

Case Study 7-2

A creative COTA responsible for treating an adolescent who was chemically-dependent recently learned the latest fad for painting striped fingernails. The assistant taught this skill to a female patient, and the patient proceeded to teach the technique to her peers. Through teaching the patient a new skill, the therapist developed a closer relationship with the patient that helped her to discuss her problems more openly. The patient's relationships with peers were also improved through this single activity.

Case Study 7-3

A male patient who was in the midst of a divorce was admitted to a hospital for depression. He could not cope effectively because his wife had always taken care of so many of his daily needs. Occupational therapy personnel taught him basic cooking, washing, and cleaning skills. After discharge, the patient informed the staff of his successes, one of which was cooking dinner for six guests.

Program Planning

The reduction in in-patient hospital insurance coverage for psychiatric care influences decisions about the nature of treatment and changes in the therapist's and assistant's roles. These budgetary constraints have caused a rethinking of traditional occupational therapy rehabilitative services and new planning and structuring to assure the most cost-effective delivery of services.

Occupational therapy personnel frequently plan and implement a **group approach** to patient treatment. This approach involves the provision of therapy to three or more people at the same time. Task-oriented groups, which focus on a particular skill or set of skills, are often referred to as daily living groups. The focus may include the following topics:

1. Personal hygiene and grooming
2. Laundry and clothing care
3. Budgeting
4. Personal care shopping
5. Menu planning
6. Grocery shopping
7. Cooking and table setting
8. Kitchen and household safety
9. Home management and housekeeping
10. Seasonal dressing

Within the structure of such a group the leader may use specific methods to assist patients in developing skills. These methods include behavior modification using a token reward system; individual patient contracts regarding goal achievement; or shaping, which uses prompts to promote desired behavior.

Group experiences are also used to provide opportunities for patient interaction while activities are performed. A primary goal is to enhance social interaction skills relative to the patient's potential and the conditions of home and community environments. This overall goal may also include reinforcement of socially acceptable behavior, fostering of effective communication skills, encouraging self-awareness, and strengthening interpersonal confidence.

For example, a patient may be assigned to participate in a group where the members must cooperate in planning a holiday party. Through the planning and decision-making experience, each member learns to recognize the ways in which his or her behavior affects the achievement of tasks and the members of the group. Greater awareness is often gained after the task has been completed and members discuss their observations and feelings openly. Such discussions are often termed *processing the group*. Occupational therapy personnel are skilled in using activities and group process as structures to develop healthy interpersonal relationships. This topic is discussed in detail in Chapter 9.

The patient experiencing problems in reality orientation is an ideal candidate for task and activity experiences. Persons who are unable to distinguish reality are given concrete examples through activities that require the use of the five senses: sight, hearing, smell, touch and speech. The occupational therapy program helps individuals work toward recognizing and reacting to reality in both work and social relationships.

Community Involvement

The profession of occupational therapy is committed to patients returning to their communities and successfully managing life tasks and roles at the end of hospitalization or rehabilitation. The occupational therapist and the assistant may visit the patient's home or workplace to assure that these environments provide adequate safety and sufficient functional freedom.

Many patients do not progress smoothly through mental health care. In some cases it is necessary to provide the patient a longer adjustment period for successful reentry into community life. Community involvement refers to the patient interacting with others and understanding the social norms. Activities must be planned to introduce the patient to more complex scheduling, organizing, and executing of personal daily life activities. These activity experiences may include budgeting time, social role management, independent housing arrangements, and assessing and using community resources. The latter is encouraged by teaching techniques such as how to take a bus, how to use an instant cash machine, and how to follow the rules of organized meetings and to participate in such meetings.[11]

Occupational therapy plays an important role in reestablishing community support systems for patients. Support groups such as family, friends, church, and day program and community centers are important links in the patient's total rehabilitation. The recognition and positive responses furnished by the patient's support systems are crucial to the resumption of life tasks and roles.

PLAY

In medieval Europe, there was no concept of childhood as it is conceived today. Even among some contemporary societies, nearly all community resources are devoted to the business of survival, and little time is allotted to the needs of children. Play as a concept has evolved considerably in the last 20 years. The earlier neglect of play as meaningful activity is perhaps attributable to the perception that it was thought peripheral to the mainstream of individual development. The modern individual views play as an activity engaged in primarily by children.[12]

Play is a difficult concept to define because it is so broad in scope and includes many forms of behavior. However, it may be classified in several meaningful ways, including simple to complex, evolutionary, and developmental. Play can also be dichotomized into the following:[8]

1. Social or asocial
2. Cooperative or competitive
3. Imitative or original
4. Repetitive or novel
5. Overt or covert
6. Active or passive
7. Organized or spontaneous
8. Peaceful or boisterous

Scholars define play in various ways. As a process, play lies at the core of human behavior and development.[12] Play is an intrinsic activity done purely for its own sake rather than as a means to an end. It is spontaneous and voluntary, undertaken by choice and not compulsion. Play involves enjoyment and activity that leads to fun.[12] One author suggests that play is what children do when they are not eating, sleeping, resting, or doing what parents tell them to do. The preschool child's play is "serious business." It is his or her work; a means of discovering the world.[13] In 1916, a Swiss scientist, Karl Goes, proposed that play is the way children rehearse roles they are destined to fill in adult life. Play gives us permission to make mistakes.[12] Scholars emphasize life preparation, recapitulation, and surplus energy in explaining play activities. Although these notions have changed in recent years, they are still considered important features of play. Contemporary researchers focus on the spontaneous, voluntary, active and pleasurable aspects of play.[14]

It is generally accepted that play makes a substantial contribution throughout life and affects every aspect of human behavior. This view presumes that adults play and that such activity involves both work and recreational activity. These activities serve both conscious and psychological purposes.[14]

How Play Contributes to Development

Play contributes to physical, intellectual, language, social, and emotional development.

Physical Development. Play is closely associated with physical development at all ages. Infants respond by squirming and wiggling their bodies when adults play with them. As toddlers, their play involves gross motor activities such as climbing, running and jumping. Sports become important during middle childhood, with football, basketball, and swimming being common activities. Physical ability finds an outlet in play, and such activities lead to further refinement of physical ability.

Intellectual Development. As a form of symbolic expression, play can be a transitory process that takes the child from the earliest form of sensory-motor intelligence to the operational structures that characterize mature adult thought. Because play is cummulative, it has both immediate and long-range effects on development. Play leads to more complex, sophisticated cognitive behavior, which affects the content of play in a continuous, upward spiral. In the cognitive domain, play functions in four ways:[14]

1. It provides access to more avenues of information.
2. It consolidates mastery of skills and concepts.
3. It promotes and maintains effective functioning of the intellectual abilities through the use of cognitive operations.
4. It promotes creativity through the playful use of skills and concepts.

Language Development. Language and play are mutually reinforcing. Where play preceded the advent of language play, it formed a language embodying symbolic representation. Hence, some scholars suggest that the ability to represent objects, actions, and feelings in symbolic play is paralleled by a corresponding ability to represent those phenomena in language.[12]

Social Development. The primary goal of childhood is to allow socialization into active and productive adult roles in the culture. When social relationships pose problems for children, play is often a way to prevent frustrations and act out possible solutions without fear of reprisals. In learning and practicing socially desirable behavior, such as cooperation and sharing, the child uses play as a foundation for adult behavior.

Emotional Development. Much of the social learning occurring in childhood involves a balance between individual needs and the demands of social behavior. Play is an important medium for learning this balance, and children deprived of play will find it difficult to adapt to social demands in the future.

Types of Play

Play can be classified primarily as *physical* or *manipulative*. In physical play, action and boisterousness are the focus. The child attempts to gain control over the environment in manipulative play. Two additional types of play are *symbolic play* and *games*. Symbolic play includes pretending, make believe or fantasy play, and nonsense rhymes. Pretend play is exhibited as early as 18 months of age. It increases steadily with age into middle childhood and then disappears. Children rarely engage in pretend play after puberty; instead, they daydream.[12] When play is governed by rules or conventions, it is called a game. Games have two important characteristics: 1) They involve mutual involvement in some shared activity; and 2) the interactions are identified by alternating opportunities to play, repetition, and succession in chances to play.[12]

In a classic study in 1932, Mildred B. Parten observed the play of children in nursery school settings. She identified six types of play, based on the nature and extent of the children's social involvement:[15]

1. *Unoccupied play:* Children spend time watching others.
2. *Solitary play:* Children play with toys and make no effort to play with others.
3. *Onlooker behavior:* Children watch other children play but make no effort to join in.
4. *Parallel play:* Children play alongside other children but not with them.
5. *Associative play:* Children interact with each other, borrowing or lending material.

6. *Cooperative play:* Children integrate their play activities, and group members assume different roles and responsibilities.

Psychologists believe play contributes to childhood development. In 1952, Piaget emphasized the importance of exploration and play behavior as vehicles of cognitive stimulation. Ultimately play allows children to develop a sense of self-identity and objectivity. More information on the work of Piaget may be found in Chapters 5 and 8.

Play is an essential phase in childhood. It is critical to healthy development and useful to the individual and society in explaining roles. Play activities are a key to developing sound minds and bodies. Table 7-1 shows some of the play activity behavior patterns from ages six months to six years.

Different developmental disabilities such as mental retardation, cerebral palsy, or disorders characterized by difficulties in organizing and interpreting incoming stimuli (such as learning disabilities) may result in the level and proficiency of the child's play skill being directly related to mastery of a specific domain. A child may be unable to become involved in all of the many social interaction skills of play such as sharing, taking turns, asserting self, recognizing the feelings of others, and showing awareness of rules. Without the acquisition of these social skills, many forms of play (such as competitive play, small group play, and social play) cannot occur.

The relationship of psychomotor skills to play skills is also interdependent. Without the development of certain gross motor, fine motor, and coordination skills, the child will have difficulty engaging in midline hard play, object play, frolic play, or exploitive play (see Chapter 5). Perceptual skills are needed to fully participate in imaginative play, pretend play, dramatic play, means-end play, or creative play.

Children's play skills are related directly to behavior they have learned. Their proficiency, interaction, and understanding of how and why to carry out play activities is based on mastery of developmental stages.

Case Study 7-4

Jason. Jason is a shy, withdrawn four-year-old boy of African American heritage. He weighed two pounds, five ounces at birth and was born 3.2 months premature. His mother was a cocaine addict and had pneumonia at the time of delivery. Jason has been placed under protective custody by the Michigan Child Protection Services agency since age two and one-half years because his mother and father, both drug addicts, were unable to care for him properly.

The child has lived with foster parents for two years. He appears to be very attached to these people who have provided him with excellent care, but who have also unnecessarily indulged him. They have no other children and have petitioned for formal adoption.

At age three, Jason was diagnosed as having cerebral palsy with moderately involved spastic quadriplegia. Before diagnosis, the child's foster mother observed that Jason appeared to be "slow" and did not use his hands and arms, particularly the right, to reach out and grasp during normal ADLs or while playing with toys. He was referred to occupational therapy to develop skills in daily living activities, including head, trunk, and extremity control; feeding; and dressing: Lack of motor functioning interfered with play skills, so the following activities were used to address the problems: therapy balls, coloring, bead stringing, pull toys, computer games, obstacle course games, barrels to climb on or roll in, soft and lightweight foam toys, and inflatable toys. Emphasis was placed on dyadic or small group play activities and games requiring interaction with peers.

Progress was slow but steady. Jason used his right upper extremity to reach and was able to grasp some objects. Because his cognitive functioning was within normal range, he was accepted in the public school system in a traditional classroom setting.

LEISURE

As individuals progress from childhood to adulthood, activities once described as play become leisure activities. Leisure is an integral part of a balanced American lifestyle. Just as children learn about themselves and the world through structured activity (play), so do adults. Through work and leisure, individuals learn about themselves and their environment. This learning process is perpetual and continues throughout life.

By the year 2000 life expectancy is anticipated to increase by five to ten years. Alternative work patterns are being proposed to provide greater worker flexibility and to improve the quality of life. The quality of one's life is determined by, among other factors, the combination of work and nonwork activities. Numerous studies have shown how repressive working conditions and impoverished social environments create a meager existence for many workers.[16] The quality of life is greatly influenced by leisure activities.

Leisure is a subjective term. Individuals define leisure by their perceptions, taking into consideration their values and cultural orientation. One commonly used conceptualization in sociology literature is leisure as discretionary time. That is, leisure is the time remaining after the basic requirements of subsistence (work) and existence (meeting daily needs) are met.[17] Leisure may also be viewed as "nonwork activity" engaged in during free time.[18] Actually, leisure is not a category but rather a style of behavior that may occur in any activity. For example, one can work while listening to music, thus providing a leisure aspect.[19] Leisure is free time where content is oriented towards self-fulfillment as an ultimate

Table 7-1
Play Activity Behavior Patterns

Typical play activity behavior patterns of children from 6 months to 6 years are indicated in the following chart.

AT SIX TO SEVEN MONTHS

He holds toys and plays actively with a rattle.
She looks at herself in a mirror, smiles, vocalizes, and pats the mirror.
He watches things and movements about him.
She can amuse herself and keep busy for at least 15 minutes at a time.

AT NINE MONTHS

He bangs one toy against another.
She imitates movements such as splashing in the tub, crumpling paper, shaking a rattle.

AT TWELVE MONTHS

He responds to music.
She examines toys and objects with eyes and hands, feeling them, poking them, and turning them around.
He likes to put objects in and out of containers.

AT EIGHTEEN MONTHS

She purposefully moves toys and other objects from one place to another.
He often carries a doll or stuffed animal about with him.
She likes to play with sand, letting it run between her fingers and pouring it in and out of containers.
He hugs a doll or stuffed animal, showing affection or other personal reaction to it.
She likes picture books or familiar objects.
He scribbles spontaneously with a pencil or crayon.
She plays with blocks in a simple manner—carrying them around, fingering and handling them, gathering them together—but does not build purposefully with them. It takes many trials before she can make three or four stand in a tower.
He imitates simple things he sees others do, such as "reading" a book or spanking his doll.

AT TWO YEARS

She likes to investigate and play with small objects such as toys, cars, blocks, pebbles, sand, water.
He likes to play with messy materials such as clay, patting, pinching and fingering it.
She likes to play with large objects such as huggies and wagons.
He can snip with scissors but is awkward.
She imitates everyday household activities such as cooking, hanging up clothes. These are usually activities with which she is closely associated and things she sees rather than remembers.
He plays with blocks, lining them up or using them to fill wagons or other toys.
She can, with urging, build a tower of six or seven blocks.

AT THREE YEARS

He pushes trains, cars, fire engines, in make-believe activities.
She cuts with scissors, not necessarily in a constructive manner.
He makes well-controlled marks with crayon or pencil and sometimes attempts to draw simple figures.
She gives rhythmic physical response to music: clapping or swaying or marching.
He initiates his own play activities when supplied with interesting materials.
She likes to imitate activities of others, especially real-life activities.
He likes to take a toy or doll to bed with him.
She delays sleeping by calling for a drink of water or asking to go to the bathroom.

AT FOUR YEARS

In playing with materials such as blocks, clay, and sand, the 4-year-old is more constructive and creative. Such play is often cooperative.
He uses much imagination in play and wants more in the way of costumes and materials than formerly.
She draws simple figures of things she sees or imagines, but these have few details and are not always recognizable to others.
He can cut or trace along a line with fair accuracy.

Used with permission of Wayne County Community College, Occupational Therapy Assistant Program.

Table 7-1
Play Activity Behavior (continued)

AT FIVE YEARS

 She plays active games of a competitive nature, such as hide-and-go-seek, tag, and hopscotch.
 He builds houses, garages, and elaborate structures with blocks.
 She likes dramatic play—playing house, dressing up, cowboy, spaceman, war games—and acts out stories
  heard. This is more complicated and better organized than at age **4**.
 He uses pencils and crayons freely. His drawings are simple but can usually be recognized.
 She enjoys cutting out things with scissors—pictures from magazines, paper dolls.
 He can sing, dance to music, play records on the phonograph.

AT SIX YEARS

 The 6 -year-old can learn to play simple table games such as tiddly-winks, marbles, parchesi, and dominoes.
 He likes stunts and gymnastics and many kinds of physical activity.
 She wrestles and scuffles in a coordinated manner with other children.
 At this point the play interests of boys and girls are different.

---

end. This time is granted to the individual by society when he or she has complied with occupational, family, spiritual and political obligations.[19]

Leisure is progressive rebirth, regrowth, and reacquaintance with oneself, renewing, refulfilling, and recreating.[20] It should be compatible with physical, mental, and social well-being. Most scholars agree that leisure is characterized by a search for a state of satisfaction. This search is the primal condition of leisure. When leisure fails to give the expected pleasure, when it is not interesting, "it is not fun."[21] There are two dimensions of leisure: the satisfaction inherent in the activity itself and the relations of the activity to external values, or social well-being.[20]

In 1960 Dumazedier[19] identified periods of leisure, including the end of the day and during retirement. During such times, leisure covers a number of structured activities connected with physical and mental needs defined as artistic, intellectual, and social leisure pursuits, within the limits of economic, political, and cultural conditions in each society.

Purpose and Function

The fundamental purpose of leisure is to provide an opportunity to develop talents and interests. Leisure also meets the following needs:[20]

1. Belonging
2. Individuality (through interests and abilities that distinguish the individual)
3. Multifunctional purposes in behavior (Some activities offer a wide dimension of function.)
4. Multidimensional effects of behavior (Some activities serve additional persons in society at the same time they serve the participant.)
5. Activities and created objects as projections of the person (providing expression of feelings, projection of self-knowledge and objects for future pleasure)

Classification

There have been many attempts to classify leisure. In a study of leisure in Kansas City in 1955 Havighurst[22] distinguished 11 categories:

1. Participation in organized groups
2. Participation in unorganized groups
3. Pleasure trips
4. Participation in sports
5. Spectator sports (excluding television)
6. Television and radio
7. Fishing and hunting
8. Gardening and country walks
9. Crafts (sewing, carpentry and do-it-yourself)
10. Imaginative activities, music, and art
11. Visits to relatives and friends

Developmental Aspect

Leisure patterns are also related to developmental tasks and issues individuals face at different stages in the life cycle. In many cases, these tasks and issues will be shaped by preoccupations, culture, and needs at each stage.[23] Because infants cannot distinguish between obligatory and nonobligatory activity, it is doubtful whether the concept of leisure is relevant to them. Socialization through play, however, influences the child's ability to cope in interpersonal relationships and is the beginning of adult leisure behavior.[24] Leisure activities help to socialize adolescents to adult attitudes and roles.[26] During adolescence, leisure time activities are an important preoccupation. Activities may represent an extension of a school subject or may be extracurricular. Among young adults, leisure is important for marital satisfaction, as it provides an environment for personal communication, sharing of experiences, and family cohesiveness. These joint activities encourage interaction and shared commitments.

Work and family continue to be the dominant themes in early maturity (ages 30 to 40). Leisure activities in this category are often home- and family-centered and provide a means of increasing the growth and stability of marriage and the family. At full maturity (age 45 to retirement), leisure activities may become less home and family centered, as there are fewer family responsibilities in many instances. There often are increased economic resources to provide opportunities for more evenings out, travel, and other less home-oriented leisure.

Leisure and Retirement

Individuals sometimes need to rediscover or develop new leisure interests as work diminishes and retirement approaches. Retirement can result in a relinquishment of social involvements. Leisure can provide a context for autonomous decision-making and social integration with meaningful other persons whose support and encouragement is very important to life cycle transition at old age.[23]

Because of improved medical science and social welfare, more people are living long past retirement age. Prime predictors of retirement adjustment are adequate retirement income and retired friends with whom to share leisure time. The loss of income, rather than employment, accounts for the negative retirement effects for many. Activities that build skills and interests of preretirement should provide a foundation of personal adjustment and life satisfaction after retirement.[23]

How do elderly people use the time freed from work? Time budget surveys have demonstrated that leisure takes most of the spare time enjoyed by the elderly, even more time than the personal, household, and family care activities. The amount of leisure activities increases with age. Eighty percent of those age 65 and over have at least five hours of leisure time per day according to Dumazedier.[19]

Retired persons often face the problem of what to do with extra time. The problem may affect men more because women may find that retirement from their responsibilities is replaced, to some extent, by activities related to their grandchildren.

The impact of retirement is considerably different between social classes and cultures. Men in professional occupations are often able to continue some form of work after official retirement. This is less possible for those in blue-collar or service occupations. Middle class women who reach retirement status are more likely to be members of voluntary organizations than working class women. Among Americans, church is an important and approved medium of social activities and entertainment for the elderly. The church is a place to meet and relate with friends. In addition to ministering to spiritual needs, the church sponsors activities such as bazaars, dinners, bowling teams, travel clubs, special lectures, and picnics as well as other activities that constitute a rich offering of social opportunities.

The influence of preretirement leisure activity patterns on retirement planning and attitudes toward retirement was investigated by two occupational therapists. Sixty male retirees were surveyed to determine the degree of preretirement planning and the type and extent of leisure participation before and after retirement. The results showed that a high degree of preretirement leisure participation correlates with a high degree of preretirement planning.[25] If the patterns that predict satisfaction among retirees can be identified, they can be used in activity planning to structure the healthful use of time for retirees. Further, if one or more characteristic activity patterns can be associated with retirement satisfaction, then occupational therapy personnel could implement preretirement programs accordingly.

Recreation

Recreation is a term often used to suggest leisure. In its literal sense, re-creating is seen as one of the functions of leisure—that of renewing the self or of preparing for work. Thus recreation is characterized by the attitude of a person when participating in activities that satisfy, amuse, direct, relax or provide opportunities for self-expression. It is generally associated with arts and crafts, outdoor activities, hobbies, literary activities, culture, clubs, and other organized groups.[26]

Leisure Activities

The physically disabled and patients with mental illness have a need for leisure. Today these individuals participate in nearly every sport and craft activity and also engage in other forms of leisure such as drama, dance and music. Participation in these activities is both enjoyable and therapeutic. Persons with physical disabilities are recreating more and more with the nondisabled, thus integrating into the mainstream of society. The need for adaptations often dictates that many disabled train and compete with others of similar functional abilities, particularly in sports.

Occupational therapy personnel are not recreation specialists; however, OTRs and COTAs are adaptation specialists and are often called on to evaluate the need for adaptation with a particular leisure activity. In many instances the patient is more skilled at the activity than the OTR or the COTA; however, as adaptation specialists, occupational therapy personnel can adapt equipment and teach compensatory movements so that the patient can engage in the leisure task as independently as possible. This could range from instructing the visually impaired to thread a needle to adapting a tripod for the photographer in a wheelchair. The following questions should be considered in making adaptations:

1. *Cost:* How much can the patient or family afford for the adaptation needed?
2. *Use:* How frequently will the equipment or aid be used? Does the frequency of use justify the cost?
3. *Expense:* What expense will be required each time the patient engages in the activity?

4. *Maintenance:* Will the adaptation be primarily maintenance free? Are replacement parts readily available?
5. *Location:* Will the leisure activity be easily accessible?
6. *Appearance:* Is the adaptation so prominent that the patient will be embarrassed to use it, or is the activity so altered that it no longer resembles its original form?

In psychiatry, individual activity patterns are often lost with the onset of mental illness. Because these activity patterns are the expressions of the individual's proper use and appreciation of time, the loss of these patterns can result in reality disorientation with others, the environment and time.[27] Consequently, many patients have difficulty engaging in play and leisure activities. There is also an inability to identify satisfying leisure-time interests. Fidler[27] notes several possible factors that may contribute to these deficits.

1. Limited self-awareness concerning one's strengths, skills, present and past accomplishments, personal goals, beliefs, and values
2. Lack of adequate planning skills
3. Pragmatic barriers to participation, such as locked wards, insufficient finances, lack of transportation, lack of equipment, and lack of opportunity
4. Limited knowledge of resources and how to use them
5. Lack of underlying competencies in sensorimotor skills, cognitive skills, and/or interpersonal skills needed to participate and experience pleasure

The activity histories of many members of the patient population receiving psychiatric occupational therapy treatment generally reveal a sparse repertoire of childhood play experiences on which to base adult leisure experiences. Play is widely recognized as the child's arena for learning and practicing rules and social skills necessary for subsequent roles in school, work and recreation. Play and leisure competencies are developed along with other daily living skills and may, in fact, facilitate the development of other functional roles, such as work.[27]

The patient's use of leisure time can be measured by having the individual complete a schedule of a typical day and a leisure questionnaire. An example of the latter is shown in Figure 7-5. It may be found that a patient's television viewing consumes 90% of leisure time. Exploring patient talents and interests and providing opportunities to experiment with and experience some of them might lead to more gratifying activity patterns.

Goals of Leisure Activity

Leisure activity can assist in developing **psychomotor** and **affective skills,** both of which can lead to helping the patient reestablish his or her role in society. Psychomotor goals include the following:

1. Improve visual perception
2. Improve range of motion
3. Improve muscle strength
4. Improve balance
5. Improve physical tolerance and endurance
6. Improve coordination
7. Increase attention span

Affective goals include the following:
1. Improve self-esteem
2. Improve interpersonal skills
3. Improve social skills
4. Improve communication skills
5. Aid in acceptance of disability
6. Develop friendship/comradeship
7. Improve self-discipline

Case Study 7-5

A "hard driving" professional man, who rarely had any time for leisure was admitted to a psychiatric treatment center with the diagnosis of major affective disorder. While in occupational therapy, he developed an interest in making clay pots on the potter's wheel. The occupational therapy assistant who was responsible for carrying out his treatment encouraged him to continue his work after discharge. She maintained a resource file of community leisure resources and drew on this material to locate a nearby art association that held classes as well as periodic exhibits. By sharing this information with the patient, an avenue was provided for him to continue to pursue his interest and develop a new area of leisure.

A knowledge of activities and interest groups within the community is essential for all occupational therapy personnel who treat patients.

Leisure Task Groups

The use of **task groups** is a common way to treat patients in occupational therapy. The types of patients who could benefit from task groups are the following:

1. A large variety of patients except the very young
2. Those with neurologic disorders or physical or mental impairments
3. Those who need to increase their levels of independence
4. Those with inadequate social skills
5. Those unfamiliar with community resources
6. Those who make poor use of free time
7. Those who have an inability to identify leisure interests
8. Those who have poor leisure planning skills

Common treatment goals for the task groups are the following:

1. To develop knowledge of and skills in using community resources
2. To develop new leisure and interest options

Name _____ Date _____

Ward or Room _____ Age _____ Sex _____

INSTRUCTIONS: Put an X before the activities you know and would like to do.
Put an O before the activities you do not know, but would like to learn or take part in.
Write, under "Other," any activities not listed that you would like to do.

QUIET GAMES
_____ Bridge
_____ Canasta
_____ Checkers
_____ Chess
_____ Pinochle
_____ Dominoes
_____ Rummy
Other:

_____
_____

ACTIVE GAMES
_____ Ring toss
_____ Billiards
_____ Horseshoes
_____ Darts
_____ Croquet
_____ Bowling
_____ Basketball

_____
_____

SOCIAL ACTIVITIES
_____ Game nights
_____ Bingo
_____ Parties
_____ Folk dancing
_____ Square dancing
_____ Dancing
_____ Picnics
_____ Trips and tours
Other:

_____
_____

ENTERTAINMENT
_____ Amateur nights
_____ Variety shows
_____ Puppet shows
_____ Quiz programs
_____ Plays
_____ Pageants
_____ Festivals
Other:

_____
_____

_____ Baseball
_____ Boccie
_____ Football
_____ Golf
Other:

_____
_____

DRAMA
_____ Acting
_____ Stagecraft
_____ Script writing
_____ Costuming
_____ Makeup
Other:

_____
_____

NEWSPAPER
_____ Writing
_____ Reporting
_____ Artwork

Figure 7-5. Leisure interest checklist. Used with permission from Wayne County Community College, Occupational Therapy Assistant Program.

3. To increase independent functioning
4. To develop transition skills for readjustment to the community
5. To further develop the ability to make decisions and follow through
6. To demonstrate basic skill in selecting activities for use during free time

Sample Activity Tasks. Trips to places of interest, such as art and historical museums, zoos, theaters, parks, cider mills, shopping centers, and movies, can be planned. Ideas for such trips may be suggested by either the group leader or the participants. A decision may be made by concensus or majority vote. Once a decision has been made, additional procedures or rules may be established by the task group,

Name _____ Date _____

Ward or Room _____ Age _____ Sex _____

INSTRUCTIONS: Put an X before the activities you know and would like to do.
Put an O before the activities you do not know, but would like to learn or take part in.
Write, under "Other," any activities not listed that you would like to do.

MUSIC

_____ Community singing
_____ Quartet
_____ Choir
_____ Chorus
_____ Instrument instruction
_____ Instrument playing
_____ Rhythm band
_____ Orchestra
_____ Listening
_____ Music appreciation
Other:

_____ _____
_____ _____

ARTS AND CRAFTS

_____ Drawing and painting
_____ Leathercraft
_____ Woodcarving
_____ Ceramics
_____ Jewelry making
_____ Shellcraft
_____ Basketry
_____ Weaving
_____ Needlework
_____ Party decorations
Other:

_____ _____
_____ _____

HOBBIES AND CLUBS

_____ Photography
_____ Discussion groups
_____ Magic
_____ Nature lore
_____ Stamp collecting
Other:

_____ _____
_____ _____

_____ Creative writing
_____ Model building
_____ Gardening
_____ Reading
Other:

_____ _____
_____ _____

List other special interests: _____

What kinds of books do you like to read? _____

What kind of movies do you like to see? _____

What kind of music do you like to hear? _____

What kind of songs do you like to sing? _____

How do you spend your leisure time? _____

Figure 7-5. Continued.

depending on the nature of the activity. For example, if the activity of going to a particular movie is decided on, the following rules could be established:

1. Each patient must sign up on the van transportation form in the occupational therapy office.
2. Each patient must be dressed appropriately for the outing.
3. Each patient must be at the van pick-up site at the designated time.
4. Each patient must purchase his or her own ticket and be responsible for obtaining correct change.
5. Each patient must purchase his or her own refreshments and be responsible for obtaining correct change.

Outside Meals. Meals can be planned at restaurants. If the task group decides on this activity, rules 1, 2, and 3 of the preceding would apply. The group may also wish to establish additional requirements which might include learning proper use of a menu, how to place an order, use of correct table manners, use of appropriate tableware, paying the bill and tipping.

Table Games. A number of suitable table games can be chosen. When task group members determine a game or games to be played, a member may volunteer or be appointed to be responsible for obtaining the needed supplies and equipment. Another group member could be in charge of explaining the rules of the game. Depending on the specific nature of the particular game chosen, additional tasks might include awarding prizes to winners or teaching the game to nongroup members.

Kitchen Activities. Kitchen activities can involve many tasks depending on the scope of the activity. Some of these might include planning the menu, obtaining the necessary supplies and equipment, making copies of the recipes to be used, inviting guests, cooking, table setting, serving, and clean-up. Some of the rules that could be established include the following:

1. All patients will wash their hands thoroughly.
2. Patients working with food will wear hair nets.
3. Everyone in the group will be responsible for carrying out at least one task.

After each group activity, the group leader or leaders can discuss the event with the patients in the task group. Topics should include positive and negative aspects, with patients being given constructive feedback on their behaviors. All members also should have an opportunity to discuss their personal feelings. More information on task groups may be found in Chapter 9.

Case Study 7-6

John. John was 30 years old when he was referred to the occupational therapy department after surgical removal of a brain tumor. He had been living in a group home before the surgery and had worked as a factory foreman up until the previous year. He began having seizures, which ultimately interfered with his job responsibilities, and he was terminated from his position.

Family members reported that John withdrew from social and physical activities after learning of his tumor and losing his job. He became extremely depressed. After an occupational therapy evaluation, the following goals were established in collaboration with the patient:

1. Develop social skills necessary for active community participation after discharge from the hospital
2. Demonstrate independence in ADLs and productive occupation
3. Exhibit improved self-esteem and feelings of self-worth

4. Demonstrate increased personal involvement in leisure activities
5. Demonstrate increased ability to structure leisure time
6. Provide evidence of ability to use resources to aid in transition from hospital to community

The COTA responsible for supervising John's treatment activities in relation to leisure goals used a supportive and flexible approach, offering John encouragement and reassurance as appropriate. Among other activities, the patient participated in a number of day trips, very reluctantly at first. He enjoyed the parks and particularly the beautiful fall colors of the trees. The COTA provided him with a city map and assisted him in locating parks near his home. She also pointed out the availability of guided nature hikes. John took his family on one of these hikes during a weekend leave from the facility.

As John became involved in meaningful activities, including leisure, his depression disappeared and self-esteem improved. He became interested in community activities again and expressed a desire to return to the cider mill as well as a museum he had visited with a patient group.[28]

Included in Appendix B is a list of recreational organizations for disabled individuals located throughout the United States. Many can provide the names and addresses of individual contacts in the patient's community.

WORK

In 1909 R.C. Cabolt, a professor of medicine at Harvard University, wrote an article entitled "Work Cure," suggesting that work is best of all psychotherapies. In a later book, *What Men Live By,* he discussed the relationships among work, play, love and religion and called for a balance among them. He believed work caused greater physical and emotional health. The relationship between a healthy body and work is also suggested throughout occupational therapy literature. Work can provide a source of satisfaction and emotional well-being.

Occupational therapy views work as skill in socially productive activities. These activities may take place in the home, school, or community and include home management, care of others, educational pursuits and vocational activities.[8]

Public opinion surveys reveal that work, in addition to its economic function, structures time, provides a context in which to relate to other people, offers an escape from boredom, and sustains a sense of worth. Moreover, work affects the individual's freedom, responsibility, social position, attitude, mental capacities, achievements, friends, self-concept and "chances in life."[20] As one writer suggests, work is not a part of life, it is literally life itself.

Studs Turkel[29] wrote that "the job" is a search for working Americans to find daily meaning as well as "daily bread" for recognition. Turkel clearly recognized the linkage between mental health and meaningful work, pride in accomplishment, recognition, hunger for beauty, and a need to be remembered by "the job."

Significance of Work

Work provides an opportunity to associate with others. Through membership in work organizations, individuals gain a fundamental index of status and self-respect. The relationship to work influences one's use of time and leisure, the nature of the individual's family, and the state of one's mental health.[30]

The importance of work is pervasive; it determines what is produced, what is consumed, how individuals live, and what type of society is created and perpetuated.[30] Human motivation ranges beyond the drive for satisfaction of essential and discretionary materialistic needs. Higher needs must be satisfied to approach the fullest potential of human existence through the activity of work.

Parker[21] categorized life space as the total of activities or ways of spending time. In considering the various definitions of work and leisure, to allocate all the parts of life space either to work or to leisure would be a gross oversimplification. It is possible to use the exhaustive categories of work and nonwork, but it is still not possible to draw a line between the two categories. Parker analyzed the 24-hour day in five main groups:[21] 1) work, 2) working time, 3) sold time, 4) semileisure time, and 5) leisure.

When analyzing life space, work is usually identified with earning a living, even though work has a wider meaning than employment. Homemaking, parenting and child care as well as the student's work of achieving an education are examples.

Apart from actual working time, most people have to spend a certain amount of time traveling to places of work and preparing for work. At least part of the traveling time may be regarded more as a form of leisure than as work related, such as time spent reading the newspaper or a book, knitting, or chatting with fellow travelers. Other activities related to working time involve husbands and wives sharing in household tasks that were considered to be solely "women's work" in the past, voluntary overtime or having a second job, reading related to one's job while at home, and attending work-related conferences and meetings.

Parker's use of the term *sold time* refers to meeting the person's physiologic needs. The satisfaction of these self-care needs includes sleeping, eating, bathing, eliminating, and sexual activities. Beyond the time necessary for reasonably healthy living, extra time spent on these tasks may become a leisure activity, such as eating for leisure, or attending to one's appearance before going to a party.

Domestic work such as making beds, caring for a pet,

gardening, and odd jobs in the home are examples of semileisure tasks. Semileisure arises from leisure, but represents the character of obligations in differing degrees. These obligations are usually to other people but may be to pets, homes, and gardens as well.

Leisure is free time, spare time, uncommitted time, discretionary time, and choosing time.[21] It is time free from obligations either to self or others, a time to do as one chooses.

Analysis of life space based on the majority, those who are employed full time, would be incomplete. Those who do not work at full-time paid positions must be considered as well. People in these groups include housewives, prisoners, the unemployed, and, in some instances, the rich.

For example, the life space of a prisoner is much more constricted than that of the average citizen in terms of both time and activity. Although some prisoners are employed outside the prison, the choice of work is severely restricted and the motivation for it is rather different. Insofar as some prison work may be more or less voluntarily undertaken to relieve boredom or satisfy a physiological or psychologic need to work, it may resemble the "work obligation" of the average citizen.

Doing housework is often the housewife's work. When compared with the husband's paid employment, it usually offers less scope for interest and less social contact. There is no real difference between work obligations and the responsibilities of the household.[21]

Many unemployed individuals develop feelings of uselessness and may be driven to occupy themselves with trivial tasks and time-filling routines. They lose the companionship and social support of co-workers. Lack of money produces a restriction on the range of leisure activities, thus narrowing the scope of life experiences. The retired are similar to the unemployed, except that absence of employment is normally planned and permanent.

Worker Satisfaction

The highly productive economy of the 1970s reduced the moral value of work. There is much discussion today about worker dissatisfaction. Although the degree of job satisfaction differs, studies reveal that substantial numbers are dissatisfied with their jobs because the job does not meet their need for self-actualization, that is, their chance to perform well, opportunities for achievement and growth, and the chance to contribute something personel and unique.[31] Scholars have identified six elements that bring satisfaction on the job:

1. Creating a product that reflects the individual's input
2. Using skill
3. Working wholeheartedly
4. Using initiative and having responsibility
5. Mixing with people
6. Working with people who know their job

The most desirable work-related outcomes are as follows:

1. To feel pride and craftsmanship in one's work
2. To feel more worthwhile
3. To be recognized and respected by others
4. To require little direct supervision
5. To have contact with others in the same type of work, both on and off the job

Women and Work

The American family has undergone many changes in recent years. One significant change is the increase of women working outside the home. Women now represent nearly 46% of the national labor force.[33] If one spouse must stay home to care for the children, however, it is almost always the wife who does so.[21] In interviews with house-wives in one community study, some women thought that leisure came when all the household chores were done and children were in bed.[20]

Growth of the female work force can be traced to many factors, which include the increasing availability of contra-ceptives, a preference toward smaller families, inflation, a rising divorce rate, an increasing number of equality-oriented college women, expansion of the service-oriented economy, and changing attitudes toward careers for women.[31] Although a greater number of women are em-ployed outside the home, a majority are in low-paying occupations or in service industries. Like homemakers, they teach children, care for the sick and prepare food.[32]

Types and Phases of Work

Aristotle believed that there were two types of work: bread and labor, or work for the purpose of subsistence; and leisure work, or labor that was interesting in and of itself. In today's society, individuals do not work solely for economic self-interest, but also because work is psychologically necessary. Work is important to human dignity. The major-ity of the poor do not want to remain idle and accept welfare. Eighty percent of the labor force say they would work even if they did not need the income because work keeps them occupied and healthy. Without it, they would feel lost, useless and bored.[33]

Sociologists and psychologists identify five work phases in life:

1. Preparatory—usually school
2. Initial—first employment
3. Trial—a period of job changing as the worker tries to find work which is attractive
4. Stable—usually the longest period when there are relatively few changes in occupations
5. Retirement

One test of the importance of work in the lives of individuals is found in the activities of retired persons. Less than 20% of men drawing Social Security benefits retire to enjoy leisure. Almost three fourths of these retirements are involuntary due to the employer retiring the worker or the worker being forced to retire because of poor health.

Occupational Therapy and Work

In occupational therapy, work and related skills and performance may be defined as the functional ability and proficiency needed to carry out the task of productive activity. The occupational performance area of work may be further defined and categorized according to *Uniform Ter-minology,* Second Edition, published by the American Occupational Therapy Association. Work activities in the area of home management include the following:[8]

1. Clothing care
2. Cleaning
3. Meal preparation and cleanup
4. Shopping
5. Money management
6. Household maintenance
7. Care of others

Work activities centered around the care of others include providing physical care, communication, nurturance, and activities that are age-appropriate for one's spouse, children, parents or significant others.[8] Educational activities are also defined as they relate to the student's participation in a school environment, including school-sponsored activities such as field trips and work-study programs.[8] The final category presented in this document is vocational activities. These are categorized as vocational exploration, job acquisi-tion, work or job performance, and retirement planning.[8]

Nelson[6] has said that the concept of activity includes "activity as form" and "activity as action." Action is that part of the activity concerned with one's actual performance of the activity, that is, the specific operations needed to carry out the activity, whether it be work, play/leisure or ADLs. Activity as form denotes the cultural expectations or general procedures an individual would follow in order to do the activity well. The term *function* describes activity of form.

Because skill and performance are functional abilities, occupational therapy personnel must concentrate their ef-forts on a thorough analysis of the patient's functional abilities, along with his or her affective skills. Such an analysis could assist in determining the feasibility of the patient's chosen work. More information on activity analy-sis may be found in Chapter 17.

Function can be divided into the following categories: physical tolerance demands, sensory/perception, motor, daily living skills, cognition, and affective demands. Sub-components of each of these are enumerated in Table 7-2.

The occupational therapy assistant, under the supervision of and in collaboration with the occupational therapist, must relate each functional ability to the impact it will have on a patient's work, whether at home, in an office, or in the community. The interrelatedness of skill to the work task must be determined.

Table 7-2
Work Behavior Skills

Physical Tolerance and Demands	Sensory/Perception	Motor
Work pace/rhythm	Color discrimination	Finger dexterity
Standing tolerance	Form perception	Manual dexterity
Sitting tolerance	Size discrimination	Coordination:
Endurance	Spatial relationship	eye-hand
Performance with repetition	Ability to follow visual instruction	eye-hand-foot
Muscle strength	Texture discrimination	fine motor
Walking	Digital discrimination	gross motor
Lifting	Figure-ground	bimanual
Carrying	Form constancy	bilateral
Pushing	Visual closure	Use of hand tools
Pulling	Parts-to-whole	ROM:
Climbing	Shape discrimination	stopping
	Kinesthesia	kneeling
		crouching
		crawling
		reaching
		Balancing

Daily Living Skills	Cognition	Affective
Self-care:	Numerical ability	Attendance
personal hygiene	Measuring ability	Punctuality
grooming	Safety consciousness	Response to:
dressing	Care in handling work and tools	praise
eating/feeding	Work quality	criticism
object manipulation	Accuracy	assistance
Mobility:	Neatness	frustrating situation
transfers	Attention span	Relationship with:
travel (mode of)	Planning/organization	evaluator
transportation	Ability to follow:	co-worker
Communication:	verbal instruction	Work flexibility
with peers	written instruction	Attitude toward work
with supervisor	Retention of instruction	Behavior in structured setting
writing	Work judgment	Ability to work independently
dialing phone	Ability to learn new task	Initiative
talking on phone	Orientation	
typing		(In psychiatry, also observe for additional pathologic behavior.)

Used with permission from Wayne County Community College, Occupational Therapy Assistant Program.

Relationship of Work to Physical Disability

Whether a homemaker or a plumber, managing everyday tasks can be difficult for anyone; but for the individual with a physical disability, the need for good management and organization is essential to success. Evaluation and training for these skills can be assessed both formally and informally. Much valuable information can be obtained when the individual completes daily living skill tasks, as well as through interviews with the patient and significant others, such as close family members. Table 7-2 identifies skills that may be assessed.

Of concern to the COTA are the following questions, which must be answered before planning and implementing an occupational therapy program to meet the patient's needs in relation to home management and child care:

1. What is the extent of the patient's handicap, and what is the subsequent functional loss?
2. What is the apparent cause of the functional loss? (eg, sensory, judgment, range of motion limitation)?
3. What role in homemaking and child care did the patient have before the disability?

4. What financial resources are available to the patient for task assistance?

5. What are the patient's goals for independence?

Other principles must also be considered in planning an occupational therapy treatment program. These include:

1. *Energy conservation*—includes work simplification and time management needs for adaptive/assistive equipment including carts, chairs, and utensils

2. *Barrier free design*—ranges from simple adaptations such as removing scatter rugs, to kitchen modification of shelves and cabinets, to use of a microwave oven, to redesigning doorways, entrances, and bathrooms

3. *Physical abilities*—includes reaching, stooping, bending, balancing, walking, standing, sitting, pushing, pulling, lifting, coordination, and speed

4. *Sensory awareness*—such as temperature, proprioception, and kinesthesia

5. *Cognition*—includes attention span, judgment, organization, and memory

6. *Family expectation*—total independence or independence with assistance

7. *Community resources*—home-delivered meals, catalog shopping, child care

The COTA should stress to the patient the need for organized, planned activities. Every step saved and energy conserved is to the individual's advantage. Simulated tasks should be practiced in the occupational therapy clinic as frequently as possible before discharge. Numerous resources are available. For example, when working on home management tasks, a detailed reference, giving step-by-step guidelines for many tasks is the *Mealtime Manual for People with Disabilities and the Aging,* compiled by Judith Klinger, OTR.

Psychosocial Implications

The emphasis when working in psychiatry is quite different from that in the physical disability setting. Rather than stressing psychomotor abilities the focus is on the affective domain. Goals may include some of the following:

1. Demonstrate the ability to develop interpersonal relationships (which the patient may have lost as a result of illness or may never have acquired)

2. Exhibit improved self-esteem

3. Provide evidence of development of decision-making skills (by encouraging individual responsibility)

4. Exhibit increased skill in socialization

5. Demonstrate adequate skills in areas such as budgeting, time management, purchasing and menu planning

The hospitalized patient may never have worked, may be temporarily unemployed, or may be deprived of the work role due to the illness. The occupational therapy clinic offers a work area where the patient can learn new skills and develop existing ones. In work adjustment programs, tasks are chosen to promote and teach work skills to allow the patient to function at an optimum level. These skills might include the ability to follow written and oral directions, sustain attention to tasks, or organize work according to priority.[34] The structured activity or craft task group may be used to assist patients in learning skills as well as to assess their readiness to return to life activities such as work or school.

SUMMARY

This chapter provides information on the areas of occupational performance: daily living skills, play, leisure, and work skills, which are the primary foundations of the profession of occupational therapy. Each section focuses on theories, principles, and adaptations; illustrative case studies are provided to explain the importance of these activities in the individual's life. The goal is to assist the reader to understand not only the individual areas but also to appreciate their relationship to each other.

Daily living skills are a prerequiste for the other areas. These basic skills must be mastered before the individual can be well adapted to community life. The focus is on independence, as well as on improving the quality of the patient's life, and to assist in restoring a sense of dignity and self-esteem for many through new-found abilities.

Play as a process lies at the core of human behavior and development. It is an intrinsic activity done purely for its own sake rather than a means to an end. It is spontaneous and pleasurable, voluntarily selected, and actively engaged in. Play activities lead to more complex and sophisticated cognitive behavior. They promote creativity, enhance social and emotional development, and make a valuable contribution to the growth of the individual.

Although we live in a work-oriented society, leisure, a natural outgrowth of play, fulfills many significant human needs. It can relieve tensions, strain, and boredom that has become so much a part of modern technologic society. Leisure or discretionary time greatly influences the quality of people's lives.

Work is presented as skill in socially productive activities and, in addition to full-time employment, includes home management, care of others, educational activities, and vocational activities. It provides the individual with a source of satisfaction and emotional well-being.

Skills in ADLs, play/leisure, and work, coupled with a healthy balance among these, assist individuals in meeting their needs, adapting to society, assuming their occupational roles, receiving gratification, and reaching self-actualization.

Acknowledgments

The editor wishes to thank Louise Fawcett, PhD, OTR for her assistance in preparing the play case study and LaDonn

People, MA, OTR for overall editorial and content suggestions and general assistance with many phases of the preparation of this manuscript.

Related Learning Activities

1. Develop a card file of community resources for a variety of play and leisure activities.

2. Working with a peer, develop a leisure activities program for a group of men aged 16 to 22 who are wheelchair-bound patients in a rehabilitation hospital.

3. Make a chart in which to list all of the activities engaged in on a recent weekday according to the following categories: ADLs, work and leisure. List times of day at half-hour intervals along the left side of the chart. Evaluate these data in terms of overall balance among the activities by answering the following questions:

    a. Do you need to make some changes?

    b. Do you need to gather more data?

    c. Did you consider the time spent in rest and sleep?

    d. How does the completed chart compare with the way you spend time on weekends?

4. How do occupational therapists and assistants manipulate the environment or components of a task for a physically disabled patient? How is this accomplished for a person with psychosocial problems?

References

1. Havighurst R: Social roles, work, leisure, and education. In Eisendorfer C, Lawton, MP (Eds): *The Psychology of Adult Development and Aging.* Washington, DC, American Psychological Association, 1973, p. 805.
2. Cynkin S: *Occupational Therapy: Toward Health Through Activities.* Boston, Little, Brown, 1979, p. 6.
3. Reed K, Saunderson S: *Concepts of Occupational Therapy.* 2nd Edition, Baltimore, Maryland, Williams & Wilkins, 1983, p. 9.
4. Rogers J: Why study occupations? *Am J Occup Ther* 38:47, 1984.
5. Mosey AC: *Activities Therapy.* New York, Raven Press, 1973, p. 7.
6. Nelson D: *Children with Autism and Other Pervasive Disorders of Development and Behavior: Therapy Through Activities.* Thorofare, New Jersey, Slack Inc., 1984, p. 38.
7. Deloach C, Greer B: *Adjustments to Serve Physical Disability: A Metamorphosis.* St. Louis, McGraw-Hill, 1981, pp. 94-109.
8. *Uniform Terminology for Reporting Occupational Therapy Services.* Rockville, Maryland, American Occupational Therapy Association, 1989.
9. Shillam L, Beeman C, Loshin M: Effect of occupational therapy intervention on bathing independence of disabled persons. *Am J Occup Ther* 37:744, 1983.
10. Hopkins H, Smith H (Eds): *Willard and Spackman's Occupational Therapy,* 6th edition. Philadelphia, JB Lippincott, 1983, pp. 900-901.
11. Bradlee T: The use of groups in short-term psychiatric settings. *Occup Ther Mental Health* 3:47-57, 1984.
12. Chance P: *Learning Through Play.* New York, Garner Press, 1979, pp. 4-24.
13. Stone J, Church J: *Childhood and Adolescence.* New York, Random House, 1966, pp. 108-112, 150-156.
14. Yawkey T, Pellegrin A: *Child's Play, Developmental and Applied.* Hillsdale, New Jersey, Lawrence Erlbaum Assoc, 1984, pp. 343-360.
15. Parten MB: Social participation among pre-school children. *Journal of Abnormal and Social Psychology* 27:243, 1932.
16. Cherrington D: *The Work Ethic, Working Values and Values That Work.* New York, Amacom Press, 1980, p. 262.
17. Murphy J: *Concepts of Leisure.* Englewood Cliffs, New Jersey, Prentice-Hall, 1981, p. 26.
18. Kraus R: *Recreation and Leisure in Modern Society,* 2nd edition. Santa Monica, California, Goodyear Publishing, 1978, p. 40.
19. Dumazedier J: *Sociology of Leisure.* Amsterdam, Netherlands, Elsevier Publishing, 1974, pp. 62-71.
20. Kaplan M: *Leisure in America, A Social Inquiry.* New York, John Wiley and Sons, 1960, pp. 28-37.
21. Parker S: *The Future of Work and Leisure.* New York, Praeger, 1971, pp. 25-30, 58.
22. Havighurst R: The leisure activities of the middle-aged. *Am J Sociology* 63:152-162, 1957.
23. Teaff J: *Leisure Services with the Elderly.* St. Louis, Times Mirror/Mosby, 1985, pp. 43-56.
24. Yoesting D, Burkhead D: Significance of childhood recreation experience on adult leisure behavior. *J Leisure Rec* 5:25-36, 1973.
25. Orthner D: Leisure activity patterns and marital satisfaction over the marital career. *J Marriage Fam* 37:91-102, 1975.
26. American Association for Health, Physical Education and Recreation: *Guidelines for Professional Preparation Programs for Personnel Involved in Physical Education and Recreation for the Handicapped.* Washington, DC, Bureau of Education for the Handicapped, US Office of Education Department, Education and Welfare, 1973, p. 5.
27. Fidler G: *Design of Rehabilitation Services in Psychiatric Hospital Settings.* Laurel, Maryland, Ramsco, 1984, p. 51.
28. Berry J: *Activity Therapy Services.* North Billerica, Massachusetts, Curriculum Associates, Inc., 1977, p. 150.
29. Turkel S: *Working.* New York, Partheon Books, 1974.
30. Best F: *The Future of Work.* Englewood Cliffs, New Jersey, Prentice-Hall, 1973, p. 1.
31. Zander J: *Human Development.* New York, Alfred A. Knopf, 1981, pp. 344-355.
32. Gross E: *Work and Society.* New York, Thomas Y. Crowell Co., 1958, p. 25.
33. Evans R: *Foundations of Vocational Education.* Columbus, Ohio, Charles H. Merrill, 1971, p. 103.
34. Minnesota Occupational Therapy Association: *Description of Occupational Therapy Services,* Minneapolis, Minnesota, Minnesota Occupational Therapy Association, 1972, pp. 15-23.

The Teaching/Learning Process

M. Jeanne Madigan, EdD, OTR, FAOTA
B. Joan Bellman, OTR

INTRODUCTION

Occupational therapists and assistants teach every day. They teach the "whats," the "hows," and even the "whys" of everyday living. They have an additional task because they must teach persons who have cognitive, emotional, or motor problems or a combination of all three. In addition to identifying the assets and limitations of patients and evaluating whether patients have accomplished goals of independent functioning, occupational therapy personnel use teaching/learning principles. These principles enable their patients to accomplish tasks they were not able to perform due to birth defects, social problems, illnesses, or injuries.

For example, consider the case of Lottie, a 29-year-old woman, who is mentally retarded. She was institutionalized all her life, but has been discharged to a sheltered home situation with a court-appointed guardian. Assessment findings indicated that she was ambulatory and cooperative but highly distractable. Lottie held a spoon awkwardly, spilling food on herself and the table. She could don clothes but could not button small buttons or tie a bow. She was able to manage toileting independently, but needed assistance in hand-washing in terms of turning the faucet on and off and drying her hands. Hand function patterns were normal only for gross cylindrical grasp; thumb opposition and wrist stabilization were poor. After discussing the patient with the guardian, the registered occupational therapist (OTR) indicated that the first goal to be addressed in occupational therapy treatment was to improve independent eating. The certified occupational therapy assistant (COTA) was assigned to work with Lottie to help her achieve this task.

In this scenario, the COTA can be identified as the instructor or teacher and the patient as the learner. The teaching/learning problem then becomes threefold:

KEY CONCEPTS

Connectionist approach

Cognitive approach

Gagne's learning types

Bloom's learning domains

Conditions affecting learning

Characteristics of the learning task

Occupational therapy teaching process

---

1. What is the best way to teach the patient to feed herself?
2. What methods will best facilitate this learning process?
3. What is the process called learning?

Learning has been defined as a relatively permanent change in behavior resulting from exposure to conditions in the environment.[1] Although this definition implies observable events, learning cannot be observed directly, and it is difficult to know what has happened within the learner. However, one can find out whether the learner has acquired the knowledge by posing a problem that requires an individual to use the knowledge then observing if the learner can accomplish the task.

The **teacher's role** is to help the learner to change behavior in specified directions. To do this effectively, the teacher must not only know what is to be taught, but also the methods that will facilitate the desired changes. The first section of this chapter briefly discusses theories of learning; the second section presents some conditions that aid or impede learning; the final section outlines steps in the teaching process that are helpful when working with patients.

THEORIES OF LEARNING

There are two main theoretical approaches to learning: *connectionist* and *cognitive*. A brief overview of these two positions is given to provide better understanding of the various techniques associated with them. Information for this section has been drawn from the writings of Travers,[1] Biehler,[2] Hilgard[3] and Hill.[4]

The Connectionist School

Connectionism is also known as *reductionism, associationism,* and *behaviorism*. In this school, learning is considered to be a matter of making connections between stimuli and responses. A response is any item of behavior, and a stimulus is any input of energy that tends to affect behavior. A simple illustration would be a child who eagerly reaches for a cookie on seeing the cookie jar. An earlier "handout" from the jar brings forth memories of delectable tastes.

Ivan Pavlov was the first to study learning under highly controlled experimental conditions. In one of his earliest experiments, he gave a dish of food to a dog a few seconds after a bell was rung. After many repetitions, the dog salivated at the sound of the bell even though no food was given. This **conditioning** process was referred to as *classic conditioning,* that is, tying a reflex to a particular stimulus so that a desired response can be triggered at will. It should be noted, however, that if the bell was rung too many times without food being presented, the response tended to

disappear (become extinct). Once conditioned, the dog tended to salivate to almost any similar sound. To prevent indiscriminate salivating, Pavlov repeatedly rewarded the dog with food only after the bell sound but never after similar sounds.

John B. Watson popularized Pavlovian theory in the United States by conducting experiments demonstrating that human behavior could be conditioned. He also did much to establish the tradition of objectivity and the concern with observable behavior in psychology, and thus became known as the founder of behaviorism.

Edward L. Thorndike conducted experiments using a hungry cat in a cage that had a door with a release mechanism and food outside the cage. After repeated attempts to get at the food, the cat hit the opening mechanism by chance. After repeated trials, the cat learned to make the correct response (hitting the release mechanism) almost immediately. Thorndike concluded from this trial and error process that learning consisted of making connections between stimuli and responses and that repetition was essential to learning.

Following these traditions, B.F. Skinner conducted experiments with rats and pigeons in which he shaped their behavior by reinforcing the action he wanted with a reward. This process, the learning of voluntary responses, is termed *instrumental conditioning* and is highly dependent on the consequences of the response. Skinner referred to the process as *operant conditioning* to emphasize that a person can operate on the environment to produce an event or cause a change in an event. Instrumental conditioning involves trial and error during the learning process, but the response must be rewarded if it is to be repeated. If a response produces positive **reinforcement** or removes negative reinforcement, it will be strengthened; if negative reinforcers are produced or if positive reinforcement is removed, the response will not be repeated and behavior will be extinguished. Secondary reinforcement (such as gold stars or smile stickers) will also strengthen the behavior. Reinforcing a desired response every time it occurs is described as following a schedule of *continuous reinforcement*. When the number of responses between reinforcement varies, *intermittent reinforcement* is being used. It has been found that the fastest, most efficient learning occurs with continuous reinforcement, but learning is less readily extinguished when intermittent reinforcement is used.

Shaping is the process of changing behavior by reinforcing responses that approximate the desired response. At first, any behavior that is close to the desired response is rewarded. Gradually, only those responses that more nearly resemble the desired response are rewarded.

Behavior modification consists of reinforcing desirable responses while ignoring undesirable ones. A reinforcer may be food, praise, opportunities to perform a favorite activity, or tokens to be traded in for prizes or privileges.

Skinner applied what he discovered to the field of teaching by inventing teaching machines and programmed instruction methods. He maintained that to promote effective learning a teacher must divide what is to be learned into a large number of very small steps and reinforce the successful accomplishment of each step. By making the steps as small and gradual as possible, the possibility of errors is low, and therefore the frequency of positive reinforcement is high. The basic techniques of deciding terminal behavior and then shaping behavior have been used by some educators to develop instructional objectives used to structure learning experiences, the mastery learning approach, and performance contracting.

Thus, many educational practices in use today are derived directly or indirectly from operant conditioning techniques based on Skinner's and other behaviorists' research and theories. It is also the basis for the occupational therapy practitioner's practice of breaking down activity into component steps, praising successful accomplishments of patients, and being sure that a patient masters one process before going on to the next. It is also one of the reasons that occupational therapists and assistants grade activities. For more information on these topics see Chapter 17.

The Cognitive School

Cognitive theories, also known by the terms *gestalt, field theory* and *discovery approach,* are concerned with the perceptions or attitudes that individuals have about their environment and the ways these cognitions determine behavior. This school of thought was developed in reaction to the researchers who accepted only measurable behavior as experimental evidence and who were preoccupied with physiologic concepts. Early cognitive theorists emphasized whole systems in which the parts are seen as interrelated in such a way that the whole is more than the sum of its parts. They also studied the ways in which cognitions are modified by experiences.

At about the same time that Thorndike was developing his laws (1920s), a group of German psychologists began experimenting with chimpanzees. Wolfgang Kohler put a chimpanzee named Sultan in a large cage with a variety of objects, including sticks. Sultan discovered that he could use a stick to rake things toward himself. One day, he discovered that he could use a small stick to reach a long stick which, in turn, he used to rake a banana that was outside his cage and too far away to reach with the short stick. This "learning" involved a rearrangement of a previous pattern of behavior. It was a new application of a previous activity. This example is the essence of learning as viewed by a cognitive or field theorist: the perception of new relationships. Rather than learning by conditioning or trial and error, the problem was solved by gaining insight into the relationship between the objects. It should be recognized, however, that Sultan's previous experience with the essentials of the problem was

necessary in order for the insight to occur.

Kurt Lewin provided an important link in the development of cognitive-field theory. He used concepts from mathematics and physics to devise a system of diagramming behavioral situations, which he called the field of forces. He also defined life space, which he said consists of everything that influences a person's behavior (objects, goals, and barriers to those goals, for example). He and his followers believe that individuals behave not only because of external forces to which they are exposed, but also as a consequence of how things seem to them, what they believe them to be.

Edward C. Tolman's "cognitive map" or *sign theory* forms a bridge between strict behaviorist and gestalt theories. He said that human learning depends on the meaning that individuals attach to situations or objects in their environment. While concerned with observable evidence, Tolman hypothesized that numerous intervening variables existed between the situation and the resultant behavior; learners vary their responses according to conditions as they know them. Thus, experience is the underlying factor in insightful and cognitive learning.

Jean Piaget believed that a person organizes and adapts sensory information through two basic mental operations: assimilation and accommodation. In **assimilation,** incoming information is perceived and interpreted according to existing schema that have already been established through previous experience. **Accommodation** is the changing of existing schema as a result of new information. Piaget described four stages of cognitive development. During the first, *sensorimotor,* which begins at birth, children form the most basic conceptions about the material world. They learn the relationship of objects to each other and themselves. The *pre-operational* stage, which begins at approximately two years of age, is that stage when children are conscious of their existence in a world of permanent objects that are separate from themselves, and they realize the causal effects between them. Behavior is still directly linked to what the child perceives and does at the time. During the *concrete operations* stage, beginning at seven years, children's thinking is no longer restricted to physical objects. They are able to make inferences from verbal information that are linked with movement or other information. In the final stage, *formal-operational,* beginning at 11 years, children develop adult abilities and characteristics. They can deal with words and relationships, solve problems involving manipulation of several variables, intellectually examine hypothetical ideas, and evaluate alternatives (see Chapter 5).

Jerome Bruner, who regards learning as a rearrangement of thought patterns, stresses the importance of structure and of providing opportunities for intuitive thinking. He believes that emphasizing structure in teaching makes the subject more comprehensible, more easily remembered, and more able to be transferred. Believing that knowledge is a process rather than a product, Bruner developed techniques for teaching by the discovery method that include the following components:

1. Emphasizing contrast
2. Stimulating informed guessing
3. Encouraging active participation
4. Stimulating awareness

Proponents of the **discovery** or **reflective method** of teaching also believe that too much exposure to lectures, texts, or programs tends to make a student dependent on others and minimizes the likelihood of the individual seeking answers or solving problems independently.

Thus, learning can be considered to be either an accumulation of associations (connectionist school) or the perception of new relationships (cognitive school). Depending on which theory one adheres to, the teacher would use quite different techniques to instruct another person. It should be noted, however, that some theorists feel that rigidly adhering to a single theory is wrong and that, depending on what one wishes to teach, one should make selected use of the techniques based on different theories.

D.O. Hebb proposed two basic periods of learning: primary learning and later learning. *Primary learning* begins at birth and continues until about age 12. It consists of sensory events that impose new types of organization through classic and instrumental conditioning. *Later learning* is conceptual and involves patterns whose parts are familiar and have a number of well-formed associations. Using this line of reasoning, one could conclude that much of adult learning requires few trials unless confronted with situations in which there has been no past experience. Somewhat along this same line, Robert Gagne identified eight progressively complex types of learning:[5]

1. *Signal learning*—an involuntary reflex is activated by a selected stimulus
2. *Stimulus-response learning*—voluntary actions are shaped by reinforcement
3. *Chaining*—individual acts are combined and occur in rapid succession
4. *Verbal association*—verbal chains acquired by connecting previously acquired words and new words
5. *Discrimination learning*—varying responses to verbal associations as what is known becomes more numerous and complex
6. *Concept learning*—response to things or events as a class
7. *Rule learning*—combines or relates chains of concepts previously learned
8. *Problem solving*—combines rules in such a way that permits application to new situations

Gagne believed these kinds of learning are hierarchical and, therefore, the more advanced types of learning can take place only when a person has mastered a large variety of verbal associations based on a great deal of stimulus-response learning. According to this theory, it would be important for the occupational therapy assistant to have some knowledge of a patient's background so that he or she could select the most appropriate type of learning for that particular individual. It also suggests why it is so important for all children to have many experiences to form the foundation for higher levels of learning, particularly for those who may be restricted physically or mentally due to disease or injury.

Another quite different classification of learning was proposed by Benjamin S. Bloom and his associates. They classified all learning into three domains: cognitive, affective and psychomotor. Categories of the cognitive domain areas follows:[6]

1. *Knowledge*—remembering ideas, material, or phenomena
2. *Comprehension*—understanding material and being able to make some use of it; includes translation, interpretation, and extrapolation
3. *Application*—being able to use correct method, theory, principle, or abstraction in a new situation
4. *Analysis*—breaking down material into its constituent parts and detecting relationships of the parts and the way they are organized
5. *Synthesis*—putting together elements and parts to form the whole in a way that constitutes a structure not previously in existence
6. *Evaluation*—making judgments about the value of ideas, methods and materials

Although the cognitive domain deals with remembering, using something that has been learned by combining old and synthesizing new ideas, the affective domain deals with a feeling tone, awareness, appreciating, etc. Categories in the affective domain are the following:[7]

1. *Receiving* (attending)—being aware, willing to receive and attending to certain phenomena
2. *Responding*—actively attending to a phenomenon by acting, which implies willingness and satisfaction in the response
3. *Valuing*—internalizing a phenomenon and accepting it as having worth; preferring it and being committed to it
4. *Organization*—building a value system that is interrelated
5. *Characterization by a value or value complex*—acting consistently in accordance with internalized values and providing a total philosophy or world view

Bloom and his associates[6] identified the psychomotor domain as including muscular or motor skill, manipulation of material and objects, or some act that requires neuromuscular coordination. However, they did not go on to develop a classification or taxonomic system for it. A number of individuals have proposed schemas that have not received the wide acceptance accorded to the two previously outlined taxonomies. However, since the psychomotor domain is of great importance in occupational therapy because many of the profession's concerns relate to neuromuscular actions, it is important to consider some classification of this domain. Harrow classifies the psychomotor domain as follows:[8]

1. *Reflex movements*—includes segmental, intersegmental, suprasegmental, and postural reflexes or movements that are involuntary in nature and are precursors of basic fundamental movement
2. *Basic-fundamental movements*—includes locomotor, non-locomotor and manipulative movements
3. *Perceptual abilities*—includes kinesthetic, visual, auditory, and tactile discrimination as well as coordinated abilities
4. *Physical abilities*—includes endurance, strength, flexibility and agility
5. *Skilled movements*—includes simple adaptive skill, compound adaptive skill and complex adaptive skill
6. *Non-discursive communications*—includes expressive and interpretive movements

These classifications could aid in planning learning experiences for teaching skills and activities to patients by identifying levels of ability and specifying graded objectives in one or more of the three domains. Since they are all hierarchical in nature, the occupational therapist would have to assess the patient to be sure that a previous level is in good order before attempting subsequent ones. For example, patients should not be expected to apply a principle before they can recall it and know what it means; nor should they be expected to respond to the therapist if they have not attended to the therapist.

CONDITIONS THAT AFFECT LEARNING

What individuals bring to the learning situation in terms of personality traits, motivation and general background has an important influence on what they are willing to learn, what they can learn, and how efficiently they will learn it.[9]

The basic motivation for learning is found in the human being's normal tendency to explore and make sense of the environment. Gradually, this general exploratory tendency is differentiated in terms of specific needs, interests, and goals, so that individuals are motivated to learn some things but remain relatively uninterested in others. If curiosity is discouraged or punished, as it may be by some parents or societies, the natural inclination for learning is greatly dulled. If what is to be learned bears little relationship to the learner's immediate interests and purposes, motivation may have to be induced by manipulation of rewards and punishments.

An individual's frame of reference (assumptions and attitudes) determines in large part what one sees and learns. The range of information that will be meaningful; the way new material will be interpreted; and whether the task is perceived as a challenge, a threat, or of no importance, depends on the individual's perception of self and the world.

Usually an individual is eager to tackle learning tasks when they are seen as related to needs and purposes and appropriate to one's competence level. On the other hand, an individual usually tries to avoid those tasks that appear of little value or with which he or she feels unable to cope. For some persons, a vicious cycle may develop in which, feeling inadequate, they force themselves into a learning situation with anxiety and trepidation; they expect to do badly and they do. The resulting negative feedback then reinforces their concept of inadequacy.

A learner must also be able to tolerate immediate frustration in the interest of achieving long-range goals. Preoccupation with inner conflicts, a high level of anxiety, feelings of discouragement and depression, and other maladaptive patterns can also seriously impair one's ability to learn.

CHARACTERISTICS OF THE LEARNING TASK

Coleman[9] outlined four characteristics of the learning task itself that influence how it should be approached and how easily it can be mastered.

Type of Task

Motor skills usually require time and practice to train the muscles to function with the desired skill and coordination (an example would be learning to hammer a nail or doing a range of motion test). Meaningful verbal information results from intensive sessions, with a focus on relationships leading to the quickest learning and best retention (an example would be for the teacher to relate new information to something similar the student already knows). Unrelated data often require a spaced drill for material that must be memorized (an example would be learning the origins and insertions of muscles).

Size, Complexity and Familiarity

Generally more material needs more time, although less time is needed for meaningful material than for unrelated data that must be memorized. Added complexity tends to increase the time required for study and understanding, but may be offset if the learner is familiar with the material in a general way and has adequate background for organizing and understanding it (in this case, the teacher should try to relate new concepts to what the learner already knows).

Clarity

The less clear the task, the more time and effort needed to master it (here, the teacher should point out the essential elements of the task or the thing to be learned).

Environment

Things that make learning more difficult include disapproval by one's peers, unfavorable study conditions, lack of essential tools or resources, severe time pressures, and other distracting life demands. Ways to enhance learning include using a well-lighted, well-ventilated study place, which is free of distractions; getting an overall view of the task; and organizing the task in terms of key elements. Long-range retention is encouraged by distributed study, periodic review, and tying new material in with previous learning and real life situations. Knowing these principles should give students very helpful clues to make their study time more effective. You will be learning many things in your classes that you must not only know for the final examination, but also remember next semester because it is the foundation for later coursework. You will also need to use the knowledge for your fieldwork experiences, the certification examination, and work itself. Therefore, long-term retention is the goal of this learning.

Little is known about how previous learning affects the ease with which individuals can understand and master subsequent learning. The available evidence indicates that some transfer will occur if there are identical elements in the two learning situations or if they can be understood in terms of the same general principles. Transfer of learning seems to depend on the learner's ability to perceive the points of similarity between the old and the new information.

The return of information individuals receive about the progress or outcome of their behavior (feedback) not only tells them whether they are proceeding satisfactorily, but also serves as a reward or punishment. Learners can modify or adjust responses on the basis of feedback. Motivation, self-confidence, and learning efficiency (not having to unlearn errors) are all facilitated by frequent feedback. Praise and progress toward desired goals reinforce what has been learned and motivate further learning.

THE OCCUPATIONAL THERAPY TEACHING PROCESS

Once the patient has been evaluated and the goals of treatment specified, it is necessary to identify what is to be taught and how to teach the patient in order to best accomplish these goals. Using principles from the theories discussed in the previous sections of this chapter, the teaching process steps are outlined and applied to specific patient treatment situations.

Teaching Process Steps

The following **teaching process steps** must be carried out in the order in which they are discussed.

State Learning Objectives. Identify what the patient needs to learn. This step can be done with a great deal of specificity or in more general terms. Using Lottie, whose case was briefly discussed in the beginning of this chapter, as an example, the learning objectives could be stated as follows:

1. "Within three weeks the patient will be able to scoop applesauce with a spoon from a bowl and place it in her mouth without spilling any sauce on self, table, or floor, seven out of ten trials."
2. "The patient will be able to feed self without spilling."

It is fairly obvious that the first objective leaves no room for guessing what exactly is to be accomplished and how the outcome is to be evaluated. A new therapist or assistant may find it useful to explicitly state all objectives in similar detail until it becomes second nature to think in these terms. If one is using a behavior modification approach, it is necessary to be even more specific in identifying what the present behavior is and what are the incremental steps between that and the target behavior. This will allow reinforcement to be applied for each small behavior that represents a movement toward the desired behavior change.

Determine Content. What exactly is to be taught? In the preceding example, the motor skills of grasp, bringing the spoon to the mouth, and removing food from the spoon with the mouth must be taught. Activities related but not included in the objective as it is stated are selection of the proper eating utensil, cutting food, drinking from a glass, and using proper table manners.

Identify Modifications Necessary for the Particular Patient or Group. In planning this step, it is important to refer to the history and assessment of the patient to determine whether any physical, mental, or sociocultural findings require adjustment of methods or adaptation of equipment that will be used. The most basic consideration to assist in determining what to teach and in selecting appropriate methods to use is the patient's **developmental level.** The term developmental level refers to the process of growth and differentiation when compared to others. One will have little success teaching a two-year-old an activity that requires the neuromuscular coordination of a four-year-old, or, in the case of Lottie, using abstract reasoning with a retarded adult who is still in the pre-operational stage.

It is also important to consider the physical limitations such as loss of mobility, coordination, sight, and hearing. The presence of pain or use of medications that affect the patient's functioning must also be considered. Educational and socioeconomic levels may require the teacher to adapt the general language and the technical terms used.

Lottie is functioning at a preschool level in many ways. It would be important to use simple words and short sentences when giving her directions. Because of her grasp and prehension difficulties, a spoon handle could be built up to facilitate grasp strength and control. Using a spoon, a bowl and applesauce at first is desirable because it is easier to get the applesauce onto the spoon and less likely to spill than peas on a fork. Use of the sauce will provide a greater chance for success early in the process. As Lottie gains skill, more difficult foods and other utensils can be introduced.

Break Activity/Process into Small Units of Instruction. In the learning objective in the example, numerous skills will need to be learned, including the following:
1. Grasping the spoon
2. Scooping the food onto the spoon
3. Bringing the food to the mouth
4. Holding the spoon so the food does not fall off
5. Inserting the spoon in the mouth without knocking the food off the spoon
6. Removing the food from the spoon with the teeth and lips
7. Closing the mouth so that food does not dribble out
8. Chewing food with the mouth closed

What seems like a very simple activity actually has at least eight separate skills that will need to be taught and combined to accomplish the original objective.

Assemble Materials. To prevent delays in the process, it is important to gather all equipment and supplies that will be needed to complete the activity. If the teacher is planning to use learning aids such as diagrams, printed instructions, or samples, they should be prepared in advance. As with the learning activity itself, these materials should be modified to be appropriate for the patient or group.

Because the learning objective in Lottie's case consists of psychomotor skills, and since she is functioning at the pre-operational stage of development, visual aids would probably only confuse her. The materials needed for this activity are few. However, if one were teaching a patient copper tooling, it would be important to think through all of the steps and ensure that the necessary supplies were on hand so that the project could be carried to completion.

Arrange Work Space. Set up the table or whatever area is to be used so that needed materials are conveniently located. If the patient is easily distracted, however, anything that is not being used at the moment should be kept out of sight. Ensure that the patient is comfortable and uses good posture to minimize fatigue. Lighting that illuminates the work area but does not shine in the patient's eyes is important. Lighting is a critical concern for someone with failing eyesight. The person instructing must assume a position in relation to the patient that will be the most advantageous to demonstrate, assist and observe, being careful not to obstruct the patient's view of

the task or activity. Usually, sitting next to the patient is preferable. In this way the work will be at the proper height, angle and perspective. When teaching a group, one must assure that all participants can see what is being shown. Lottie is easily distracted; therefore, it would be important to try to reduce visible objects and eliminate sounds in the area that may divert her attention from what is being demonstrated or displayed.

Simulate as closely as possible the conditions under which the patient will have to carry out the activity. If circumstances between the learning situation and the "real" one are very different, the patient may not be able to transfer the learning, even though he or she can accomplish the task perfectly in the treatment setting.

Prepare the Patient or Group. Try to determine if the patient is ready to learn by asking the following: Is the patient alert? Is the patient paying attention to the person in the teaching role? Does the patient appear interested in what is to happen? Concerns, anxieties, or other emotions may divert the patient's attention and make it difficult to concentrate on what is being taught. The therapist or assistant may need to deal with these matters or to make a referral to another discipline to attend to them before the patient is fully ready to learn.

Does the patient need basic skills or knowledge before learning can proceed? Learning will be more successful if it can be tied to some familiar elements. Does the patient know what is going to happen and the purpose of the activity? Instruction will be more easily grasped and retained if the patient knows why he or she is doing the activity and feels that it is something needed or wanted. For example, Lottie wanted to be like "other people," which included not having to wear a bib. This was her ultimate aim—no spilling, no bib!

Present the Instruction. Once the activity has been broken into small component steps, the next phase is presentation of the first step. Begin by securing the patient's attention. Tell the person what you are going to do and what you expect him or her to do. If diagrams or other visual aids are being used, point out the salient features. Demonstrate the first step accompanied by a verbal explanation that emphasizes a few key words that provide "word pictures," cues to the action or important signals to watch for. In this way the instructor is providing input through two senses, sight and hearing. Repeat the step and observe whether the patient seems to understand. Ask questions that will indicate the level of comprehension. Point out precautions or common errors to avoid. When teaching a motor skill to a patient who is very young or has limited cognitive skills, it may be desirable not only to demonstrate but also to physically guide the patient through the action (an example would be to place the patient's hand on the spoon, place your hand over the patient's hand, and guide the individual through the correct action several times; this will allow the patient to "get the feel" of the correct movement).

Have the Patient do a "Tryout". Ask the patient to proceed with the activity independently. If working with an object, give it to the patient and do not assist in the task at hand. If help is needed, repeat the verbal cues. Have the patient repeat the step several times, gradually decreasing the cues until he or she is doing it independently without any assistance. Correct any errors immediately so that the patient does not learn the incorrect method, as it will be difficult to unlearn the wrong way before relearning the correct way. In Lottie's case, self-feeding had been accomplished in a very sloppy manner, so it will be difficult for her to overcome a set habit pattern and to learn a new way of eating.

Observe whether the patient gives nonverbal clues that he or she understands or does not understand; the individual may not want to admit confusion. Invite questions. Allow the patient to perform independently several times to provide assurance that the individual knows the correct procedure and did not just happen to do it correctly by chance. Offer sincere praise for correct work. Look for indications of fatigue, pain, or waning attention. A rest or redirection may be necessary.

Lottie was eager to please others and so responded well to praise when she accomplished one of the component skills. Good performance was also rewarded by adding new foods that she liked, especially ice cream.

Evaluate Performance. Decide how many times, how far apart, and in how many different circumstances the correct performance should be observed to assure that the patient has mastered the skill or skills that have been taught. Carry-over will be greater if the patient has repeated the activity several times and made it a habit.

If the activity is composed of several steps, present each one, making sure the patient has learned one step before going on to the next. Retention will be aided if each previous step can be practiced as each new step is added.

The therapist and assistant should ask themselves the following questions:
1. Does a caretaker need to be instructed in the particular process to increase the likelihood that the activity will be done correctly when the patient returns to the ward or home?
2. Does the patient have a sense of accomplishment?
3. Is the activity accomplishing the desired effect or goal?

The following brief case study is presented as a contrast to the profile of Lottie; it presents quite a different teaching/learning situation:

Case Study 8-1

Mildred. Mildred is a 57-year-old woman with a diagnosis of degenerative joint disease. She complains of low back pain when performing many household chores. She lives at home with her husband, who is receiving disability benefits because of a heart condition. He is unable to assist with heavy housework. Mildred is of average intelligence but has a high level of anxiety about keeping her home neat and clean. She is also afraid of pain. The occupational therapy goal was to enable Mildred to perform household work within a tolerable level of discomfort.

In this case, the COTA identified the learning objective: "The patient will apply principles of body mechanics and energy conservation to carry out household tasks." The content includes, for example, 1) the correct method of lifting heavy objects and 2) reducing the amount of bending and stretching. Because this patient has a high school education, is of average intelligence, and has no limitations other than the arthritis for which she is receiving treatment, no special modifications in teaching methods are necessary.

The COTA prepared charts that illustrated each principle. The principle was printed at the top of each chart and a stick-figure diagram showed how the principle is applied in a particular cleaning or cooking task. The COTA discussed each principle with Mildred, pointing out how the illustration of the figure in the diagram made use of the principle. She then demonstrated several times how to perform the task correctly, noting precautions. Next, she asked Mildred to perform the same task, correcting errors as soon as they occurred. Mildred was asked to repeat the task until she could carry it out correctly three consecutive times.

Because the objective was to have the patient apply the principles rather than just learn specific techniques, the COTA could not conclude instruction at this point. She continued by asking Mildred to identify a chore that she did in her home that could be accomplished by using the principle that she had learned. At first, Mildred was at a loss to associate the principle with another task, so the COTA asked her to describe how she washed clothes. When Mildred described carrying the clothes basket from the bedroom to the washing machine, the COTA suggested that she could use the principle of lifting objects by keeping her trunk erect, bending at the knees, and holding the object (the clothes basket) close to her body. Mildred showed recognition that this task used the principle. The COTA again asked Mildred how the same principle could be used with another, closely related task. Mildred identified carrying a scrub bucket of water. A similar process was used in identifying chores that required the patient to bend and stretch and, as a result, Mildred has altered how she carries out many household tasks. For example, she rearranged her cabinets and cupboards so that commonly used items would be within easy reach.

She now uses a long-handled feather duster to dust her bookcases and china cabinet, and cleans the kitchen and bathroom floors with a sponge mop with a squeeze attachment at midshaft on the handle.

Once Mildred had mastered a principle (by correctly doing the task during the treatment session and identifying another task that used the same principle), she was directed to incorporate it into her home routine. She was also asked to look for ways to use the same principle with other chores. During the next treatment session, the COTA asked Mildred to list the tasks that she had identified since the last treatment session and to demonstrate how she applied the principle taught during the previous session. In this way, the COTA determined that the patient had understood the principle and could easily apply it to her everyday functioning. As Mildred demonstrated that she understood and was using a principle, the COTA introduced additional ones. She made up a little booklet with principles and diagrams so that Mildred could refer to it and continue to modify tasks in the future.

It should be noted that the COTA used some of the same teaching principles with Mildred that she used with Lottie (eg, immediate correction of errors), but other techniques were not necessary. Praise of work well done and use of extrinsic rewards were not necessary because Mildred understood what was being accomplished, and the ability to keep up her house according to her standards while suffering less pain was reward enough. The COTA was able to use the modified discovery approach by having Mildred reason out how she could use the principles she had learned. This meant she would be able to apply the principles daily and not have to rely on the COTA to teach her the modified method for every task she needed to carry out.

SUMMARY

Much of what occupational therapy assistants hope to accomplish through their treatment relates to patients actively carrying out certain activities as independently as their condition permits. Thus, the COTA becomes a teacher, the patient must become the learner, and the treatment planning process must include consideration of the most effective and efficient methods to facilitate the learning process.

Knowledge of how learning occurs and of conditions that aid or impede learning will improve the COTA's ability to help patients change their behavior in specified directions identified through evaluation and goal selection. Two main approaches to learning are connectionist theory and cognitive theory. The former, a result of Pavlov's classic conditioning experiments, proposes that learning is a matter of making connections between stimuli and responses; careful

attention to reinforcing desired responses will result in accomplishing behavioral changes. Cognitive theorists, on the other hand, regard learning as a perception of new relationships. Emphasis is on providing the basic knowledge and structure of a subject and motivating the learner to actively explore and discover concepts related to the subject at hand.

These views are shunned by some individuals who maintain that neither of these theoretical views adequately explains all learning. They propose a hierarchical progression of learning, which uses different teaching methods for different levels and domains of learning. Other important considerations include the learner's previous experiences, motivation to learn, and personal and environmental conditions that aid or hinder the learning process.

Related Learning Activities

1. Use the following scenario to plan learning experiences and methods: The long-term goal for a group of five patients is to improve interpersonal social skills. The short-term goals are learning to take turns, to share materials, and to respond appropriately to one another.

Make two separate plans, one using the connectionist school of learning approach and the other using the cognitive school approach. List differences and similarities.

2. Select a craft activity and prepare a plan outlining how you would teach it to a classmate or a peer. Be sure to consider all ten steps in the teaching/learning process.

3. Using the plan developed in item two, teach a classmate or peer the craft. Ask the person to give you feedback on the teaching session.

4. Select a different activity than the one used in item three, and prepare a plan for teaching it to a group of six classmates or peers. Again, use the ten steps, but be sure to adjust your plan to accommodate six different individuals instead of one. Present the activity to the group and have them critique the experience.

5. Make a chart illustrating the steps in making a pizza.

References

1. Travers RMW: *Essentials of Learning,* 4th edition. New York, Macmillan, 1977.
2. Biehler RF: *Psychology Applied to Teaching,* 2nd edition. Boston, Houghton Mifflin, 1974.
3. Hilgard ER, Bower GH: *Theories of Learning,* 4th edition. Englewood Cliffs, New Jersey, Prentice-Hall, 1975.
4. Hill WF: *Learning,* 3rd edition. New York, Thomas Y. Crowell, 1977.
5. Gagne RM: *The Conditions of Learning,* 3rd edition. New York, Holt, Rinehart & Winston, 1977.

6. Bloom BS (Ed): *Taxonomy of Educational Objectives Handbook I: Cognitive Domain.* New York, David McKay, 1956.

7. Krathwohl DR, Bloom BS, Masia BB: *Taxonomy of Educational Objectives Handbook II: Affective Domain.* New York, David McKay, 1964.

8. Harrow AJ: *A Taxonomy of the Psychomotor Domain.* New York, David McKay, 1972.

9. Coleman JC: *Psychology and Effective Behavior.* Glenview, Illinois, Scott, Foresman, & Co., 1969.

Interpersonal Communication Skills and Applied Group Dynamics

Toné F. Blechert, BA, COTA, ROH
Nancy Kari, MPH, OTR

INTRODUCTION

Understanding oneself and learning how to live and work with others in satisfying relationships are goals for healthy living. Occupational therapy personnel teach skills that lead to improved interpersonal relationships. The teaching and reinforcement of these skills can happen within a one-to-one relationship or within a group setting. The registered occupational therapist (OTR) makes this choice based on the patient's needs and skill levels.

Working effectively with people, whether on a one-to-one basis or within a group, requires that the occupational therapist and the certified occupational therapy assistant (COTA) develop specific intrapersonal and interpersonal skills. Intrapersonal skills are related to developing a clear and accurate sense of self. These skills allow the individual to cope effectively with the emotional demands of the environment. Interpersonal skills are communication skills that help occupational therapy personnel to interact effectively with a variety of people. One must be able to identify, assess and strengthen skills in both areas. These skills are prerequisites to group work.

Group work is an effective and powerful medium for planned change in occupational therapy treatment. The group creates an environment that enhances the individual's abilities to gain new insights and increased self-awareness. Within a therapeutic group, a controlled environment is carefully designed to provide opportunities for patients to identify and practice specific skills. Members establish peer relationships that can support and

ESSENTIAL VOCABULARY

Self-awareness

Sentient

Active listening

Paraphrasing

Reflection

Genuineness

Group process

Task roles

Group-centered roles

Self-centered roles

Initial dependence

Conflict

Interdependence

Community

KEY CONCEPTS

Intrapersonal and interpersonal skills

Group role functions

Group norms

Group growth and development stages

Leadership preparation, attitudes, and approaches

Activity qualities and examples

strengthen self-confidence and encourage risk taking. Members can experience conflict and personal struggle in a supportive setting. When resolution occurs, a heightened sense of affiliation with others emerges. In this way, the occupational therapy group becomes a "living laboratory" where members learn about themselves in relation to others.

It is strongly recommended that all entry-level occupational therapy personnel begin group work under the supervision of an experienced therapist. Co-leading a group provides an opportunity for the beginner to learn and refine group facilitation skills. Team leading is also a benefit to group members, as it provides role models of appropriate interaction. This chapter offers a summary of the key factors involved in effective intrapersonal skills, interpersonal communication and applied group dynamics.

INTRAPERSONAL AND INTERPERSONAL SKILLS

The establishment of a relationship among the therapist, the assistant and the patient is the first step in the process of facilitating any change in a therapeutic setting. Specific skills in effective communication and skills related to forming helping relationships are discussed in detail in later sections. These are prerequisites to effective group leadership. Their importance cannot be overemphasized.

A COTA must first develop the skills to relate to others on a one-to-one basis. This level of interaction is defined as a *dyad*. People are relating when each is responding to the other as a person instead of an object. An example of the latter would be to say, "Hello, how are you?" when passing someone on the street without stopping to hear the reply. Relating to another individual as a person involves time, interest, energy and interpersonal skill. The ability to relate effectively to another is an art that can be learned and improved with experience and practice.

An effective COTA demonstrates four characteristics: self-awareness, self-acceptance, awareness of others, and the ability to communicate that awareness.[1] A person need not develop these competencies in sequence; they are singled out as important attributes. A COTA needs to achieve and integrate all four areas. One cannot become self-aware and accepting in isolation. These abilities are developed and refined simultaneously through interaction with others.

Self-Awareness

The ability to recognize one's behaviors and emotional responses is **self-awareness.** As one plays and works with other people, personal strengths and weaknesses emerge. Feedback is received from others and from the environment. Self-concept emerges from this dynamic, continuously developing process of interaction. Self-concept refers to the individual's overall picture of self. Both positive and negative qualities are a part of this self-concept. The more experience one has with others, the clearer the picture becomes. Accompanying these pictures is a set of judgments and evaluations of one's self that have been accumulated over a long time. Examples of these judgments include competent or incompetent, effective or ineffective, and intelligent or dull. Feelings about self come from these evaluations and judgments. These feelings help form self-esteem. Self-esteem can be influenced by many feelings including guilt, confidence, shame, and security. Self-concept and self-esteem usually remain relatively stable but can fluctuate at times. For example, one may feel basically good about self but feel embarrassed or shameful about a specific action.[2]

For the COTA to communicate and relate effectively with the patient, he or she must have an awareness of self and an acceptance of individual limitations and strengths.

Self-Acceptance

Acceptance of one's own feelings is an important step in gaining self-respect. When a person dislikes himself or herself, feelings of worthlessness may occur and interfere with personal growth; however, people often make their greatest strides in personal growth just when they begin to see themselves realistically and recognize their limitations.[1]

Part of self-acceptance is learning to understand the difference between self-concept and self-ideal. Self-ideal refers to the way one would most like to be seen by others. Self-ideal may differ considerably from one's true self-image. Self-acceptance does not mean that a person is resigned to his or her self-image. It means that one does not dislike oneself. There is a recognition and acceptance of strengths, limitations, and the feelings that accompany these.

Awareness of and acceptance of one's own feelings enable a person to express those feelings more openly to other people. Verbal expression of feelings helps one gain a fuller understanding of them, as well as emotional relief. Openness, when appropriate, is a positive signal to others that can create opportunities to develop more meaningful interpersonal relationships.

Awareness of Others

To be highly sensitive and responsive to another person's feelings is to be **sentient.** Sentience is a quality that is difficult to describe. The COTA who learns to be keenly aware of the feelings of other people is more likely to gain the trust and cooperation of patients as well as co-workers. Sentience enables the COTA to enter empathetically into the lives of others. This does not happen on an intellectual level; instead, it occurs on a feeling level. One must behave in such a way that the patient can feel the concern being expressed. When the patient senses this interest and caring, a bond is created.[3]

People are motivated to take action and make changes in many different ways. Healthy people have need-satisfying environments, supportive friends and family, and energy reserves. Those who are suffering from emotional or physical trauma are sometimes lacking these supportive elements. Through affiliation with a sentient individual, a patient may receive the support and energy that is needed to make positive changes.

Demonstrating Acceptance and Awareness

Although it is important to have a clear understanding of oneself and of others, this alone is not sufficient to establish a therapeutic relationship. The purpose of a therapeutic relationship is to facilitate change and collaborative problem solving while maintaining or promoting the patient's autonomy. To accomplish this goal, the effective COTA must be able to communicate awareness of others. In a therapeutic environment the therapist and assistant assume a variety of important roles. For example, he or she may be a catalyst creating challenges for the patient, a solution giver, a resource person, or a process helper by assisting the patient to identify his or her own needs and choose appropriate solutions. These roles are all legitimate and necessary to facilitate change. In the initial phases of the relationship, however, the most important role is that of the listener. It is essential to clearly understand the patient's point of view and to be able to communicate understanding. This goal is achieved most effectively through active listening. There are a variety of listening responses; some are actually blocks to communication, whereas others enhance understanding. The following four common responses can become barriers to communication in initial patient relationships.

Giving Advice. One way that people try to be helpful is by *giving advice.* Many times people do not really need or want advice at all. They have already thought through options and may even have the problem solved. What they need instead is a listener who can demonstrate true understanding. Giving advice tells a person that the primary interest is in the content rather than in the feelings expressed. Here is an example:

> *Patient:* I'm worried about telling my friends I've been in the hospital for treatment. I don't know if I want to tell them I've decided not to use drugs anymore.
> *Assistant:* The way I would handle that is to be as clear about it as possible. Make an announcement as soon as you are back in school that you are through using drugs.

In this situation the assistant ignores the feeling of concern expressed by the young patient. The response might imply a lack of confidence in the patient's ability to find his or her own solution. Although COTAs may need to assist the patient by giving advice at some point, it is an ineffective response when the individual is trying to communicate a feeling.

Offering Reassurance. Another common response in conversations is *offering reassurance.* Reassuring another person is usually well intended but can limit further communication. When one gives reassurance, the person talking tends to feel that he or she ought to discontinue discussing the problem. This can minimize the uncomfortable emotion expressed by the patient. Here is an example:

> *Patient:* I feel so confused and overwhelmed now, I don't know where to start.
> *Assistant:* Don't worry so much; things always work out in the end.

In this example, offering reassurance is a kind of emotional withdrawal from the patient. It does not acknowledge the feelings expressed. Encouragement and assurance are often important verbal responses in a therapeutic relationship. Reassurance used as a response to another's expression of a feeling is not effective.

Diverting. A third response choice, referred to as *diverting,* involves relating what the patient has said to one's own experience.[4] This is sometimes done in an effort to communicate understanding, or it can be used to change the subject when the topic of conversation becomes uncomfortable. Sometimes people find it difficult to talk about topics such as anger, death, divorce, or violence because they create an inner tension. Changing the subject or shifting the focus of the conversation may reduce tension, but it does not communicate to the patient that the message has been heard. Here is an example:

> *Patient:* One of my biggest problems right now is feeling so lonely. That is worse than going through the divorce itself.
> *Assistant:* I know how you feel. My sister just had a divorce and she talks about that often. She's joined a ski club though, and is meeting all kinds of people. Do you like to ski?

In this example, the focus of the conversation is shifted by the assistant to his or her own experience; therefore, the assistant is not making a clear response to the feelings the patient has shared. The patient may feel as though the message had not been heard.

Questioning. A fourth response that is sometimes used ineffectively is *questioning.* To try to understand the details of an individual's situation, the COTA might ask questions that relate more to the facts than to the feelings expressed. Although it is important to have a clear picture of the patient's situation, excessive questioning or responding with an immediate question can limit the patient's opportunity to clearly describe the experience. In this regard, questioning is not a useful response to another's expression of feelings. Here is an example:

> *Patient:* The doctor told us our daughter's problems are caused by rheumatoid arthritis. We were so hoping it was just growing pains.
> *Assistant:* How old is your daughter?

The question asked by the assistant in this example does not respond to the emotion shared by the patient.

ACTIVE LISTENING—NONVERBAL AND VERBAL COMPONENTS

Active listening is a term given to a set of skills that allows an individual to hear, understand and indicate that the message has been communicated. It is an effective listening response. Active listening is a necessary component in the relationship between the COTA and the patient. It is fundamental to effective communication and basic to the occupational therapy process. Active listening enables the assistant to understand more objectively and accurately the meaning of the verbal and nonverbal messages communicated by the patient. It is important and sometimes difficult to achieve a balance between too little and too much listening. However, if the therapist and the assistant do not understand the meaning of the messages communicated by the patient, inappropriate treatment goals and treatment activities may be chosen. If the interview or treatment session is entirely unstructured and the therapist or assistant "listens" to whatever the patient wishes to say, valuable and expensive treatment time may be lost. Active listening on the part of a COTA is a combination of the verbal and nonverbal behaviors and skills that communicate an attitude of acceptance. These are discussed in terms of the following nonverbal components: appropriate body posture and position, eye contact, facial expression, and a nondistracting environment. Paraphrasing and reflection are also important elements in this process.

Body Posture and Positioning

The most effective body posture includes facing the patient in an open, relaxed manner and leaning forward slightly. Arms should not be folded across the chest; legs should not be crossed. Tightly crossed arms and legs can be interpreted by the patient as rigidity or defensiveness.[5] Extraneous body motions such as swinging legs or tapping

fingers do not indicate a relaxed posture and should be avoided. It is better not to sit behind a desk but to position oneself directly across from the patient. In an occupational therapy clinic it is acceptable and often desirable to use a table during the interview. In this instance sit across from or beside the patient. Optimal communication usually occurs when the participants are three to five feet apart.[6] Cultural differences may dictate variations. It is always useful to watch for and respond to nonverbal cues given by the patient regarding a comfortable distance for communication.

Eye Contact

An effective listener maintains good eye contact with the speaker. Eye contact is thought to be an effective way of communicating empathy.[7] Avoiding another's eyes in an interaction can communicate disinterest, discomfort, or preoccupation.[6] At the same time, staring intently can make the speaker uncomfortable. It is important to look directly at the patient without staring.

Facial Expression

One's facial expressions are an important component of non-verbal communication. A frown, a smile or raised eyebrows send a specific message to the other party that indicates disapproval, approval or questioning.

Environmental Considerations

To actively listen to another, the interaction must take place in a nondistracting, pleasant environment. It is important to hold group sessions or dyadic interviews in quiet, uncluttered areas. Avoid interruptions from others or the telephone. It is sometimes useful to use "Do Not Disturb" signs and to ask that telephone calls be held.

Paraphrasing and Reflection

Two verbal techniques related to active listening include paraphrasing and reflection. **Paraphrasing** is repeating in one's own words the verbal content of the message received. **Reflection** is a summary of the affective meaning of the message and may include the patient's verbal and nonverbal communication. These techniques are used to ensure understanding by checking the accuracy of the message received. A paraphrasing response might begin with "Do you mean that. . ." or "I understand you to say. . ." and then rephrasing the content of the message. Message content includes information about an event or situation: who, what, when, where, how. The affective meaning is the accompanying feeling or emotion that is stated verbally or implied in nonverbal cues. It is important to listen to both aspects of the message. The following patient statements are provided as examples:

> *Patient 1:* I haven't had time to get used to the idea that I'll soon be leaving, and I'm scared to death of this change.

In this example, "I haven't had time to get used to the idea that I'll soon be leaving" is the content because it provides information about the situation. "I'm scared to death" is the affective message because it describes the emotion.

> *Patient 2:* I'm disappointed with the way this turned out. I guess I didn't read the directions thoroughly.

In the second example, "I'm disappointed" is the feeling response and, therefore, the affective message. "I didn't read the directions thoroughly" is the content because it describes the "what" in the situation.

When the patient does not directly state how he or she feels about the situation just described but expresses this nonverbally through body movements, facial expression, or tone of voice, the assistant can reflect what the patient may be feeling by naming an emotion. To practice using reflection as a listening tool when the patient does not directly state the feeling one can 1) listen for the feelings inferred by the overall tone of the message, 2) observe patient body language, or 3) ask, "How would I feel?" Putting oneself in another's place allows one to guess another's reaction. This technique is sometimes helpful but it must be remembered that each person's response is unique.[4] Following are examples of a COTA's response to the feelings implied by the patient:

> *Patient 1* (an elderly woman who recently moved to an apartment): When my husband was alive he did everything for me. Now not only do I have to take care of things myself, I have no one to talk to.

The assistant recognizes that the patient is feeling lonely.

> *Response:* It must be an empty feeling to suddenly find yourself without your spouse.

> *Patient 2* (a patient who is recovering from severe burns over the upper half of her body. The patient's hair is gone and she is trying on the wig for the first time. She adjusts and readjusts the wig. Finally she says): There, I can almost stand to look at myself again.

The assistant observes the patient's frustration and depressed manner and thinks that the woman feels unattractive, anxious and depressed.

> *Response:* This recovery period must be a very difficult time for you. I can tell your appearance is important to you and that you are anxious to look yourself again.

> *Patient 3* (a woman whose ten-year-old daughter is having trouble in school states that): Nancy has never

had problems before. She seems discouraged, and her teacher appears disinterested in her.

The COTA thinks the patient is expressing anxiety or concern about her daughter and anger or frustration with what she thinks is the teacher's disinterest.

> *Response:* It's worrisome to see your child struggle, and it's irritating when the teacher doesn't seem interested.

OTHER IMPORTANT COMMUNICATION COMPONENTS

Other components of effective communication incorporate both verbal and nonverbal responses. These include communicating respect, warmth and genuineness.

Communicating Respect

The COTA must be able to effectively communicate respect to the patient. Respect means to believe in the value and the potential of another person. When respect is communicated, a person feels more capable of self-help. Attention must be focused on the patient's interests and needs instead of the therapist's concerns. The COTA attempts to help the patient meet his or her needs without dominating the situation or the patient.

Communicating respect involves the process of affirmation. To affirm means to reinforce the worth of an individual. This process allows the patient to begin to value himself or herself. The COTA must develop the capacity to recognize quickly the strengths in the patient, and these must be communicated to the patient whenever possible. A sense of timing is needed, however, because sometimes patients are not ready to hear their strengths and the feedback may be threatening. Communicating respect is associated with the ability to communicate personal warmth and genuineness.

Communicating Warmth

Warmth is the degree to which the therapist communicates caring to the patient. Warmth by itself is not adequate for developing a therapeutic relationship or for assisting someone in problem solving; however, it can facilitate these positive outcomes.

Warmth may be demonstrated in tone of voice, facial expression, or other body language, as well as in words and actions. Touching, for example, is an effective way to communicate concern and empathy. Touching a patient's hand or shoulder may offer reassurance, approval or encouragement. It is important to remember, however, that not all people like to be touched, and in some situations touching may be contraindicated.

Communicating Genuineness

Genuineness, also termed *authenticity,* is a human quality that greatly enhances communication and the establishment of therapeutic relationships. Individuals who communicate genuineness respond in an honest, unguarded, and spontaneous manner. This means the therapist is willing to appropriately share reactions to what she or he experiences within a group or dyadic relationship. The ability to communicate genuineness as well as respect and warmth through effective use of listening skills, body language, and feeling centered messages enables the COTA to give and receive feedback in a responsible manner.

FEEDBACK

Giving and receiving feedback are important interpersonal skills necessary for the COTA when working with groups.

Giving Feedback

The purpose of giving another person feedback is to describe as specifically and objectively as possible one's perception of another's behavior. It is essential that therapists and assistants know the guidelines for responsible feedback, because they must frequently teach this skill or serve as role models when working with groups. Following are five rules for responsible feedback:[8]

1. Feedback represents an individual perception. It is therefore necessary to own what is said by making "I statements."

Response 1: I'm upset when I see you come late to work as you did this morning.
Response 2: We're all getting frustrated with your frequent tardiness.

Note that the second response is general in that it tries to represent everyone's reactions. This kind of statement is not responsible and can leave the receiver feeling defensive. The message can also be distorted.

2. Be specific rather than general; give examples of the behavior described. It is often difficult to respond accurately to a broad, nonspecific statement.

Response 1: When you came in the room just now you slammed the door. I feel upset when you express your anger that way.
Response 2: You are always going around expressing your hostility by banging things and slamming doors. I'm tired of it.

Phrases such as "you always" or "there you go again" are too general and become blaming statements. It is difficult not to react defensively to feedback worded in this way.

3. Be descriptive rather than evaluative. This means that the behavior should be described rather than labeled. Avoid making judgments about another's behavior, as this is also likely to elicit defensiveness.

Response 1: I heard you speaking to your friend in an abrupt manner. I thought you were not responding to his question seriously and it bothered me.
Response 2: I've always thought you were too flippant, and when I heard you speak to your friend like that, I thought you were a fool.

The words "flippant" and "fool" are labels and imply a judgment in this example.

4. Give feedback as soon as possible after the specific event occurs. This technique is called *immediacy.* Giving feedback immediately avoids problems caused by built-up feelings, which are often expressed out of proportion to the incident if they have been held back for a long time.

Response 1: I feel frustrated and uneasy today because I don't know where you stand. You said nothing during this session.
Response 2: This is the third week you have sat here and not made a response. I'm getting frustrated with you, and I don't trust you at all.

Because giving feedback requires risk taking, group members are often reluctant to state how they feel at the time. The second response is much angrier than the first and, therefore, harder for the receiver to hear. The assistant needs to help group members express feelings as they arise; this helps the group build trust.

5. After giving feedback, check to see that the feedback has been heard accurately. This is a critical part of the feedback process. To do this one might say, "I want to make certain you understand what I've said, could you tell me what you've heard?"

Responding to Feedback

Receiving feedback is one way people learn how they are perceived. It is a valuable tool in making behavioral change. Because giving feedback to another person requires risk taking, it is necessary to avoid misunderstanding. When feedback is given, the receiver should indicate what message was heard. It is not necessary to decide immediately what to do about it, but the person giving the feedback needs to know that the message was heard accurately. The receiver might say, "I don't know how I feel about what you've just said, or what I'll do. I need some time to think this over. This is what I heard you say to me. . ."

Giving and receiving feedback in a group can initially create tense situations because of the risk taking involved, and it is a skill many people do not have. It is a necessary part of learning about oneself and making change. COTAs can help facilitate this process by teaching the skill using the guidelines listed in the preceding discussion. It is useful to provide groups or individuals with specific activities that elicit and reinforce these skills.

UNDERSTANDING HOW GROUPS WORK

A group is three or more people who establish some form of an interdependent relationship with each other. In occupational therapy groups, the activity usually provides the common ground for these relationships. This definition, however, does not include that human quality that is brought to an effective group by the leader and group members. This quality helps provide each individual with a sense of belonging and sharing which in turn facilitates and reinforces learning. The word *community* is also used to describe the desirable outcome of member relationships. Implied in this definition is *union with others.* At their best, groups form true communities in which members are able to give and receive support and insights, which in turn encourage personal growth. To achieve this degree of group cohesion, the COTA must understand how groups work.

Group process refers to how members relate to and communicate with each other and how members accomplish the task. Group process might be described in terms of the way the group solves problems, makes decisions, or manages conflicts that arise. This process perspective of group assumes a holistic view that describes how different group functions fit together to determine the ongoing development of the group. To better understand how groups work, the following characteristics will be considered: group role functions, group norms and developmental group stages.

Group Role Functions

Analysis of individual roles assumed within a group is one of the most familiar ways people use to understand how groups work. Bales[10] suggested the presence of two main areas in all groups based on types of communication that describe the particular behavioral roles: task roles and maintenance or group-centered roles. **Task roles** refer to those behaviors that facilitate task accomplishment. **Group-centered roles** refer to those behaviors that enhance relationships among members. The COTA needs to be

versatile in the roles that he or she assumes during group work. Role flexibility refers to an individual's ability to take the action necessary to accomplish a task and, at the same time, maintain cohesiveness in the group. Balancing task and group-centered roles is an important goal for effective group work. In examining a group with a definite leader, one finds that the leader initially assumes multiple roles. As groups mature, leadership is distributed among the members who are able to play the following functional roles: task roles, group-centered roles and **self-centered roles.**

Task Roles. Task roles are concerned with the accomplishment of the group task. Following is a summary of group task roles:

1. *Initiator/Designer:* This role involves starting the group and providing direction. The person who assumes this role plans activities and suggests learning experiences.
2. *Information Seeker/Information Giver:* This role is assumed by asking for or offering facts related to task accomplishment.
3. *Opinion Seeker/Opinion Giver:* The member who assumes this role asks for reactions from others or states his or her own beliefs and values.
4. *Challenger/Confronter:* This role involves asking for clarification about what is communicated. A member who assumes this role also raises issues that are being avoided in the group.
5. *Summarizer:* The member who acts in this role stops the group occasionally to state what is being accomplished. This role serves to keep the group on track.

Group-Centered Roles. Group-centered roles are concerned with keeping the group together by maintaining relationships and satisfying the members' needs. The most important of these roles are the following:

1. *Encourager:* The member who assumes this role is meeting the esteem needs of individuals in the group by offering praise in response to what members do or say.
2. *Gate Keeper:* This role involves facilitating and regulating communication by spreading participation among the members. It involves drawing out quiet members and managing conversation monopolizers.
3. *Tension Reliever:* The member who assumes this role is sensitive to the frustration level of self and others. It is a role involving the use of appropriate jokes, kidding remarks, or suggestions for compromise that dissipate anxiety or hostility in the group.
4. *Harmonizer:* This role is focused on the feelings group members may have. The harmonizer demonstrates caring by naming feelings, thus acknowledging their importance. Harmonizing can help promote positive relationships among group members.

Self-Centered Roles. The roles just described are considered *functional* because they support task accomplishment and the people within the group. Other roles are considered *nonfunctional* because they interfere with group process. These roles are termed self-centered.

Self-centered roles are common in groups and occur because an individual is primarily concerned with satisfying his or her own needs and lacks the adaptive skills needed to function effectively. It is necessary for the COTA to learn to recognize and deal with these roles, which interfere with individual and group progress.[9] Some of the most common self-centered roles include the following:

1. *Withdrawer:* This member does not participate in the activity or discussion at any time. A person may withdraw because of feelings of insecurity, fear of rejection, anger, or lack of interest. A distinction should be made between a withdrawer and an active listener. The listener may be quiet for a time while absorbing information. The active listener does not remain passive for the entire session. To help a member who is withdrawn, the COTA may sit next to him or her, ask open-ended questions, take time at the beginning of the session to establish a greater comfort level among members, or take the individual aside and try to identify the reason for the withdrawal.

2. *Blocker:* This individual may consistently raise objections or insist that nothing can be accomplished. A common phrase used by a blocker is "We've already tried this" or "It won't work." To help a person who is blocking progress in the group, the COTA must let the individual know how this behavior is affecting other members and task accomplishment. Direct feedback is necessary and may be provided within or outside the group depending on the skill level of the group members.

3. *Aggressor/Dominator:* This member tries to take over the group by interrupting when others are speaking, deflating the status of others, insisting on having his or her own way, or telling other members what to do. To help members deal with an aggressor/dominator one may provide and encourage feedback by directing the discussion to identify feelings or call for "time out" to discuss what is happening in the group.

4. *Recognition Seeker:* A recognition seeker tries to get the attention or approval of other members in inappropriate ways. He or she may make distracting jokes or comments, engage in "horse play," boast about accomplishments, or seek pity or sympathy. The COTA may be helpful to a recognition seeker by offering approval of the member's strengths and discouraging inappropriate behaviors.

Group dynamics research is clear regarding the outcome of self-centered behaviors. Initially, considerable leader and group effort is directed to the member who behaves in the manner(s) described previously. If the leader or group perceives that there is a reasonable chance of changing the behavior this effort may go on for some time. If, at some point, it becomes clear that the inappropriate behavior cannot or will not change, communication toward the individual declines. Group members may begin to exclude the member, and he or she may have to be asked to leave.[10] All members of the group are responsible for dealing with disruptive behavior; however, if the group is unsuccessful, the formal leader must intervene. If issues are not resolved, members may lose confidence and commitment to the group.

Group Norms

Group norms are standards of behavior that can be stated or unspoken. They define what behaviors are expected, accepted and valued by group members. Group norms serve several purposes. They allow groups to function in an organized manner; they define ways in which members respond to conflict, make decisions or solve problems; they help define ways in which members relate to each other and to the leader. They define "reality" for the group. Norms can change as the group evolves and as expectations of member behavior changes. Those attempting to understand how groups work must carefully examine group norms. Sometimes it is useful for the members to identify their own group norms and to determine whether or how these norms should be changed. In this way, implicit norms, or those that influence member behavior but are unspoken, can be made explicit. Some examples of implicit norms might include manner of dress, attitudes toward authority, or group response to change.

The group leader can influence group norms when the group is forming. The norms that the COTA encourages influence the behaviors that will lead to trust, group cohesion and goal attainment. Norms that might be facilitated by the COTA include the following: 1) Each member is valued, 2) expression of feelings is important, 3) making mistakes is expected, and 4) disagreement is desirable. A group that demonstrates these qualities creates a social support system. This quality is important in a therapeutic setting. Social support systems consist of meaningful, often long lasting, interpersonal ties that one may have with a variety of groups of people. A system like this may be found at home, church, or other settings where friendships form. The people in these groups think and behave in accordance with shared values and offer each other support and assistance when needed.

Social support systems are crucial to an individual's well-being. They serve as a buffer to stress in one's life. The effects of exposure to difficult situations can be minimized by social support; conversely, the effects of stress will often be made worse if these systems are not in place.

Group Growth and Development

A third consideration in learning about how groups work is understanding the developmental phases of group life.

Researchers who study groups agree that common, predictable, sequential and developmental stages emerge as the group matures. Group phases are best observed in closed groups in which membership is stable over time. These stages often overlap, and earlier stages may be repeated with the introduction of new tasks or change in membership. For this reason, some theorists describe group evolution as a developmental spiral.[11]

Many theorists have studied and described phases of group development. Bales[12] describes three stages: orientation, or defining the problem/task; evaluation, or how the group feels about the task; and control, or how the task will be completed. Tuckman[13] summarized the literature available on group development and determined four stages:

1. *Forming* deals with orientation issues of coming together.
2. *Storming* represents conflict and power struggles that relate to the issue of control.
3. *Norming* is the stage in which members determine how they will relate to one another.
4. *Performing* represents how the task will be accomplished.

It is important to use a developmental frame of reference when working with groups. This approach can help give meaning to events occurring within the group and can assist the leader in choosing an appropriate intervention.

For the purposes of this discussion, two dimensions of group development will be examined. Mosey's developmental framework lists and describes levels of group interaction.[14] Those groups are parallel group, project group, egocentric cooperative group and mature group. A group at any one of these levels, if together long enough, can also mature. The predictable maturation phases possible for each group are named by the authors as initial dependence, conflict, and interdependence.

Initial dependence describes the first phase of group maturation. Members are concerned about their place within the group. Feelings can be manifested in different ways depending on the developmental level of the group; however, each newly formed group, regardless of developmental level, experiences an initial dependency phase.

The second phase of maturation within each level is characterized by some **conflict** and struggle. The important issue in this phase is control—control of self and control of others or of the environment. This struggle is a necessary and normal part of group development. It should be recognized and encouraged because learning usually requires some degree of labor. It is necessary for groups to experience and resolve this issue before interrelatedness is achieved.

The final phase, **interdependence,** emerges through successful resolution of control issues. This stage is characterized by a high level of affiliation. Members relate at a deeper interpersonal level. It is at this point, when members experience a sense of community with each other, that greater risk taking can occur, thus enhancing the opportunity for greater personal growth. The potential for learning and behavioral change may vary among patients, especially those with cognitive limitations; but even in low level groups, the opportunity for this phase of interdependence is present.

APPLICATION TO DEVELOPMENTAL GROUPS

This section details the application of interpersonal communication skills to various groups. Specific examples are provided to illustrate the developmental progression in terms of level of independence and interpersonal competence of participants. Emphasis is placed on characteristics of the group as well as leader preparation, attitude and approach. Qualities and examples of various group activities are also delineated. It is important for the reader to have an understanding of the following basic concepts:

Leader preparation refers to those activities the group leader completes prior to convening the group to assure that it will run smoothly. Examples include learning as much as possible about the group members and their goals; reviewing instructions and gathering materials for group activities; and arranging the environment to assure maximal interaction.

Leader attitude and approach refers to the affective qualities exhibited by the leader to enhance overall group effectiveness. Examples include showing warmth and genuineness by greeting each member of the group by name; establishing structure, consistency and routine as required by the level of the group; and acting as a role model for effective behaviors.

Activity qualities and examples refers to the selection of group activities that have attributes that will assist group members in achieving their goals. Types of activities include mosaic tile work with limited supplies to encourage sharing; quilt making to encourage cooperation; and planning and implementing a party to encourage consistent interaction over time.

The Parallel Group

The first and most basic group in terms of independence and interpersonal competence of the members is the parallel group. There are usually five to seven members who work side by side but on individual projects. The leader assumes total leadership and responsibility for meeting the group members' needs for security, love and belonging, and esteem while assisting them with their activity.[14] Treatment goals of this group are to develop work skills, experience mastery over a simple task, and develop basic awareness of others. Craft projects are designed to offer opportunities to meet these goals.

At first, the group members exhibit anxiety and total dependence on the leader(s). Members may express uncertainty about why they are together, appear passive, laugh nervously, or seem confused. The activity presented in the parallel group provides a means of focusing a person's attention away from self and onto other objects in the environment. The conflict phase in a parallel group is seen in the patient's struggle for control over the materials, tools, and the process of the task. For mastery to occur, the COTA must make certain that activities provide a manageable challenge. To do this, the occupational therapy assistant serving in this role must have a clear understanding of each person's limitations. Mastery must be strongly reinforced as the patient works.

Interconnectedness or **community** can occur even at this group level if the COTA helps to create the connections among members. One way to achieve connections is to have individuals work on similar kinds of projects.[14] As the assistant helps patients recognize their success, self-esteem begins to build. A reinforced sense of self enables a person to begin to experience others.

Another means of providing individual identity to group members in a parallel group is through *sentient role recognition*. The COTA, serving as a group leader, learns to observe members carefully and to recognize and reinforce personality qualities that may have brought the individual recognition at one time. The leader may notice evidence of nurturing qualities, sociability, or a sense of humor in particular members. Once identified, the personality quality may be described to the patient in positive terms and its use directed. For example, a patient with nurturing qualities may be asked to sit next to a new member and told that his or her warmth and manner would make the new person feel more comfortable. If this quality is recognized by the patient and has given meaning and uniqueness to his or her self-concept, it will be strengthened by providing a special role for that person in the group.

It is ideal to work with an occupational therapist, sharing leadership responsibility and providing members with a parental team. OTRs and COTAs, working together as a complementary team, model appropriate and caring interaction skills.[15]

Leader Preparation, Attitude and Approach. Before the group arrives, it is important for the COTA to attend to the following:

1. Know as much as possible about the individuals beginning the group to provide members with meaningful activities.
2. Preplan and organize the activities and instructions carefully so that energy is used most efficiently during the group itself.

After group members arrive, the leader is responsible for carrying out the following tasks with particular attention to affect and attitude:

1. Greet each member individually and use names frequently (name tags are visual reminders).
2. Project warmth, friendliness, and calmness through facial expression, words, and actions to promote comfort and trust.
3. Provide consistency in approach and routine through assignment of permanent seating and storage space for each individual.
4. Explain the purpose of the group and the activity.
5. Give clear and structured directions.
6. Sit down and spend time with each individual.
7. Stimulate members to perform at their highest level by offering activities that provide a manageable challenge with help from the leader.
8. Offer approval and recognition of members' efforts as well as their completed projects.
9. Establish a nurturing milieu. The leader's ability to demonstrate a warm, caring attitude is important. Meaningful objects present in the environment can also be helpful. Sometimes serving food or beverages can create this feeling of hospitality.
10. If members become disruptive, take them aside for feedback.
11. Encourage interaction among group members by expressing and modeling concern if individuals are absent or ill.
12. Direct positive use of personality strengths to create opportunities for interaction.

Activity Qualities and Examples. The following activity qualities and examples must also be given consideration by the group leader. Activity length depends on the attention span of the members (from 15 minutes to 45 minutes in most cases). Efforts should be made to structure the activities to minimize the need for personal decision making and to assure success. Equally important, activities should be meaningful and have a recognizable end product or provide a sense of identity. With this goal in mind, the COTA should provide projects that do not require heavy concentration, as this allows the opportunity for participants to develop an awareness of others in the group. Most any craft can be adapted to meet the needs of the parallel group. Examples include textile stenciling, mosaics, simple leather work, needlecraft, papercraft, simple weaving, copper tooling, and ceramics.

Project Group

A project group requires higher level social and work skills. The larger group is broken down into subgroups of two and three people and a short-term task requiring some interaction and sharing is provided. Member interaction is secondary to the activity and primary interest is in task completion.[14]

The dependence phase of the group presents itself in much the same way as the parallel group. Members view the group leaders as protectors and authorities who define limits and goals and satisfy needs. The COTA allows this dependence but begins to encourage reliance on others.

The conflict emerges as dependency shifts from the leader to peers in the subgroup. Members may struggle as they attempt to establish trust in other members and cooperate in the shared activity. Members may seek out the leader for help instead of working with their partners. Some individuals may express dissatisfaction with the activity and the ability of peers. Members may appear overwhelmed by the task.

Interrelatedness begins to occur as the patients' sense of community encompasses the small work group. Patients are now able to share completion of the task, but this group level still will rely on the group leader or leaders to create connections or at least strengthen them through questions, comments and summarizing activities. For example, after completion of a subgroup activity, a sharing session may be used to display completed projects. Members could be asked to name those with whom they worked. Each subgroup could be given a symbol or name to help members identify themselves as a member of a team. A short and competitive game between "teams" could be encouraged at the end of each session to reinforce the concept of belonging.[16]

Leader Preparation, Attitude and Approach. The following approach should be taken:
1. Gently encourage members to rely on others in the group.
2. Answer some questions but redirect questions to other members when possible.
3. Help members examine ideas and problems by asking pertinent questions.
4. Assist individuals in asking for help from partner or group by helping them to phrase questions.
5. Reinforce positive behaviors and relate them to *successful task completion.* (At this level the activity provides a concrete reference.)
6. If members appear overwhelmed, restructure a specific part of the activity and offer repeated contact and support.
7. If individuals in the group display negative behavior, intervene; help identify the problem and suggest possible solutions.
8. If negative behavior is persistent and if it interferes with task completion, remove the person from the group to discuss the problem.

Activity Qualities and Examples. The projects should be short-term, lasting from 20 minutes to one hour. At first, projects should have easily divided components so that cooperation and contact is not constantly required among members. The following activities can be used at this level:
    planning menus
    "no bake" cookies
    stir and frost cakes
    simple dips for snacks
    pizza
    making holiday or other decorations
    assembling party favors
    decorating bulletin boards
    potting plants or planting a terrarium
    making collages
    making mobiles
    dyeing eggs
    making ice cream
    games, including relays
    team bowling
    cards

Egocentric Cooperative Group

In the egocentric cooperative group, members work together on a long-term activity requiring substantial interaction, cooperation and sharing. Members are primarily self-centered at this level and are able to recognize and verbalize their own needs. Members are beginning to identify the esteem needs of others because of a developing awareness of the effect of their behavior on individuals in the group. The members begin to assume responsibility for selecting, planning and implementing the activity.[14]

The dependence phase will be seen as ambivalence. Members may exhibit heavy reliance on authority at times and then shift to an attitude of disregard. Although this tendency is sometimes difficult for the therapist or assistant to deal with, it may be regarded as a positive behavioral sign, as it signals the members' growing sense of self.

Conflict occurs within individuals and externally among members as the group struggles with the increased complexity of the activity and the interpersonal demands of the expanded group. Competition will be evident. Some individuals may have difficulty following established norms and may arrive late or ask to take frequent breaks. This testing behavior is an attempt to identify boundaries, and the COTA must offer guidance, identify feelings, and stress each individual's value in the group. The group leader must avoid power struggles and yet reinforce cooperation and adherence to the rules, as they pertain to successful task completion and interpersonal relations.

To help this group achieve interrelatedness or community, one must assist members in understanding what occurred as they worked together. Work time may be followed by discussion that focuses on the behavioral strengths that have enhanced group progress and also on the group norms that have been established.[14] A sense of community can be identified when individuals receive recognition from other members.

Leader Preparation, Attitude and Approach. The following steps should be taken:

1. Reinforce autonomy by demonstrating respect and concern for the feelings and rights of each individual through direct verbal statements and acknowledgment of contributions
2. Provide structure as the group begins by clarifying directions or plans for each session.
3. Assist the group in establishing implicit and explicit norms by clarifying behavioral expectations, modeling desired behaviors, and complimenting positive behaviors observed in peers.
4. Assist members in recognizing the progress they are making by asking individuals to describe their own strengths and weaknesses after the activity is over.
5. Manage conflict between members by facilitating understanding of one another's perspectives.
6. Help members discuss whether they feel accepted and appreciated because they are learning to recognize esteem needs in others.
7. Model empathy and concern for the feelings of members.
8. Encourage members to provide support for each other.
9. Provide members with a decision-making process that encourages participation by all. Brainstorming or taking turns can be used as procedures.
10. Provide constructive feedback within the group because members are learning how their behavior effects others.

Activity Qualities and Examples. Activity time may be expanded to 45 to 60 minutes, and the task may take more than one period to complete. Activities should require consistent interaction among all members. The following are some examples:

newspaper layouts
planning and implementing parties
planning picnics or outdoor cooking activities
refinishing furniture
painting murals
planning and presenting skits and videotaping the performance

Cooperative Groups

The cooperative group is most often homogeneous; that is, members share similarities of age, sex, values, and interests.[16] Because of these likenesses and the members' increasing ability to identify and articulate their own needs, they begin to recognize the multiple needs of other people as well. At this level the task becomes secondary and a vehicle for interaction. Interpersonal relationships become the primary focus.

Initially members will depend on the leader(s) for structure, support and guidance as new group roles are learned and trust is established. Members will need help in identifying and responding to the needs of others as well as expressing positive and negative feelings. Members will also depend on the COTA to help maintain cohesiveness.

Conflict occurs as members attempt to learn the balance of task and group-centered roles. Some members will see conflict or disagreement as bad and will need help in understanding that disagreement is a positive element and a sign of growth.[17] Members must learn to deal with conflict as it occurs and then to give and receive feedback responsibly. At this level, members are capable of learning many new communication skills but may have difficulty as they practice new roles and behaviors.

Affiliation potential is very high as members experience a stronger belief in themselves. Individual strengths are validated by others, and members begin to feel accepted and understood. In this phase, members are able to share leadership and a sense of equality, which strengthens bonds among people. Members are able to identify problems, propose solutions, and have an improved sense of how the group as a whole functions. The group begins to deal openly with conflict and members experience cohesion. Warmth and caring are evident even when members disagree.

Leader Preparation, Attitude and Approach. The following steps should be taken:

1. Assist members in establishing trust with one another by modeling openness and a willingness to be vulnerable. (This means that the COTA should openly admit shortcomings and mistakes to the group.)
2. Ask the group to decide what new skills members would like to learn.
3. Clarify the purpose of the group by emphasizing that although participation in the task is essential, the purpose of working together is to learn group and communication skills.
4. Offer skill building resources to the group and provide structure and information as necessary.
5. Monitor verbal and nonverbal communication to facilitate processing when the activity is over.
6. Encourage risk-taking behavior.
7. Provide group with activities that teach group processes such as problem solving, decision making, and conflict management.
8. Assist members in taking on new leadership roles.
9. Provide activity choices that encourage the development of ability to give and receive feedback responsibly.
10. Provide encouragement and suggest activities or assignments for members to practice new skills outside of the group.
11. Teach members how to process their own group.
12. Disengage self from the authority position as affiliation emerges.

Activity Qualities and Examples. A variety of suggestions may be offered to the cooperative group so that members may plan and implement an activity that could last through multiple periods. The process of choosing and planning the project provides an excellent opportunity for learning. It is useful to provide suggestions of shorter term tasks intermittently so that newly learned skills can be applied and gratification is immediate. This process reenergizes the members. The following are some examples of long-term cooperative projects:

banner design and construction
quilt making
plays and talent shows
outdoor gardening
camping trips

Among the short-term cooperative projects that may be used occasionally are activities such as meal preparation, writing a group poem, designing a group symbol, and planning an outing.

Mature Groups

Mature groups function at the highest interpersonal level. They are heterogeneous, meaning that members vary in age, sex, values, interests, and socioeconomic or cultural background. Individuals able to function at this level are comfortable with a variety of people and are flexible in performing group roles. This is a skill level attained by healthy people and may be difficult to achieve in a hospital or rehabilitation setting. A COTA may more likely encounter a group at this level in a community setting, such as adult education groups, senior citizen centers, and neighborhood and special interest groups.

Dependency on occupational therapy personnel or any appointed leader will be minimal even in the initial meetings of this group. There may be an expectation that the COTA will make necessary physical arrangements for the meeting place or initiate discussion.

Members may experience conflict or ambivalence toward acceptance of increased responsibility and leadership roles. Issues related to the use of personal power may arise as members attempt to discover the extent of their influence over each other. Members struggle as they learn to draw on their own assets more consistently and look inward for answers rather than relying on others. Another phase of conflict may occur when the group loses members or comes to closure. This occurrence may cause the members to return to a brief dependency phase as they experience disequilibrium. These tensions usually last only briefly.

Members develop a strong social support system and experience a satisfying sense of community with others. Genuineness is evident in the sincere communication patterns. Openness and honesty become established group norms. Members respect and value each other. Each individual feels a sense of worth and importance in the group.

Individuals feel deeply understood owing to empathetic communication. Risk taking occurs as members challenge each other and gain new personal insights leading to fuller awareness and social integration. Group members at this level not only accept diversity but seek it out and enjoy gaining new perspectives of self through understanding difference.

Leader Preparation, Attitude and Approach. The following approaches are appropriate:

1. Facilitate formation of group and establish a conducive environment for meetings.
2. Relinquish leadership and allow the group to be self-directed.
3. Become an equal member of the group.

Activity Qualities and Examples. The group will determine its own direction and will choose activities related to the purpose of the group. As an activity specialist, the COTA will serve as a resource person to the group. Some possible activity categories would include the following:

community service activities
academic/intellectual activities
creative thinking/problem-solving activities
self-help activities, such as grief encounter groups and parenting

CONCLUSION

Although group phases and characteristics are somewhat predictable, every group develops a unique process and profile. Occupational therapy personnel seldom find a group that fits the developmental levels exactly as they have been described. These descriptions are intended as a guide in assessing individual and group levels and for planning appropriate activities to encourage growth.

A patient group is more likely to become cohesive and contribute to one another's growth if the members have been selected for their ability to function at a particular level. Too much variance in the members' abilities will interfere with individual and group progress.[17]

Many patients will never function at the cooperative or mature levels. It is important, however, to recognize that through the effective use of interpersonal and group skills, the COTA can assist even low-functioning groups to achieve a measure of interrelatedness or community. This sense of belonging will help satisfy basic needs, develop adaptive skills, and contribute to maintenance of physical and emotional health.

Groups that function at the higher developmental levels present more complicated patient issues, behaviors and interactions. Entry-level COTAs need to work with groups

Table 9-1
Roles and Functions of Occupational Therapy Team Members in Group Work

Task	OTR	COTA
Screening	Determine appropriate screening information; initiate referrals; interpret findings; document recommendations	Collect information from patient, family and other resources; report findings to supervisor
Assessment	Determine patient's level of ability in cognitive, psychological, social and sensory areas; determine appropriate group level	Determine dyadic and general work ability through interview, observation and structured tasks

Collaborative Roles

Task		
Treatment planning	Plan patient's placement in a specific group and examine profile of the total group, including such factors as ages, backgrounds, interests and treatment goals. Collaborate with patients to set individual goals for each group member. Explore task and activity options. Analyze component parts of activity choice. Consider environmental factors to provide a meeting room and seating that satisfies the physical and security needs of the patients. Determine the role, attitude and approach of team members, maximizing the use of personal strengths. Document the overall plan.	
Treatment	Introduce the activity; explain the purpose of the activity and reinforce individual goals. Engage the group; assume leadership roles as determined by the group level. Process the group; enable the members to achieve the maximum amount of learning from the group experience by providing time at the end of the session to discuss problems that occurred as members worked together; discuss progress the group is making, feelings related to problems and progress, and reaffirm or establish new group goals.	
	Summarize and analyze each patient's progress; document response to program; reassess and modify program	Document patient performance as directed; assist in determining need for program change

over an extended time to develop and refine the necessary skills. Forms appropriate for use by a COTA in assisting with the assessment of patient work and social skills, as well as patient exercises, may be found in Appendix C.[14,18]

Entry-level personnel are advised to seek supervision and guidance from advanced clinicians. Table 9-1 provides an outline of the roles and functions of OTR and COTA team members involved in cooperative group work.

SUMMARY

This chapter described the need for COTAs to be interpersonally competent. To become competent, one must gain an awareness of self and others and be able to demonstrate that awareness through the use of verbal and nonverbal communication skills. Active listening, a necessary communication skill used to help establish therapeutic relationships, was described.

A general knowledge of group leadership roles, group norms, and the maturation phases of small groups helps the COTA develop a basic understanding of how groups work. This information can be applied to the use of groups in occupational therapy treatment. Groups used in this context can help the patient develop self-esteem, work skills and interpersonal competence.

Mosey's developmental group levels identify group characteristics related to patient skill levels. Maturation phases of the group at each of the levels were described to help the COTA recognize group and patient issues. This information allows the appropriate choice of an activity as well as structuring it to appropriately challenge group members. A skilled group leader will be able to help a group at any developmental level to work toward some form of community, also referred to as relatedness. The leader must allow for an initial dependency and help members resolve the personal struggles and interpersonal conflicts as they arise within the group. From the successful resolution of these experiences, members are able to risk interaction on a deeper, more personal level. Group cohesion is strengthened, and members then have greater opportunities for insight and personal growth. Interpersonal skills are thus improved.

Related Learning Activities

1. Attend a small party and spend some time observing nonverbal forms of communication. Identify those that enhance communication and those that do not.

2. Invite a small group of people to your home to plan a shower, a birthday party, or other social event. Practice leadership skills and roles appropriate for a cooperative group. Determine the factors present or not present that would allow mature group functioning.

3. Working with a peer, volunteer to conduct two short-term craft groups for children who are mentally retarded. Establish both parallel and project groups using the same activity. Co-lead both groups and seek feedback about your effectiveness.

4. Role play a conflict situation with peers. Identify your strengths and weaknesses in this situation.

5. View a segment of a television "soap opera," involving three or more people, with a small group of peers. Identify and discuss functional and nonfunctional group roles noted.

6. Identify ways that a COTA group leader can effectively interact with a group member who is demonstrating the behavior patterns of a blocker.

References

1. *Basic International Relations: A Course for Small Groups.* Atlanta, Georgia, Human Development Institute, 1969, pp 15-21.
2. Miller F, Nunnally E, Wackman D: *Couple Communication: Talking Together.* Minneapolis, Interpersonal Communication, 1979, pp 144-145.
3. Curran CA: *Counseling Learning.* New York, Grune & Stratton, 1979, pp 20-27.
4. Bolton E: *People Skills.* Englewood Cliffs, New Jersey, Prentice Hall, 1979.
5. Smith-Hannen SS: Affects of nonverbal behavior on judged levels of counselor warmth and empathy. *J Counseling Psychology* 24:87-91, 1977.
6. Cormier WH, Cormier LS: *Interviewing Strategies for Helpers—A Guide to Assessment, Treatment and Evaluation.* Monteray, California, Brooks Cole, 1979, p 44.
7. Hasse RF, Tepper D: Nonverbal components of empathetic communication. *J Counseling Psychology* 19:417-424, 1972.
8. *Basic Interpersonal Relations—Book 2: A Course for Small Groups.* Atlanta, Human Development Institute, 1969.
9. Miles M: *Learning to Work in Groups,* 2nd edition. New York, Teachers College, Columbia University, 1981, pp 241-245.
10. Bales RF: Task roles and social roles in problem solving groups. In TM Newcomb, EL Hartley (Eds): *Readings in Social Psychology,* 3rd edition, New York, Holt, Rineholt & Winston, 1958.
11. Sampson DD, Marthas MS: *Group Process for Health Professions.* New York, John Wiley & Sons, 1977.
12. Bales RF: Adaptive and integrative changes as sources of strain in social systems. In AP Hare, EF Borgatta, RF Bales (Eds): *Small Groups.* New York, Alfred Knopf, 1955.
13. Tuckerman BW: Developmental sequence in small groups. *Psychol Bull* 63:384-399, 1965.
14. Mosey AC: *Activities Therapy.* New York, Raven Press, 1973.
15. Napier R, Gershenfeld M: *Making Groups Work.* Boston, Houghton Mifflin, 1983, pp 108-109.
16. Hopkins HL, Smith HD (Eds): *Willard and Spackman's Occupational Therapy,* 5th edition. Philadelphia, JB Lippincott, 1978, pp 293-295.
17. Loomis ME: *Group Process for Nurses.* St. Louis, CV Mosby, 1981, pp 101-109.
18. Fidler G: The task oriented group as a context for treatment. *Am J Occup Ther* 1:43-48, 1969.

Chapter 10

Individualization of Occupational Therapy

Bonnie Brooks, MEd, OTR, FAOTA

INTRODUCTION

One of the foundations of occupational therapy theory is that humans have a need to be active and participate in various occupations. Occupation is essential for basic survival and optimal mental and physical health. **Occupation** is also an integral part of survival and a basic drive of every person. Within this individual frame of reference, a person's activities and occupations enable him or her to function as a central part of a larger whole. It is the difference between existing and actively participating. Participation and optimal functioning within a person's environment provide an individual with feelings of purpose and self-esteem throughout his or her life span.

What does the word occupation mean? To those in occupational therapy, it means engaging in purposeful activity. Occupations are effective in preventing or reducing disability and in promoting independence through the acquisition of skills, as the following examples illustrate:

1. The occupation of a preschool child with a disability is learning the motor skills necessary to enter school.
2. The primary occupation for a young adult may be planning for a career or vocation.
3. Occupation for others may be providing for financial security through employment, which may require a variety of activities.
4. Occupation for an individual with serious cardiac problems may include learning to conserve energy while doing daily activities.
5. An occupation for the elderly may be prolonging participation in rewarding activities and maintaining personal independence.

KEY CONCEPTS

Uniqueness of the individual

Internal environment

External environment

Sociocultural considerations

Impact of change

Disuse syndromes

Misuse syndromes

ESSENTIAL VOCABULARY

Occupation

Individualized

Self-image

Phobia

Climate

Community

Economic status

Customs

Traditions

Superstitions

Disruptions

Prevention

An occupation may require a variety of activities and skills. For example, the occupation of self-care includes the activities of bathing, shaving, dressing, and feeding, each of which requires varying degrees of skill in gross and fine motor coordination and judgment.

Occupational therapy is the art and science of directing an individual's participation in selected tasks to restore, reinforce, and enhance performance. Occupational therapy facilitates learning of skills and functions essential for adaptation and productivity, for diminishing or correcting pathology, and for promoting and maintaining health. The word occupation in the professional title refers to goal-directed use of time, energy, interest and attention. Occupational therapy's fundamental concern is developing and maintaining the capacity to perform, with satisfaction to self and others, the tasks and roles essential to productive living and mastering self and the environment throughout the life span.[1]

Three main types of occupation are necessary for the achievement of optimal performance and quality of life: activities of daily living, work and leisure. These areas are discussed in greater depth in Chapter 7. Acquiring and maintaining skills in these areas enable a person to interact successfully with the environment. Activities and skills also enable a person to engage in a variety of occupations that result in the establishment of the individual's lifestyle.

Occupational therapy provides service to those individuals whose abilities to cope with tasks of living are threatened or impaired by developmental deficits, the aging process, physical injury or illness, or psychological and social disability.[2]

Intervention programs in occupational therapy are designed to enable the patient to become adequate or proficient in basic life skills, work, and leisure, and thereby competent to resume his or her place in life and interact with the environment effectively. With these goals in mind, this chapter focuses on case studies and examples of how occupational therapy intervention can be **individualized** in relation to the environment, society, change and prevention.

CASE STUDIES IN INDIVIDUALITY

The profession of occupational therapy recognizes that the level of optimal function to which a patient may aspire is highly individual and determined by all of the circumstances of the individual's life.[3] No two patients are alike, even if they are the same age and have identical problems or disabilities. Intervention programs should be individualized and focus on the uniqueness of the individual. To understand the multitude of factors that create an individual lifestyle, a description of John and Darlene follows. They will be referred to later in this chapter to illustrate various content areas.

Case Study 10-1

John. John is a 24-year-old obese man. He smoked two packs of cigarettes a day for four years and recently quit. He appears in good health.

Family Information

John is the oldest of three children. His sisters, aged 19 and 21, are away at college. His mother is 53 years old and in good health. His father is 57 years old and has high blood pressure. Three years ago the father experienced two severe heart attacks and was hospitalized both times. The following year the father had three minor attacks. He had generalized weakness and has been very depressed; however, he exhibited significant improvement recently.

Vocational Information

John graduated from college two years ago. He returned home to manage the farm because of his father's illness. The crop farm is located 25 miles outside a rural town in southern Minnesota. Employment opportunities were very limited for John in that particular region of the state, and he had just accepted a job to work as an accountant in Duluth. He plans to move there in four months.

Leisure and Socialization

During the winter, John watches television a great deal and plays cards. Recently, he decided to take half-hour walks twice a day to lose weight. In the summer, John plays softball on a local team, goes swimming, and meets socially with friends.

Case Study 10-2

Darlene. Darlene is a 35-year-old woman in good health. She is slightly underweight because of constant dieting.

Family Information

Darlene is an only child. She was married for five years, lived in California, and divorced two years ago. She had no children. Her mother is 62 years old and her father is 65 years old and retired. They are healthy and travel extensively, spending most of their time in Florida. Darlene lives in her parent's home located in a wealthy suburb of New York City.

Vocational Information

Darlene worked for a short time prior to her marriage at age 27. Before that time she took classes at a local college periodically and worked in her father's office part-time. Darlene completed a computer course three years ago and now works as a full-time programmer for a moderate salary. She pays no expenses while living in her parents' home; however, she does buy groceries and presents for her parents periodically. Her parents recently decided to sell their home and move to a condominium in Florida.

Leisure Information

Darlene is very active. She goes out every evening and frequently takes weekend trips. She is very fashion-conscious, often attending fashion shows, and identifies shopping as a major interest. After shopping sprees, she and her friends frequently go to art galleries or the theater. Darlene belongs to a health spa, racquet ball club and country club. She enjoys golf and swimming.

John and Darlene have been introduced to provide a context to examine some of the factors that have impact on the development of their present lifestyles. These include the effect of the environment, sociocultural aspects, local customs and economic implications. All of these factors must be considered to gain an understanding of an individual's current lifestyle, who they are, what roles they have, what they want and expect, and what they need.

ENVIRONMENT

A person's environment is comprised of all of the factors that provide input to the individual. The environment includes all conditions that influence and modify a person's lifestyle and activity level. Environmental considerations vary significantly in complexity. They can be as simple as climate, geographic location, or economic status or as complex as considering the sociocultural aspects of traditions, local customs, superstitions, values, beliefs and habits.

Every individual has two environments that constantly provide input: internal and external. These environments are so closely integrated in an individual's life that it is often difficult to consider them separately. Both internal and external environments must be considered in designing treatment intervention that will allow a person to function at maximum capacity. This coordinated approach is the essence of total patient treatment in occupational therapy.

Internal Environment

One method of separating the internal and external environments is by considering the physiologic feedback provided by the various body systems. This feedback is the body's way of informing a person of his or her ability to respond to the daily requirements of the external environment.

Some common examples of this feedback occur when an individual has not had enough sleep the night before or has eaten something that was not agreeable. Often, there is a generalized feeling of unresponsiveness of the body. This commonly happens before the development of a cold or flu. It can be a temporary condition (such as muscle cramps, indigestion, or premenstrual syndrome), or it can be a warning signal of early symptoms of disease such as diabetes or ulcers.

Moods and emotional states can be considered parts of an internal environment that influence the way a person responds to the external environment. Depressed persons frequently respond more slowly to their environment and may decrease social activities. Some may further restrict the environment by remaining at home.

A person's mood is often the direct result of something that has occurred in the external environment. Grief is an internal reaction that can result from the loss of a loved one through death, divorce, or the termination of a relationship. Euphoria and states of elation and happiness can result from a promotion, salary increase, falling in love, or inheriting money. These moods affect an individual's ability level and daily occupations.

Moods and emotional states can also be totally unrelated to the external environment. Some people complain of loneliness. These feelings can persist even when a person is with a group of people he or she knows. Such individuals complain of shallowness in relationships and interactions, and can feel lonely even in a crowd.

Self-image is another example of previous feedback from the external environment that creates an *internal set* or environment. These internal environments can exist long after the external environment has changed. One can encounter a person who has lost a significant amount of weight and yet still feels "fat" and dresses to camouflage weight that no longer exists. Conversely, others may gain weight and dress as they did when they were thin. Persons who have been demoted from high authority positions or have changed jobs to assume lesser positions may still present themselves as authority figures and dress accordingly. They maintain the same nonverbal body language that they had in their previous status. Periodically one encounters an individual who graduated from college 30 years ago and still wears a Phi Beta Kappa key in an effort to maintain a self-image that was appropriately achieved three decades before.

Phobias are yet another example of adverse internal environments. They are defined as abnormal fears or dreads and are as illustrated in the following case:

Case Study 10-3

Mrs. Anderson. Mrs. Anderson is 45 years old, married, and the mother of two children, aged 13 and 17. Her husband's job as an industrial consultant requires periodic travel for up to four consecutive weeks at a time. He is generally at home one week at a time between trips.

Approximately eight years ago, Mrs. A began to decline social invitations from friends when her husband was at home. She would excuse herself for some minor or nonexistent complaint or say that their time together was so limited that they needed to be alone as a family. Eventually, she reached the stage where she encouraged her husband to attend events without her because of headaches.

Mrs. A no longer liked driving the car. She complained about heavy traffic, crowded grocery stores and rude clerks in department stores. She located a small grocery store that would deliver orders, and she began buying mail-order clothing. Cosmetics and other items were ordered through door-to-door distributors. Her family became concerned and began encouraging her to go for rides or have an occasional dinner out. Mrs. A was very uncomfortable and obviously in a state of anxiety. Finally she simply refused to leave her home.

Mrs. A was exhibiting symptoms of *agoraphobia,* a Greek term meaning fear of the marketplace which, in current usage, refers to a fear of open or public places. In all probability, her agoraphobia had occurred as a result of previous environmental feedback; however, once the condition developed, it then became an internal environment affecting her occupation and effectiveness as a member of her family unit.

External Environment

The external environment is comprised of a number of factors, including climate, community and economic status. One of the most obvious external environmental factors is the **climate.** Some climates are warm or cold for most of the year and offer extremes in temperatures and weather hazards during several months. Many regions experience four seasons. In general, spring and fall are periods of transition. Whereas winter and summer exhibit extremes in weather such as floods, hurricanes, tornadoes, or blizzards. Individual responses to climates and weather conditions vary. Many people dislike the winter months and restrict their activities. It is very common for some people to gain weight during these months and then lose the added pounds when the weather permits them to resume their outdoor activities.

The Effects of Climate on John and Darlene. The impact of winter weather is greater for John than for Darlene. Darlene's work and leisure activities occur within a much smaller geographic area than those of John. Her suburban environment offers a variety of transportation options. The winter months impose more restrictions on John. This period of snow storms and icy conditions usually limits his transportation, which in turn restricts his opportunities for socialization. During severe weather, John restricts his leisure activities to watching television and playing cards, and he frequently gains weight during this period.

Summer also affects John more than Darlene. Although Darlene experiences some changes, these have minimal impact on her activity level. John's farm work requires heavy labor as soon as the soil is workable, beginning with the first sign of spring and continuing well into the fall. He completely changes his leisure, recreation, and social activities, which include playing on a softball team, swimming and meeting with friends.

Case Study 10-4

Special Splint Consideration. A patient living in Georgia was required to wear a basic cock-up splint. During his monthly visits to the clinic, his splint always needed significant adjustments. It was discovered that he would frequently leave the splint on the back shelf of the car. The internal temperature of the closed car in a hot climate was excessive. The splint had been fabricated from a low temperature material, which tended to change shape in the high heat. A new splint was made from a heavier material that would withstand high temperatures, thus solving the problem.

Severe cold can also affect the selection of splinting materials. Some are made of plastic, which can become brittle and shatter on impact in extreme cold. Metal braces and splints can also be very uncomfortable in extreme temperatures. Special attention should be given to lining the splint to protect the skin that comes into contact with the device.

Community

Another important environmental consideration is the type of **community** in which the person lives. There are three basic types of communities: rural, urban and suburban. Each type has different characteristics that can affect an individual's occupations, activities and lifestyle.

Rural communities have small populations distributed over large geographic areas with a somewhat denser population near the town center. Resources can vary greatly in rural communities. Public transportation is often extremely limited or nonexistent. Social activities often revolve around community groups (such as Rotary and Lions Clubs) and socials and dinners sponsored by churches and schools.

Urban communities contrast sharply with rural areas. They are densely populated in small geographic areas. There is usually a variety of public transportation such as buses, taxis and subways, and a wide range of resources are available. Material goods (such as groceries, clothing and furniture) and services (such as car repair and medical care) must be selected from a wide variety of options. Urban areas may still offer activities designed by community members and groups; however, these represent a much smaller component of the overall offerings. There is usually a wide variety of leisure activities to choose from, including theater, museums, dance, galleries, concerts and sporting events. Crowding affords individuals anonymity and privacy in contrast to the rural communities where individuals seem to know each other and come into contact with one another more frequently.

Suburban communities are often a blend of their rural and urban counterparts. They are less densely populated than cities and have larger lots for homes, parks and some recreational activities. Public transportation is somewhat limited but is generally available. Necessary services are available; however, there are fewer options from which to choose than there are in cities. Fewer choices exist for leisure activities compared with those in the core city, and contact with neighbors and other community members is variable.

The Effects of Community on John and Darlene.   John is well known in his small farming community. His neighbors know that he completed college and returned home to help his father. John knows the grocer, auto mechanic, drug store clerk, dentist and physician personally.

Darlene shops and receives necessary services in a variety of places and therefore does not know many of these people personally. She knows the names of two women who work in her favorite boutiques. Personalized service and recognition can be status symbols if deliberately developed.

Economic Environment

The economic environment of the community and the **economic status** of individuals must also be considered. Values and standards vary greatly and affect occupational therapy treatment, as shown in the three case examples that follow.

Case Study 10-5

Susan. Susan was 16 years old when she was diagnosed as having juvenile arthritis, which was affecting her right hand. The rheumatologist referred her to occupational therapy to have a splint fabricated, which would block metacarpophalangeal (MCP) flexion of all four fingers. A variety of splints were presented to the patient and her family. All were visually unacceptable. The patient agreed to wear the "ugly" splint when she was at home, but adamantly refused to wear it in public. Her family supported her in this decision, even though they understood the medical benefits that could be achieved by a regular wearing schedule. The parents requested that the occupational therapist work in collaboration with their local jeweler to design something more attractive.

Working with the jeweler, the OTR designed rings for each finger, which were connected by chains to a large medallion on the back of the hand. The medallion was then connected by chains to a snug, wide bracelet. The design proved to be highly workable, although not ideal medically. The final product was made of 14-carat gold and studded with rubies and pearls. The patient wore it constantly and several of her friends requested similar jewelry. It seemed that the "splint" had become a status symbol in her social group.

Case Study 10-6

Mrs. K. A diagnosis of rheumatoid arthritis had far reaching implications for Mrs. K, a 36-year-old woman employed as a bank clerk in a small community. Weight bearing had become very painful, and a total hip replacement and bilateral knee surgery had been recommended.

Several months before the diagnosis was made, persistent pain and stiffness had forced Mrs. K to give up her job in the bank, even though her salary was important to maintain the family's modest standard of living. She had allowed her health insurance coverage to lapse and was in the process of applying for coverage under her husband's policy when her condition was diagnosed. As a result, she was denied coverage.

Mrs. K was referred to occupational therapy for homemaking training and self-care activities before surgery. The evaluation revealed the need for a variety of adaptive equipment, including a wheelchair and a ramp to access her home. She also needed a commode, as the only bathroom was upstairs. A utility cart would be needed for basic kitchen activities.

When these recommendations were presented, Mrs. K began to cry. She explained that the family had already remortgaged their home to pay for her medical bills and the planned surgery. There was no money for the necessary equipment. She felt that in less than a year she had gone from being a contributing member of society to becoming a burden on her family. She was worried about the effects of financial stress on her husband and her inability to care for their two small children. The mere mention of possible sources of community assistance brought a fresh flood of tears.

The COTA working with Mrs. K had grown up in a small community and knew how important it was for people to maintain their pride and sense of self-worth. She also knew that friends and neighbors would welcome the opportunity to help Mrs. K and others like her who might need assistance. She suggested to the occupational therapist that they contact the local Kiwanis and Lions Clubs to propose the development of a community adaptive equipment bank. She also recommended that Mrs. K be asked to serve as coordinator of the equipment bank, receiving requests from physicians and family members, arranging for purchase and delivery of equipment, and maintaining records and inventory. The occupational therapist approved the plan, which was put into action within two weeks. Mrs. K was pleased to have an opportunity to use her office and managerial skills and to have the use of the equipment until she recovered from her surgery.

Case Study 10-7

Mr. J. Mr. J had recently experienced a stroke with resultant right side hemiparesis and severe disarthria. He also exhibited overt personality and behavioral changes and was very hostile. Mr. J was a very wealthy, prominent public figure. Once he had been medically stabilized, he refused to stay in a hospital room and instead rented a penthouse suite in a hotel across the street from the hospital.

An occupational therapist received a referral to evaluate the patient's functional level and to begin remediation treatment including self-care activities. When seen for the initial evaluation, a male companion was feeding Mr. J a sandwich. Although eating a sandwich is a one-handed activity, he preferred to be fed.

The evaluation began with a discussion of Mr. J's functional level with his companion. The companion explained that he had signed a two-year contract to see to all of Mr. J's basic needs. While providing neuromuscular and other remediation treatments, occupational therapy intervention also included treating the patient indirectly by advising and training the companion in transfer techniques, dressing techniques, and identifying one-handed activities. The occupational therapy assistant was primarily responsible for carrying out this aspect of the program.

SOCIOCULTURAL CONSIDERATIONS

Many communities contain diverse ethnic groups. People from the same cultural background have common traditions, interests, beliefs and behavior patterns that give them a common identity. Frequently these individuals tend to cluster in geographic areas to preserve their customs, values, traditions, and (at times) their native language. The ethnic neighborhood can be viewed as a society within a society. These clusters or environs provide individuals with opportunities for perpetuation of their culture and lifestyles.

Some cultures are *matriarchal,* or female controlled, whereas others are *patriarchal,* or male controlled. The roles and performance expectations of the oldest, middle or youngest child can also vary among cultural groups. In some societies, the number of male children may determine the financial security of the parents in later life.

Customs

A **custom** is a pattern of behavior or a practice that is common to many members of a particular class or ethnic group. Although rules are unwritten, the practice is repeated and handed down from generation to generation. Cultural implications can have a significant impact on designing occupational therapy intervention techniques that enable a person to function at his or her maximum in the specific environment, as shown in the following case study:

Case Study 10-8

Mrs. F. Mrs. F was a 61-year-old Italian woman who had recently had a stroke. Her primary residual deficit was mild, right-sided hemiparesis. Mrs. F was also slightly disarthric and difficult to understand, as her native language was Italian.

When she returned home from the hospital, Mrs. F was depressed, unmotivated, and not interested in beginning any activities of daily living. When cooking activities were suggested, she became very upset and burst into tears. This behavior was discussed with one of her sons, and it was discovered that the entire family routinely gathered at the parents' home for Sunday dinner. Mrs. F greatly enjoyed this custom. She made all of her own pasta and canned home-grown tomatoes for sauce. She did not want her daughters-in-law to bring food or assist too much in meal preparation. Convenience foods and ready-made pastas had never been used, and the suggestion was totally unacceptable to the family.

In occupational therapy at the rehabilitation center, Mrs. F was encouraged to regain her cooking skills, which required some minor adaptations. Her family bought her an electric pasta machine since she was no longer able to knead and roll her own pasta. Her heavy cooking pots were replaced with new, lightweight styles.

Once Mrs. F regained her cooking skills and resumed a role that was very important to her, she became receptive to relearning other aspects of daily living skills.

Traditions

Traditions are inherited patterns of thought or action that can be handed down through generations or can be developed in singular family units; they also may be perpetuated through subsequent generations. Many families develop their own special traditions during holidays, birthdays, vacations, and other occasions.

Customs and traditions may also occur on a daily basis and can be highly individualized. Their origin may be unknown and not related to any particular sociocultural custom or event, as illustrated by the following case:

Case Study 10-9

Mr. W. Mr. W, who is 50 years of age, was admitted to the Veterans Hospital with a diagnosis of multiple sclerosis. He was confined to a wheelchair and exhibited severe weakness of the upper extremities. His wife was 45 years old and they had six children all living at home who ranged in age from four to 16 years.

In occupational therapy, Mr. W participated in dressing activities, bathing and transfer techniques and was actively experimenting with a variety of adaptive equipment that would assist him in returning to his previous employment. Although he was a very quiet, nonverbal person, he seemed highly motivated and always carried through on any requests made as a part of his treatment.

When the occupational therapy assistant suggested that he begin shaving techniques, Mr. W said that it simply wasn't necessary and told the assistant not to worry about it. The COTA reminded him of the accomplishments he was making in independent living skills and pointed out that this was one more activity in which he could achieve independence. He acquiesced and went along with the program to please the COTA. One day, when Mr. W had successfully shaved himself, the COTA asked him if he didn't feel better shaving independently. Mr. W replied that "it felt okay"; however, in his family it was a tradition for the wives to shave their husbands. Mr. and Mrs. W felt that this daily activity reaffirmed their commitment to each other and was a daily declaration of their devotion.

Superstitions

Superstitions can be difficult to identify and define. They can be customs, traditions, and beliefs of a very small population that may be geographically localized. They can also be highly individualized and border on mental or emotional pathologic states. Webster defines them as "beliefs and practices resulting from ignorance and fear of the unknown."[4] They are also viewed as a statement of trust in magic. Superstitions are further defined as irrational attitudes of the mind toward supernatural forces.

It can be very difficult for occupational therapy personnel to deal with superstitions. It may be easy for a therapist or an assistant to point out how "ridiculous" superstitions are and to present facts that disprove such "ignorant" notions. The personal environment, standards, values, traditions and beliefs of the COTA and OTR can, at times, be in direct conflict with those of the patient. Occupational therapy personnel must realize that the ultimate goal of occupational therapy is to return the individual to his or her lifestyle with all of its implications. The following case illustrates this point.

Case Study 10-10

Mrs. C. Mrs. C is an 82-year-old woman who was admitted to the hospital with severe circulatory disturbances in her left leg. This condition resulted in surgical amputation of the lower left extremity.

The patient was referred to occupational therapy for generalized strengthening activities, cognitive stimulation, and reality reorientation. Although she frequently did not know where she was, past memory appeared to be intact. Mrs. C presented herself as a very pleasant person with a warm, personable manner.

During one of her initial treatment sessions it was noted that she wore a small bag of coins tied tightly around her right thigh with several strips of gauze. When the occupational therapist questioned her about this, she explained that the bag of coins "kept evil spirits away" and made a person happy. She elaborated further saying that she had always worn the bag on her left leg, but since the doctors had to remove that leg, she would now have to tie it to the right one. This situation had not been noted during prior medical examinations, as Mrs. C always removed the bag when she disrobed.

Occupational therapy intervention consisted of introducing a six-inch wide cohesive, light woven, elastic bandage, applied lightly on the thigh, with the small bag of coins attached with a safety pin. This solution was accepta-

ble to Mrs. C. She also reported that all of the other family members also observed this practice. Therefore all 12 family members were also instructed in this new method.

Values, Standards and Attitudes

Values, standards and attitudes are other aspects of an individual that develop through environmental transaction and influence lifestyle. These facets of a person's life usually result from feedback received from other people within one's work and leisure environments, as well as from the individual's sociocultural and economic status and self-image. They are very personal and become an important part of a person's internal environment. The presence of disease or injury can be very disruptive and require reassessment of all aspects of an individual's life and lifestyle, requiring some temporary or permanent adaptations. It is important for occupational therapy personnel to use intervention techniques that can be adapted to minimize the stresses that occur when the patient's values, standards, and attitudes are in jeopardy or must be compromised to some extent. Two case examples are presented to elaborate on these points.

Case Study 10-11

Mr. H. Mr. H, a 50-year-old farmer living in a rural community in Indiana, had sustained a nerve injury to his left wrist. When his wrist was maintained in 50° hyperextension, he could perform most prehension patterns and his hand was functional.

All standard splints were unacceptable to Mr. H, who stated that he would "feel like a sissy" and wouldn't wear any of them in front of his friends. The solution was to fabricate a splint from a tablespoon, which was bent and angled to the correct medical alignment. The spoon was then riveted to a wide leather wrist band. Mr. H wore the splint daily and enjoyed joking with his friends that he was "always looking for a meal." This adaptation was the change that convinced the patient to wear the appliance.

Case Study 10-12

Mrs. B. Mrs. B was 60 years old when she had a stroke, which resulted in left hemiparesis. She had slight subluxation of the left shoulder. Shoulder subluxations are very common, as the pull of gravity on the paralyzed or weakened limb frequently causes the ligaments surrounding a joint to stretch and the head of the humerus to pull out of the socket. Hemiplegic arm slings are almost always recommended to prevent this condition. These slings are very noticeable and not very attractive.

The patient was a very well-dressed, fashion-conscious woman of financial means. She frequently met with friends for luncheons and other social gatherings at her country club. Wearing the sling was an embarrassment for her. The solution involved adapting a leather shoulder bag to wear on these occasions. The bag was strong and large enough to support her forearm, and the strap was adjusted to a length that would support the humeral head in the shoulder joint. A wooden handle was attached to the bag, which maintained Mrs. B's wrist in hyperextension and held her thumb in opposition.

Consideration of these individual values and self-images enabled the occupational therapist to use everyday objects to fabricate necessary medical appliances in a form that was acceptable to both of the patients and compatible with their lifestyles.

Each occupational therapist and assistant has values, standards and attitudes that may be in direct conflict with those of the patient, thus making it difficult to work with some individuals as noted in the example that follows.

Case Study 10-13

Mr. S. An occupational therapist was working one-half day per week in a very small, rural general hospital. When she reported for work she found four treatment requests for one patient, Mr. S. Two were referrals from physicians requesting immediate initiation of feeding and toileting activities. There were also memoranda from the Director of Nursing and the Hospital Administrator requesting the same services. Mr. S had been admitted for prostate surgery. He refused to use the toilet in his room, preferring instead a small, rectangular, plastic-lined wastepaper basket.

The patient was seen for an initial evaluation during the lunch hour. The meal consisted of cube steak with gravy, mashed potatoes, carrots, and a dish of sherbet. Mr. S used no utensils; he ate with his fingers and licked up some foods. This behavior, together with his lip-smacking and belching noises, was in total violation of the therapist's standards and values, as well as those of two female aides who cleaned up the food scatterings on the bed.

Limited information was available in Mr. S's medical record. In addition to the problems discussed previously, nursing notes indicated that his behavior was that of a very hostile and angry person. It was difficult to determine whether Mr. S was experiencing mental changes that required psychiatric intervention, whether his behavior was a reflected form of his personal lifestyle, or whether a combination of both was involved. Intake records revealed that Mr. S refused to state his age or financial status.

Since there was no social worker available, the occupational therapist was requested to gather additional information from neighbors and the community. Mr. S was described by his neighbors as an antisocial recluse. He had lived for at least 40 years in a large old toolshed on the back acres of a farm, which was a long distance from town. There had been windows in the building; however, he had covered them with roofing material many years ago. His home had

no electricity or running water. He was always piling up wood and rubbish, so the neighbors felt certain that he had some sort of stove for cooking and heating.

The therapist visited a small grocery store nearby to see if Mr. S bought food there. It was learned that he had indeed shopped there as long as the elderly owners could remember. Mr. S would slip a grocery list under the door and specify when he would pick up the items. He always paid in cash and requested that no females be present when he came to the store. He would talk with the male owner and periodically try new products that he recommended. If the owner's wife or other females were present, Mr. S would slip in the back entrance, grab his groceries, pay, and leave hurriedly. With this information, the therapist made the following changes when she returned to the hospital:

1. A male orderly was assigned to the patient.
2. Mr. S was informed that he could eat in any manner he chose; however, he would have to change his own linen. (He began to cover himself with a large towel when eating and folded it neatly when finished).
3. A portable commode was placed in his room. (He liked it and stated that he had disliked the coldness of the toilet seat and the loud rushing of water. He also disliked two females taking him to the bathroom).

If Mr. S had recently developed this lifestyle, intervention techniques may have been different. When a therapist or an assistant encounters a lifestyle that has existed for over 40 years, it requires different consideration. At times it can be difficult to understand how persons living in the same general environment respond in such highly individualized manners.

CHANGE AND ITS IMPACT

Changes in lifestyles, roles and activity levels occur throughout the life cycle. Normal changes are expected at various ages. For example, a child is expected to walk and talk at a certain age, and a young adult is expected to begin a career when he or she has completed the necessary education.

Changes can be self-imposed or superimposed on an individual. Self-imposed and superimposed changes and their resulting influence on the individual can occur over a prolonged period or they can be very sudden. The length of time and timing of such change have an impact to varying degrees on lifestyles, roles, self-image and activity levels.

Retirement, whether self-imposed or superimposed, is a change that affects most aspects of a person's life. Many professionals are becoming involved in preretirement planning. These programs are designed to help people consider the various aspects of their life and plan ahead. The emphasis is on all important areas, not just financial planning.

Stress

The potential for stress is inherent with any change. Individuals react very differently to what appears to be the same stress situation. People who have explored different environments and adapted to change may have some sense of mastery over their environment. They can recall and apply previous actions and thoughts that either worked successfully or were ineffective. This provides them with more resources and information to plan an action and respond appropriately.

John and Darlene: Follow-up.   Both John and Darlene will be experiencing significant changes in their environment. These changes will effect their activities, roles and lifestyles. John's decision to relocate in Duluth is a self-imposed change. He has given a lot of thought to this decision to move and start a new career. This cognitive planning has prepared him for the changes in his environment, new roles, and a markedly different lifestyle from the one he has established on the farm.

Darlene's future change has been superimposed on her by her parent's decision to move. She must now identify and evaluate alternatives and make a decision. She could locate a place of her own or move to Florida with her parents. These two alternatives offer very different considerations in terms of finances, employment, social status, and activities, as well as the total physical environment.

As these changes occur, they will create stress for both John and Darlene. Individuals who have made significant changes in the past often find that they can draw on these past events in terms of future decision making and adjustment.

Severe Disruptions

Disruptions are sudden changes in a person's environment that require immediate attention and response. They are usually superimposed on an individual. Disruptions can be as simple and temporary as a common cold or loss of a job, or as complex and permanent as a stroke or death of a loved one. Most disruptions are high stress situations for the individual directly affected, and they can also directly affect and cause stress for other persons in the individual's environment.

Case Study 10-14

Michael. Michael, a mentally retarded young man functioning at about a five-year-old level, had a severe disruption when his parents were in an automobile accident. Due to multiple injuries they both sustained and the length of time needed for rehabilitation, it was necessary to move Michael from his home to an institution. Michael's reaction to this abrupt change was evidenced by withdrawal and frequent tantrums. The OTR at the facility visited the parents in the hospital to gain information that might assist in helping Michael to adjust to his new environment. She learned that Michael had particular food preferences and favorite television programs and enjoyed hearing short bedtime stories. Other details of his daily routine were discussed. The therapist then made the appropriate changes in Michael's daily regimen, and Michael discontinued his tantrums and began relating to others again.

Case Study 10-15

John. John was recently discharged from the hospital after his involvement in a tractor accident. The tractor had overturned and his left arm was almost completely severed. John also experienced a head injury and was comatose for five days.

John was seen in occupational therapy for reality orientation, daily living skills, and instruction in stump care. When first seen, he was confused, his speech was slightly impaired, and his left arm had been surgically amputated just above the elbow. John is right-handed.

John was pleasant, highly motivated, and exhibited a good sense of humor. Several of his friends came for regular visits, as did his family. He would show them some of his one-handed activities and talk about what he would do when he got his new prosthesis.

He exhibited much improvement during his five-week hospitalization. John was no longer confused and his speech was almost normal. His stump had healed well, and a prosthesis had been ordered. He became independent in most self-care activities and used minimal adaptive equipment. John and his mother were instructed in stump massage and wrapping techniques. At the time of discharge John needed minimal assistance with these activities.

John's accident had a profound effect on his parents. His father had difficulty accepting the appearance of his son's missing arm and seemed to blame himself for the accident. He became very depressed and cried about his son being disabled for life. John's mother appeared exhausted from the daily drives to the hospital. She seemed to feel burdened with the needs of her son and her husband, who both required so much help and attention.

As John developed his ability to perform self-care activities, his parents were encouraged to attend occupational therapy sessions. They soon began to realize that he would be independent again. John's mother observed some of her son's struggles to learn to perform various self-care activities. As a result, she decreased the amount of assistance she had been providing, offering verbal encouragement and praise instead. After watching John engage in various activities, his father seemed more accepting of his son's disability. He became intrigued with adaptive equipment and spent hours with John discussing devices he could invent. His depression began to subside.

The family minister visited John and also attended a treatment session. He said that the neighbors were working the farm while John's parents were at the hospital. The occupational therapist explained that John would need to be seen as an out-patient three times a week for an extended time. She indicated that this was very difficult and exhausting for the parents, as the hospital was 60 miles from their farm. The minister said that other church members would be happy to provide transportation twice a week so that John's parents could return to their work at home.

Case Study 10-16

Darlene. Darlene had been admitted to a hospital several months ago. She had been cooking when grease caught fire and exploded. She had first-degree burns on the lower left side of her face and neck, the dorsum of her left hand, and distal third of her left forearm. There were possible second-degree burns on the anterior portion of the left glenohumeral area and upper arm.

The patient received occupational and physical therapy on an out-patient basis for exercises and activities to maintain range of motion at the shoulder. The first-degree burns healed very quickly, and the skin was only slightly pink, which was barely noticeable. The second-degree burn areas were healing and would not require skin grafting.

When seen in occupational therapy, Darlene was wearing a scarf draped across the lower third of her face and a long-sleeved blouse. She adamantly refused to remove the scarf due to her disfigurement. She also refused to believe that there were no visible markings on her face and neck. This situation was discussed with her parents who indicated that Darlene was seeing a counselor.

The accident had occurred about six weeks after Darlene had moved to Florida. She was just beginning to explore the area and establish new relationships. Since her release from the hospital, she had refused to go anywhere and stayed in her room when her parents entertained guests. Darlene's parents felt guilty whenever they went out and left her alone. It was also awkward for them to have friends at their home.

The occupational therapist contacted the counselor and recommended a referral to vocational rehabilitation. Eventually, Darlene was encouraged to work part-time and assist a boutique in opening a central office. Darlene convinced them to purchase a computer. She is now a partner in the firm, has her own apartment, and no longer wears scarves or feels deformed.

Case Comparison of Change. In comparing the cases of John and Darlene, it is important to note that John was still at home when the disruption occurred, whereas Darlene had just changed her environment. Darlene had no friends and no job and was not familiar with the area when her accident occurred. The only constant element in her environment was her parents, who were also in the process of change and adjustment to their new surroundings.

John and his parents had a strong support system in their community. The people knew of their problems and offered their help in a variety of ways. Fortunately, John was comfortable with his role in the family, the community, and working on the farm. He had been apprehensive about moving to the city and working regular hours on a new job. He knew what was expected of him in his home environment. He could work toward achieving familiar roles, lifestyles, and activity levels before exploring a new environment.

On the other hand, Darlene was not only adjusting to a new environment, but was also entering a new role with her parents. When she had first moved back home, her parents traveled a great deal. Her presence at home was quite independent of them. They appreciated the fact that her presence made the home look "lived in," and she was also available if anything went wrong. This arrangement had been mutually beneficial. Now she was simply living with them. Darlene's disruption occurred at a time when her stress was paramount in relation to the external environment, and the potential disfigurement was an assault on her self-image and her relationship with the external environment.

John's body image and internal environment was also disrupted. Although he was concerned about his appearance, his values and standards placed a priority on performance. He had made achievements while in the hospital and knew he would be independent again with the prosthesis. Although the changes brought about by John's disruption seemed more severe than Darlene's, both individuals required therapeutic intervention to resume successful performance in their environments and to successfully adjust to change.

PREVENTION

Humans strive to achieve a balance between their internal and external environments. This is an ongoing process occurring throughout an individual's life span. This same principle can be applied to the structure and function of the human body. No body part, system, or organ functions in isolation. Physiologically, the body works to achieve a homeostatic balance among all of its parts. It is of the utmost importance to remember that any change in the structure or function of one part results in a corresponding impact or change of other parts.

At times, the change in the structure or function of a part may have a healthy and positive influence on another part. For example, a person who begins an exercise program may increase the strength and range of motion of a muscle group; improve vital capacity; and increase heart rate, general circulation, and activity tolerance. Changes in the structure and function of a part can also result in pathologic responses of other areas. Such responses are usually referred to as misuse or disuse syndromes. Health care personnel need to be knowledgeable about these syndromes to include prevention techniques in their treatment programs.

Prevention may be defined as taking measures to keep something from happening.[5] It is a global subject that has numerous components, which must be considered. In health care fields these include adequate environmental shelter and safety; preventive health care (such as inoculations and regular medical checkups); a diet that provides adequate nutrients; moderation in the use of alcohol; abstinence from tobacco; regular exercise; and (particularly in occupational therapy) a healthy balance between work, play/leisure, self-care, rest, and sleep activities.

Many studies confirm that activity is necessary to the well-being of an individual. Activity enhances health and promotes mental abilities, while reducing stress. It provides individuals with feelings of self-control and mastery of their environment, which is necessary for self-satisfaction.

Studies have also documented the impact of inactivity on an organism. Complications arising from inactivity are called hypokinetic diseases and are a direct result of inactivity or lack of use of a part. Hypokinetic diseases are more commonly referred to as disuse syndromes.[6]

Disuse Syndromes

Many disuse syndromes are preventable and reversible; however, some become irreversible. Prolonged inactivity without preventive intervention can create disuse syndromes or secondary complications, which can lead to morbidity. When prevention measures are not initiated, these common disuse syndromes frequently become secondary complications that can be more disabling and life threatening than the primary diagnosis or disability.

A primary disability is the presenting diagnosis and the direct result of pathologic change or injury. Secondary complications are frequently created by the primary disability. These complications can be the result of superimposed activity restrictions that occur as a direct result of the disease process or injury. Examples include the patient who must spend weeks in traction due to a back injury, or the depressed, suicidal patient who must be kept under constant surveillance on a small locked unit.

Prolonged disuse is inherent in a multitude of different diagnostic categories. It is important for health care team members to recognize this problem and to initiate appropriate prevention and health promotion techniques. Consider the individual whose primary diagnosis is a stroke with paralysis on one side of the body. If preventive techniques are not initiated within a few weeks, secondary complications can develop, such as bed sores (decubitus ulcers), contracted joints, deformities of upper and lower extremities, urinary tract infections, and incontinence. Mental health may also deteriorate as evidenced by withdrawal, dependence and depression.

The health problems that result in inactivity or disuse of a part are caused by a variety of conditions and demands. Some of these include the following:

1. Pain resulting in a protective response
2. Loss of sensation
3. Enforced bed rest
4. Restricted activity due to a primary disability, such as cardiac precautions or recent surgery
5. Immobilization of a part due to casts or braces
6. Mental disorders that result in activity level changes or self-imposed decreases in range of motion
7. Limited activity due to cultural or vocational requirements

Some restrictions are temporary and resultant complications can be reversed in a short time. A broken arm or leg that is immobilized in a cast may restrict a person's activity level until the cast is removed. Normal function usually returns after a short period of generalized weakness and decreased range of motion. Physical therapy and occupational therapy personnel frequently treat such individuals and assist in reversing any disuse limitations as quickly as possible.

Ten Disuse Syndromes

Most of the disuse syndromes discussed can be prevented by three simple, physical intervention techniques: active exercise, passive exercise or range of motion, and frequent changes in position. These physical intervention techniques will be effective only when combined with psychological considerations.

In the area of psychosocial dysfunction, it is important to provide a variety of activities within the interest area and ability of the patient. Efforts must be made to provide opportunities for decision making and control over elements of the environment. Maintaining communication with family and friends is another important factor. More specific information on the diagnostic categories and techniques outlined may be found in the case study chapters in *Practice Issues in Occupational Therapy,* SLACK Inc.

Prolonged restrictions and permanent changes require specific, ongoing intervention techniques to prevent the following ten most common disuse syndromes.

Decubitus Ulcers. Decubitus ulcers are areas of tissue necrosis (cell death) due to prolonged pressure. The ulcers frequently occur in bedridden and paralyzed patients. They usually occur around large bony prominences such as the trochanter when the patient is in a side-lying position. They can also occur around the ischial tuberosity from prolonged sitting and around the sacrum from maintaining a supine position for prolonged periods.

Prolonged pressure in these areas results initially in a red or blistered area. These areas become discolored or black and eventually the necrotic tissue sloughs off, leaving a deep open ulcer. Decubitus ulcers can be prevented by frequent changes in position and the use of special mattresses and chair pads.

Muscle Atrophy. Muscle atrophy is the diminution of muscle mass due to disuse. The two major types of atrophy are *denervation* and *disuse*. Denervation atrophy occurs when a muscle has lost its nerve supply. This is a normal physiologic reaction to some conditions and is not preventable or reversible. In contrast, disuse atrophy is preventable and usually reversible. This type of atrophy takes place when a muscle has not been contracted for a period of time. The muscle fibers gradually diminish in size and maintain the length required in their position. They lose their elasticity. Volitional contractions can occur as well; however, the involved muscles are usually very weak.

Joint Contractures. Contractures of the joints are brought about when the soft tissue surrounding the joint shortens due to a decrease in range of motion. If a joint is not moved through its full range of motion for a prolonged time, the contracture can be irreversible or require surgical intervention. These are usually referred to as "frozen" joints. Complete contractures do not exhibit increased range of motion, even when the area is anesthetized.

Orthostatic Hypotension. This condition is caused by a rapid fall in blood pressure when assuming an upright position. It is usually caused by blood pooling in the abdominal area and the lower extremities, which is a result of the loss of elasticity of the blood vessels. Persons who have been confined to bed for three or four days frequently experience dizziness or weakness when they first stand up. However, if a patient is maintained in an upright position after a prolonged recumbent position, brain damage and death can occur. People with quadriplegia and other patients are frequently placed on tilt tables and the upright position is assumed by degrees over a period of time.

Phlebothrombosis. This disuse syndrome most frequently occurs in the lower extremities from lack of motion or prolonged positioning. The stasis of blood in the circulatory system can allow the development of a venous thrombosis (vascular obstruction), which can become a pulmonary embolism, an often fatal condition.

Pneumonia. Another complication of prolonged disuse is pneumonia; it is frequently seen in bedridden persons. The decrease in vital capacity leads to an accumulation of fluid in the lungs, which causes congestion. Many persons die of pneumonia as a secondary complication of enforced or prolonged bed rest.

Osteoporosis. This metabolic disturbance can occur with immobilization. When the muscles do not pull on their origins or insertions, the bones begin losing their matrix and excreting minerals, and become porous and brittle. Osteoporosis can be painful and render a person susceptible to fractures. Calcium is the most common mineral excreted by the bone. The abundance of calcium in the system can lead to the development of stones in the urinary tract.

Kidney and Bladder Stones. These conditions can be brought about as the result of disuse syndromes. One causative factor is the overabundance of calcium circulating through the body. This problem is frequently compounded by the high calcium content of hospital diets. The patient who is in a prolonged supine position may have urine pooling in the kidneys and bladder, which encourages the development of stones.

Incontinence. Incontinence is a common complication of disuse from a prolonged supine position. It can be a result of decreased gravitational "push" against the sphincters of the urethra and colon, which, under normal circumstances, elicits sphincter contractions that permit control of elimination of body wastes.

Psychological Deterioration. The condition of psychological deterioration is perhaps the most devestating disuse syndrome. Prolonged inactivity can be catastrophic to some individuals. These persons frequently exhibit loss of appetite, decrease in communication, and lethargy. They appear to have "lost the will to live." The many personality changes that lead to psychological deterioration depend on the individual and range from withdrawl to aggression.

Misuse Syndromes

Any change in the structure or function of a part can result in the misuse and abuse of other parts. While disuse syndromes affect other body parts and systems, misuse syndromes usually occur at the primary site of assault or abuse. Some misuse syndromes develop as a result of leisure activities, some are work related, and some develop in response to a change in another body part.

Complications from leisure activities were observed during the sudden popularity of video games, which resulted in a medical condition commonly referred to as "Atari thumb." This condition is actually the development of tendonitis of the thumb due to excessive use. Tennis elbow is another example of a misuse syndrome.

Work-related conditions are very common. People who install carpet frequently have one enlarged knee. This is due to the accumulation of calcium in the knee that is used to strike the carpet stretch hammer. The quadriceps of the same leg may also be more developed than those of the other extremity.

Functional changes require special consideration. Occupational therapists and assistants frequently work with persons who have difficulty reaching a standing position from a seated position. This condition can be due to the normal aging process, arthritis in the hips and knees, or pain and other medical problems in the lower extremities. Many of these individuals have a "favorite" chair in their home. These chairs are frequently large, overstuffed, and have a bottom cushion that provides support from the sacrum to just behind the knees. These chairs may also support the calves of the lower legs and maintain the knees in 90 degree flexion. This position makes it difficult, if not impossible, for most people to easily assume a standing position.

Persons experiencing this difficulty usually put excessive strain on their upper extremities. They commonly form a tripod pattern with their thumbs and first two fingers and then push on these small joints to lift their body weight. Prevention of this misuse syndrome in the hand can be accomplished by providing instruction in using the entire length of the forearms to bear the body weight. If grab bars are available, it is important for occupational therapy personnel to instruct these individuals not to grasp the bars with their hands but rather to loop the entire forearm around the bar and then pull up.

In addition to analyzing self-care and other daily activities, the OTR and COTA may need to investigate the patient's daily use of tools, appliances and accessories. It may be necessary to check something as simple as a handbag or purse that the individual routinely carries, as these vary greatly in style, size, weight and types of closures.

Mrs. B, the stroke patient previously discussed in this chapter, agreed to use an adapted shoulder bag instead of a sling. When Mrs. B visited the occupational therapy clinic on an outpatient visit, the COTA asked her about the adapted purse. Mrs. B stated that it was effective and added that her husband also appreciated the added convenience of having her carry such extra items as his camera, extra film, maps, and tour guides when they went on their frequent day trips. The occupational therapy assistant instructed Mrs. B to keep her purse as light as possible and suggested that Mr. B purchase a separate carrying case for his equipment.

The examination of the type of purse carried by a person with arthritis can be critical in preventing damage to the joints of the upper extremity. Unfortunately, this consideration is frequently overlooked.

There is no existing list of common misuse syndromes comparable to those for disuse syndromes. Misuse and abuse problems and the potential for developing misuse syndromes need to be identified on an individual basis. These problems and preventive measures are identified through the therapists' and the assistants' knowledge and understanding of the interrelationships of the various body parts and through a thorough knowledge of the components of task and activity analysis as they relate to the individual's values and lifestyle.

SUMMARY

It is much easier for health care personnel to treat arthritis, a hand injury, a personality disorder, a suicide attempt, or an amputee than to treat the *whole* person. The latter requires knowledge and insight about the individual's development, values, lifestyles, environments, self-images, roles, and activities in planning and implementing purposeful and meaningful therapeutic intervention programs.

The goal of occupational therapy is to return the person to his or her environment with the skills necessary to resume previous occupations and roles. Occupational therapy is concerned with the quality of life, which is determined by the individual and his or her environment. The relationship between humans and their environs goes far beyond the simple stimulus and response theory. A total transaction occurs between the individual and the external and internal circumstances that make up the person's unique environment.

To effectively treat a person and not a disability, all members of the profession must know the sociocultural, economic, psychological and physical aspects and view them in relation to the standards, values and attitudes of the patient's total environment. Occupational therapists and assistants are performance specialists who design and implement highly individualized developmental, remediation and prevention programs.

Related Learning Activities

1. Identify some of the customs, traditions or superstitions in your family and discuss how they might affect therapy.

2. Working with a peer, compare and contrast how your plan for therapy might be different in each of the following instances:

Patient Condition	Patient Environment
arthritis	well-to-do matron bag lady
stroke	rancher in Texas accountant in Chicago
depression	Cambodian refugee American suburban housewife

3. Discuss common misuse and disuse syndromes with a classmate or peer. Determine what intervention techniques are likely to be most effective.

References

1. The Philosophical Base of Occupational Therapy. American Occupational Therapy Association Resolution #531, April 1979.
2. Reed K, Saunderson S: *Concepts of Occupational Therapy,* 2nd edition. Baltimore, Maryland, Williams & Wilkins, 1983.
3. American Occupational Therapy Association Council on Standards: Occupational therapy: Its definition and functions. *Am J Occup Ther* 26:204-205, 1972.
4. Guralnik DB: *Webster's New World Dictionary,* 2nd College Edition. New York, Simon and Schuster, 1982.
5. *The Doubleday Dictionary.* New York, Doubleday, 1975.
6. Kielhofner G: *Health Through Occupation.* Philadelphia, FA Davis, 1983, pp. 98-99.

Section III
TECHNOLOGY

Video Recording

Small Electronic Devices and Techniques

Computers

As a profession, we have entered an age of rapid technologic advances that impact on the delivery of occupational therapy services. The use of video recording continues to make new inroads as a tool for evaluation, treatment, patient education, record keeping and leisure enjoyment. The lightweight portability and high-quality picture of today's camcorders have added a new practical tool for occupational therapy personnel. Simple, inexpensive microswitches, easily purchased or constructed, allow individuals to interact actively with their human and mechanized environments in ways never thought possible. This single basic electrical component has afforded patients many new opportunities for achieving greater independence. The invention of the microcomputer and a wide variety of peripheral input and output devices has greatly influenced the profession and the individuals we serve. It has allowed

people with performance deficits to achieve many goals both in occupational therapy treatment and in their personal lives. It has, in many cases, revolutionized our society. The microcomputer has also greatly improved our management and communication systems by greatly reducing the time necessary to collect and process data and produce reports.

It is important for the reader to focus on specific technologies in terms of developing new skills or enhancing existing ones. After content related to basic applications is mastered, one should explore the numerous opportunities for applying technologic concepts in management and system development in health care. As we find increasing ways to use technology in occupational therapy practice, we must heed the words of Dunford who stated, "Traditional occupational therapy skills must be the basis for a practical approach to using technical aids."

Video Recording

Azela Gohl-Giese, MS, OTR

INTRODUCTION

Recent advances in technology have allowed video equipment manufacturers to market systems that are so automated and easy to operate that practically anyone can produce a video product of reasonable quality. This development has allowed occupational therapists and assistants to create ways of adapting the media for individual patients and groups.

This chapter focuses first on the video recorder as a machine. A simplified explanation of the mechanical aspects is presented, and diagrams illustrate the relationships between input and output devices. Next, the use of video recording to provide a historical library is presented. Historically referenced tapes can be of great value to the educator, researcher, and writer, as well as occupational therapy personnel involved in day-to-day treatment activities. Some recordings may "sit on the shelf" for years, whereas others that present education topics to the patient, parent, or family may be used daily. Standard treatment procedures that are used frequently can be taped for use with patients as well as new staff members as a part of the orientation process. A videotape library will be commonplace in every occupational therapy clinic in the future.

The use of video recording as a mirror that reflects an objective view of the subject on camera is then considered.[1] The intent is to provide immediate feedback to an individual or a group as to how they performed or reacted in a particular situation during a specific time interval. Replay of the videotape can assist in recalling the actions that took place as well as the feelings that may be associated with these actions. In a group situation the replay will assist in focusing the group so that the critique will be based on input from everyone. These recordings are generally not cataloged and stored.

Occupational therapy staff members seeking specific, objective feedback on skills such as interviewing or supervising can replay a videotape at their convenience, in privacy if desired. This approach can be an effective way to improve skills. Camera shy people may have difficulty using video for this purpose; however, the fact that the tape can be erased instantly may give them added comfort in using this medium for self-evaluation. It need not be an embarrassing experience.

KEY CONCEPTS

Recording principles

Maintenance and problem solving

Production techniques

Developing an historical library system

Objective recording of behavior

Projective tool applications

Creative uses

Future applications

ESSENTIAL VOCABULARY

Input

Output

Lighting

Portability

Camcorder

Maintenance

Script

Confidentiality

Video feedback

Projective technique

Psychodrama

The fourth part of this chapter describes the use of video recording as a projective tool. Segments of commercial television such as "soap operas" and news broadcasts may be used as a part of the treatment milieu. Psychodrama techniques may be added to tailor the roles of particular characters in the television program to the patient's real life situation. The psychodrama skit may also be taped for later viewing and discussion. Finally, video recording is presented as a tool for creating. The intent is to emphasize the human quality of creativity and encourage the patient to use video for this purpose. Future trends in the creative use of video recording are explored along with the importance of keeping abreast of new technologic advancements.

THE MACHINE

Over the last 20 or more years, video recording has evolved from an amateur's nightmare to a fairly common leisure activity. In the past, it seemed that only a person with a degree in electrical engineering could possibly cope with the technical maze of connecting a video camera, recorder, monitor and microphone system. Today, because of the tremendous advances made in automating video recording equipment, a person who is familiar with a 35 mm still camera and with making adjustments on a commercial television set, may feel fairly comfortable using a video camera and recorder after minimal instruction. There is a standard electrical connection system for operating video equipment. Once this basic system is understood, extra enhancements, such as use of a character generator for titles and dubbing in background music on a second audio channel, can be tried when more professional recordings are required.

The following neurologic analogy is used to provide a basic understanding of the video recording system. Consider the camera as the eye and the microphone as the ear picking up environmental sounds and actions that become **input** and travel via cables, which are the nerves of the system. The cables connect directly to the videotape recorder and store the information on tape just as the brain stores information in memory. When **output** is needed, the "play" button on the videotape recorder is depressed and the recorded information is sent to the television monitor via an output cable. Three basic principles must always be followed when using video recording equipment:[2]

1. The camera and microphone must be connected to the input terminals of the recording unit.
2. Output cables are connected to the output terminal of the recorder and the input terminal of the monitor.
3. When taping a commercial television program, the monitor is providing input; therefore, it is connected to the input terminal of the recorder.

The diagrams in Figure 11-1 show specific connecting patterns for four different uses of video equipment. Either commercial power outlets or batteries may be used.

It should be noted that the camera and the microphones provide input only. When one or both of these pieces of equipment are being used, the "record" switch on the videotape recorder must be turned on to record the information on tape and view it on the monitor. Newer camera models have built-in microphones with a fairly long range; thus the camera cable contains both the audio and video connections. When connecting the various components of the system, it is important to apply firm pressure, but never force. If force seems necessary, it is likely that an improper connection is being attempted. Consult the operation manual for possible errors in the procedure.

The quality of the video recording is determined when it is being produced. There is little that can be done to improve a flawed or inferior recording while it is being viewed on the monitor, no matter how sophisticated the monitor's tuning system may be. Therefore, at the time of recording it is important to check and recheck the functioning of the camera, recorder and monitor. By making a short "trial" tape and viewing it on the monitor, the following common problems can be avoided:

1. Poor color or black-and-white contrast
2. Improper focus
3. Inadequate lighting
4. Inaudible or unclear sound

By checking the monitor for proper contrast and "sharpness" of images, the camera can be adjusted for both focus and level of light. In some environments it may be necessary to use auxiliary lighting. Sound problems can generally be solved through the use of extra microphones and the elimination of background noise such as traffic, air conditioning, and fans. It takes several practice sessions to successfully accomplish all of these tasks and develop the skills necessary to produce a quality tape.

Video equipment in current use is designed for either a VHS or Beta cassette tape format used on a video cassette recorder (VCR), with the VHS type being the most popular. Care must be taken to use the proper size and mode of recording material that fits the specific video recorder available, as the various formats are not interchangeable. For example, a $3/4$-inch videotape cassette cannot be used on a video recorder that is designed for $1/2$-inch tape. Once the correct tape is selected, it is fairly simple to insert the cassette into the machine. When the tape is in place and the camera is connected to the recorder, the recording process may begin.

Lighting

It is important to evaluate the **lighting** in the room where the videotape is to be produced. Before recording a trial tape, the following steps should be taken to assure adequate

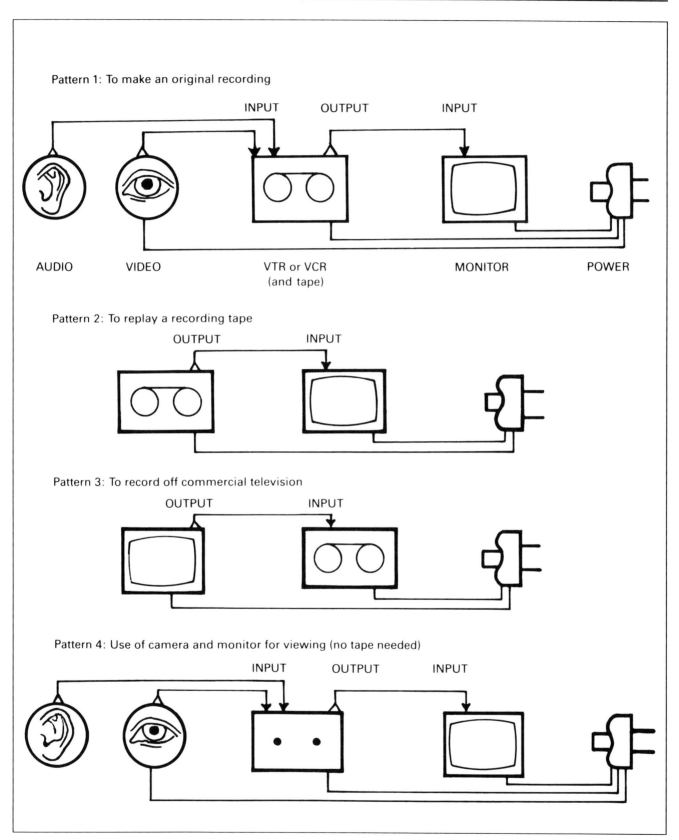

Pattern 1: To make an original recording

Pattern 2: To replay a recording tape

Pattern 3: To record off commercial television

Pattern 4: Use of camera and monitor for viewing (no tape needed)

Figure 11-1. Relationship of input and output equipment.

lighting. The subjects should be positioned so that their faces are not in a shadow. If there is bright sunlight, the camera should be placed so that the light comes from behind. Never point the camera lens into the sun or other bright light, as this can cause damage. Most clinic settings that have fluorescent lighting provide adequate illumination for videotaping. If other lighting is needed, auxiliary lamps can be used to "bounce" light off a wall or the ceiling. Place these lights so that the stands or shades do not appear on camera. Producing an outdoor videotape can be particularly difficult due to the wide range of light and shadow. Camera lens filters may provide a partial solution in this situation. Seek advice from a factory representative or a local audio-visual consultant about which style filter works best on the particular camera you are using.

Other Environmental Considerations

The more isolated the environment selected for making a videotape, the less likely background noise and interruptions will interfere with the production. It is advisable to close windows to help eliminate noise from traffic and aircraft, unplug telephones, and turn off fans and air conditioning units. Post a sign on the door or doors that states "Video Taping in Progress—Do Not Disturb!" Interruptions of any kind can mean that the work must be retaped. When a very professional tape is required, it is best to use a soundproof video studio.

Arrange all furniture and equipment that will be needed in the production to assure that the camera can be moved about the area with ease. Consider the location of electrical outlets to be used for the camera and other video equipment. If the placement of electrical cables is likely to interfere with the tape production, battery power should be used.

Focusing and Timing

The key to good videotape production is focus and timing. Most video cameras have "zooming" power. This literally means that the lens is capable of quickly moving very close to the subject for a close-up view. Many new users of a video camera will overuse this technique, which tends to distract or tire the viewing audience. It is better to try to provide a mixture of varying distances and angles, using the zoom technique occasionally for emphasis or a detailed close-up picture, to help keep the viewer interested in the subject. Record what is being communicated by the subjects both orally and physically as the person may be saying one thing, but body posture or action may be conveying a different or conflicting message. It is important for patients to see such incongruence to develop self-knowledge and to improve communication.

Timing is also essential for keeping the viewer's attention. It is important to maintain a balance; moving the camera too fast will result in the viewer missing the action; moving too slowly may cause the viewer to be bored and some important action may be missed. As you move the camera, keep the motion as smooth as possible. Avoid sudden stops and starts as the videotape will appear jerky when it is shown.

Supporting the camera securely on a tripod allows the camera operator to have both hands free to focus and move the camera smoothly about the room. There is also less danger of dropping the camera or being bumped. The one great advantage of having a small, portable camera is the flexibility of moving quickly into a narrow space or at a specific angle to the subject for a special shot. A tripod does not allow that motion in most cases. The trade-off is safety and smoothness for accuracy and immediacy.

If written material, such as titles, is included in the tape production, focus the camera on each line of print from four to five seconds to give the audience sufficient time to read the message. When in doubt, add an additional second or two. Chances of maintaining viewers' attention are better with too much time rather than not enough. Above all, try to maintain a professional approach and avoid reminding the viewer that the producer was a clever person with a brand new camera.

Portability

The elements of videotaping described to this point are standard, regardless of the brand of camera used; however, there is a great deal of difference in the degree of **portability,** or ability to be moved easily from place to place, among the various models of videotape production equipment. Heavy-duty systems tend not to be moved about too much except on carts made especially for that purpose. Portable video recorder units weighing as little as 25 to 30 pounds come in "packs" that have harness-type straps that secure them to the waist and shoulders in much the same manner as a camper carries a backpack. The lightweight cameras have various types of hand grips and shoulder rests, which provide some added stability. Their disadvantage is that they tend to be easily dropped, bumped, or shaken beyond the normal limits. For these reasons, mechanical adjusting needs to be made on a regular basis to assure proper functioning. Care must be taken to evaluate what measure of use the equipment is to withstand before investing in new equipment.

The **camcorder** is one solution to the portability problem. All functions of the video recording process are combined in one package—camera, microphone, recorder with cassette tape, miniature monitor, and battery power option. The same principles of video production presented previously apply to this video format. Although the camcorder is relatively lightweight and portable, a tripod should still be used for a precision quality production. Figure 11-2 shows a composite model of the camcorder.

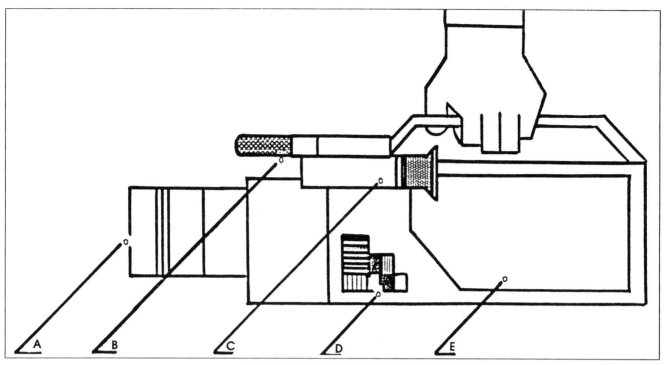

Figure 11-2. Camcorder. A. Zoom lens; B. Microphone; C. Electronic viewfinder; D. Control panel (power, focus, light regulator, fader, record/review); E. Cassette tape holder.

Maintenance and Related Problem Solving

Like any other precision tool, a video camera and recorder require a certain amount of **maintenance** to operate properly. Use of dust covers and storage in a clean area make it unnecessary to clean the vital parts of the equipment before each use. Excess dust can scratch videotape. The operation manual gives precise instructions on specific areas to be cleaned and frequency of cleaning to assure long-term service. For example, if you notice that the picture on the monitor seems "grainy" or distorted, it may be caused by an accumulation of dust and dirt on the recording heads of the video recorder. Follow the operator's manual instructions carefully when cleaning. If this technique does not solve the problem, the distortion could be caused by using a tape that was recorded in a different timing format. For example, if the video recorder being used is designed for two-hour tapes, it will not play a tape recorded in a four-hour format.

It is advisable to document when the equipment is cleaned, as well as when it is sent out for professional repair or maintenance. Information on the replacement of parts and other adjustments should be noted together with costs and may well serve as justification for replacement when necessary.

Videotapes last longer if they are stored in closed cabinets in an area where the temperature is moderate and the humidity is low. It is best to set the tapes on edge rather than flat so that the tape does not become distorted by binding to the edge of the container.

PRODUCTION TECHNIQUES

Developing Scripts

Once the user has made several short video recordings, preferably in varying environmental settings with both group and individual subjects, a taping "layout" or a **script** must be developed to explain exactly how the equipment will be used to maximize the best of its unique qualities in the production.

Initially, one must determine the objectives for using videotape recording: Why is it essential to have a visual record of the situation? Would an audiotape and still photographs or slides be just as effective? If not, then lay out a general plan to determine what equipment is to be used, where it is to be placed, and when it should be moved. Try to anticipate how the events will unfold and generate ideas on possible events so the camera operator knows what is important and what might occur. The latter is a particularly important aspect in the recording of group interactions. Realistically, all group actions cannot be recorded; however, fewer surprises will occur if careful planning takes place before the actual videotaping. The following is an example of a segment of a production script for a videotape on the topic of learning to knit:

Production Title: "Learning to Knit".
Initial Camera Location: Five feet from table and title easel.
  1. Zoom in on title for five seconds.
  2. Film presenter from waist up during introduction.

3. Zoom in on specific pieces of equipment as they are described, then back to presenter.
4. Move camera to the left and behind the presenter to demonstrate "casting on stitches."
5. Maintain this position throughout this segment, using zoom initially.
6. Change camera angle to show one or two students practicing the technique.
7. Move from presenter to students as dialogue occurs.

A videotape on this or other craft techniques can be a valuable aid in student learning. The tape can be viewed at the student's convenience, perhaps in a media center. The program can be designed to allow the student to look at one or two segments and then stop the tape to practice the required skills before moving to the next step. The student may watch the tape again, before a test, to review the material.

It is important to note that the script for the camera operator is different from a dialogue script. The latter reads in much the same way as the script for a play and is used for productions where factual interchange is the primary objective rather than spontaneous conversation. This script should also be prepared in advance and rehearsed with the participants. Once the script is finalized, the camera cues can be added directly to the dialogue pages, the goal being to give the camera operator as much information as possible to ensure a good quality production. Figure 11-3 presents an example of how a dialogue script may be written.

Since activity analysis is such an important aspect of occupational therapy, a student who is absent when this information is discussed can view the tape at a later time, thus gaining information that may not have been recorded in notes borrowed from a classmate.

Editing, Tape Reuse and Tape Transfer

Although it is fairly simple to do "add on" editing at the end of a tape, most individuals who need more sophisticated editing take their tapes to a professional studio, as most health care facilities do not have the necessary equipment to do a professional job.

Videotape can be reused by simply recording over it. As the new material is recorded, the recorder automatically erases the material that was on the tape before. The number of times this can be done successfully depends on several factors, including the original quality of the tape, the age of the tape and the number of times a tape has been used.

Both occupational therapists and occupational therapy assistants can be involved in making videotapes, depending on their individual interests and skills as well as the particular needs of the department. Helpful resouces for information on both the mechanical and production aspects of video recording are listed in the bibliography.

As technologic advances continue to improve the video recording process, new formats will be marketed. Fortunately as part of this development, techniques are available to transfer existing tapes to these new formats. When replacing video equipment, it is important to keep the old recorder until all tapes that are to be retained can be transferred from the old format to the new.

Other General Considerations

Policies for honoring patient's rights of freedom and **confidentiality** (ie, the maintenance of secrecy regarding entrusted information) apply to video recording. Each occupational therapy department should have a written policy and necessary consent and release forms on file and available to patients. The policy should outline the specific instances where videotaping will be used as a therapeutic technique, as well as the conditions under which the tapes are used for other purposes, such as student education. Some facilities require that all patients sign a consent and release form before participating in any video projects, whether used internally or externally by the facility. The right of the patient not to be videotaped must always be respected.

CAMERA CUES:	DIALOGUE:	
4 feet from teacher	Teacher:	"Knitting is frequently used as a treatment modality in occupational therapy. What are the major therapeutic strengths of this activity?"
Move to student A	Student A:	"I think knitting is relaxing now that I've learned how to do it. It might be a good activity for an anxious patient."
Move to student B	Student B:	"I agree, but my field work supervisor said that knitting could be used only in the clinic, where the patients are closely supervised. This surprised me—it looks pretty harmless."
Move to teacher Zoom in on yarn and needles	Teacher:	"While yarn does indeed appear harmless, a depressed, suicidal patient might use it to braid a noose. Knitting needles can be used to inflict personal injury."

Figure 11-3. Sample dialogue script. Production title, *Activity Analysis of Knitting.*

THE HISTORICAL LIBRARY

One of the most common uses of video recording is to make a permanent audiovisual record of the treatment of a patient over time. Due to the complexities of some treatment regimens, a visual record is essential in recording the patient's progress or lack of progress. It is a way of objectively documenting the changes and improvements that have been gained and those that have not. In some pediatric programs, a videotape record is made at regular intervals over several months or in some cases several years. Thus all pertinent details of work with the child are documented. If the therapist's memory fades, the recording maintains a firm image. A written record usually accompanies the tape and serves as a sequential index of the recorded content. The tapes are then cataloged using a convenient library system for efficient retrieval.

The key to the effective use of a videotape library is the accuracy of the index. A good index includes not only the title, producer, and date but also a detailed listing of the location of specific categories and events on the tape. These categories are referred to as "time locations." The critical measure in determining accurate time locations is to check that the timing gauge is on zero at the beginning of the recording session. Once the tape is running, begin a recorded log of the general categories and significant events. Such information will allow the user to locate quickly a particular segment when needed. When viewing the tape again, return the time gauge to zero before beginning. If tapes are frequently used in this way, an automatic time gauge can be purchased.

Occupational therapy personnel are also using videotapes to record evaluation procedures. If the same person is repeating the evaluation, the previous assessment can be reviewed to duplicate the procedures accurately. If a different person is doing the procedure, viewing the tape will help ensure consistency in administering the evaluation.

This video recording technique was used to establish rater reliability while using a checklist of behaviors designed for a research project.[3] A number of videotaped sessions were produced showing an occupational therapist testing children individually. The tapes were then viewed later by occupational therapists who were asked to observe the children being tested and record their observations on the checklist. Using the videotaped programs as part of this research allowed participants in the research project to contribute over time at different locations. They did not have to be present at the actual time or place of the testing. More important, all viewers were observing the same testing situation, thus assuring a more valid research procedure.

Holm[4] describes another use of video recording in which information was taped to be used at a specific time in a treatment program when the patient is ready for it. For example, a patient can view a tape of another patient engaged in an activity. By viewing another patient engaged in the activity, instead of watching a nondisabled therapist demonstrating it, the patient may show less resistance to attempting an unfamiliar or difficult task. A number of different tapes can be available in the clinic for this use. If new tapes are made on different patients on a regular basis, the library will be current and aid in a variety of patient informational and motivational needs. Holm also describes the use of video in providing an orientation for patients who will be having a new experience or feel uncomfortable with attempting an activity. The therapist filmed the environment in which the activity was to take place and then showed it to the patient as a means of "rehearsing" before the actual experience. This technique allowed the patient to visualize where and how to approach the unfamiliar, thus reducing anxiety and even discovering some of the enjoyable aspects of the activity.

A certified occupational therapy assistant (COTA) added another dimension to patient viewing of a videotape on home care programming by engaging the family to watch the same tape. As a result, the family members were less apprehensive about their responsibility for patient care and more enthusiastic about the patient's return home.[5]

Columbia University's program in occupational therapy also produced a videotape about home care programming. The tape consists of assessments used to evaluate levels of function for the elderly, as well as examples of group activities that will assist older adults in accomplishing the developmental tasks of aging.[6]

Another common reason for developing videotapes is for staff in-service or continuing education.[7] The Minnesota Occupational Therapy Association, Continuing Education Committee is building a library collection of videotapes for this purpose. The project was given impetus when the public service department of a local television company agreed to provide free use of their equipment and recording studio. The committee had to furnish the videotape, script and actors. Several videotapes on topics such as feeding techniques and wheelchair adaptations have been completed and are available to therapists and facilities for a modest fee to cover postage and handling. This educational method is particularly helpful for occupational therapy personnel residing outside of metropolitan areas where continuing education opportunities may be less available.

This educational service demonstrates one of the advantages of using video recording rather than 16mm film production. A video product may be produced at less cost and more quickly because the processing time is shorter, requiring only the time necessary to record the tape. The advantage of 16mm film over videotape is that the film provides sharper color distinction. The structure of film may also provide a better slow-motion mechanism because it can be moved forward one frame at a time, a feature not possible with videotape.

The educator in the classroom or the clinic can access many tape libraries nationwide. Often these libraries are found at larger universities, which may furnish catalogs of their current holdings upon request. Usually the tapes are available in more then one format, and the exact type required must be specified when ordering.

A MIRROR OF BEHAVIOR

The video camera is often compared to an eye focusing in on the action. Just as a famous individual, because of his or her degree of notoriety, can detract the viewer from the content of a television interview, the presence of a video camera in an occupational therapy clinic can detract from what would otherwise be spontaneous action. Until the subjects being taped have become comfortable with the camera and less aware of its focus on them, viewing of their actions must be tempered somewhat when interpreting the scene on the monitor.

Add to this predisposition the historical situation for most people in middle-class society; they have watched television for many hours during their lifetimes. The content viewed and the normal viewing environment will surely have an impact on how seriously they view the monitor in a therapeutic situation. If they have maintained a regular schedule of watching certain quiz shows and situation comedies, their participation in a videotaped psychodrama as part of a psychiatric occupational therapy treatment may not make a lasting impression. They may view television as primarily fantasy that can be turned on and off. Such individuals may also "turn off" a display of their anguish or hostility as they view the playback of the psychodrama. For the most part, television is passive. Nothing is required of the viewer except to select the channel and make slight tuning adjustments from time to time. This passive viewing pattern is difficult to alter due to long-term conditioning and the fact that most individuals see television as a form of entertainment.

Cater[8] suggests the presence of an additional conflict for the television viewer who happens to be left-brain dominant in mental development. Such individuals show resistance to taking the television media seriously, as it is a type of media that appeals more to the right hemisphere of the brain. It does not fit into the intellectually analytical thinking of the left-brained viewer. Thus, from a therapeutic standpoint, the right-brained individual may be more adept than one who is left-brain dominant at using **video feedback,** the information received objectively via the camera and tape. If the video feedback can be structured in a sequentially analytical manner using propositional thought, the left-brained person perhaps also will become engaged in using video feedback therapeutically.

A simple measure that helps patients reach a comfort level with this media is to demonstrate how easy it is to erase the tape used in the treatment session. Knowledge of this fact can aid the patient in relaxing and being spontaneous during the videotaping. Although few patients request erasure of a tape, knowing that erasure is possible provides continuing reassurance. Once patients recognize the value of the feedback, their anxiety over the recording is reduced. Engaging the patient in the mechanical control of the video equipment provides a sense of control over what is going to take place in the therapeutic session. The patient who feels in control is likely to make a greater investment in and commitment to changing behavior or risking new behavior. With the availability of instant replay, the patient is able to receive immediate feedback on what effect his or her behavior has in relation to the human and nonhuman environment. They also gain a perspective of how their behavior was seen by others viewing the tape.

Engaging the Viewer in the Results

Although the recording process is basically the same, the reasons for making the video recording and the manner in which the tape is viewed may differ considerably. The following examples of six situations offer methods for actively engaging the viewer in the results shown on the tape.

Example One. The video recording of a staff member or a student who wants to improve a skill, such as interviewing a patient or administering a patient evaluation, may be set up at his or her convenience. Once the tape has been made, the individual can review it at a later time either privately or with a colleague who has agreed to review the performance. By allowing these two options, the individual is able to choose the one with which he or she is most comfortable. The tape does not make any judgments; the person being taped controls how the tape will be used. Once the person has viewed the first taped experience, some confidence will be gained, and the next taping is much easier to accomplish.

Example Two. The complex situation of using video feedback in a group therapy session can be invaluable to the group. The technical aspects of filming should be accomplished with ease and in the most unobtrusive manner possible. Using two cameras and two operators is ideal because it significantly reduces the amount of camera movement. If a second camera cannot be used or operators are not available, consider having group members take turns being the group observer and operating the camera. This alternating of tasks allows the individuals to continue in their roles as group members while also contributing to the collection of objective feedback that will be shared with the group at the appropriate time. Using this type of system frees the group leader to address the immediate needs of the members as they occur. It should be noted, however, that it is best to have a nongroup member operate the equipment. An occupational therapist or an occupational therapy assistant is ideal to run the camera because he or she possesses knowledge of group process and dynamics.

Placement of the camera or cameras should minimize distraction. The type of action to be focused on should also be discussed. Usually the group's action provides clues that may suggest what should be emphasized. Because of the size of some therapeutic groups, it may not be possible to tape all activity and dialogue. Larger groups generate more background noise that may effect the clarity of the sound track. Adding extra auxiliary microphones and a second group observer may assist in providing accurate feedback.

Example Three. One form of video feedback that has been found invaluable to parents is viewing taped therapy sessions of their children. Often parents find it difficult to believe that their child acts differently in an environment away from home. With the help of tapes made over a period of weeks or months, insight may be gained as to how the child is behaving and the degree of progress that is being made to improve inappropriate behaviors. The tapes may also show the parents how specific reinforcement techniques can be used with the child at home. Since progress may be slow or very minimal at times, a tape may provide contrast if viewed again at a later time. Occupational therapy personnel have noted that the use of videotape can be an effective way of obtaining support from parents during the treatment of their child. The University of Colorado School of Nursing has developed videotaped "packages" to help parents, families and professionals who care for handicapped and at-risk infants. These include six training tapes for use on home video cassette recorders, accompanied by self-instructional lessons.[9]

Example Four. Video feedback may also be used to motivate patients to make behavioral changes on their own behalf. Patients who experience seizures or have behavior disorders may be appropriate candidates for this approach, as they are unable to control themselves and are unaware of what is happening during an episode. By viewing the specific event on videotape with a staff member present for support, the patient can gain insight into what is happening. Patients may be more willing to cooperate with the staff in taking the prescribed medication or attending the group therapy sessions that are often so uncomfortable for them.

Example Five. The use of the video camera and monitor without tape can be of great assistance in presenting information to a group of people, particularly when the content being emphasized requires close-up viewing for comprehension, and a permanent record of the material is not necessary. When demonstrating how to use small tools such as needles, be sure to focus the camera on the detail so that each member of the audience can see an enlarged view of the proper technique. This method is effective for teaching students the detailed steps in beginning or ending double cordovan leather lacing, for instance. It also could be used to show a group of patients with hemiplegia how dressing techniques can be adapted to the use of one hand or the best methods for paring vegetables unilaterally. Recording on tape may occur at the same time as the viewing, but, as stated earlier, it is not essential unless a permanent record is needed.

If the room being used is too small to accommodate both the audience and the subject and equipment, the camera and subject can be placed in a smaller room, and extension cables can be connected to the monitor or monitors in the larger room.

Example Six. Whereas some people are camera shy, others enjoy being filmed, finding it stimulating and energy generating. This increased patient energy can be used to advantage by filming the patient when he or she is exhibiting appropriate behaviors. Occupational therapy personnel must structure the experience so that the patient does not become overstimulated and lose self-control.[10] Later viewing can serve as a reinforcement and, in many cases, can enable the patient to gain greater confidence and self-esteem in attempting the unfamiliar. Use of such a reinforcement technique can help many to live more enriched lives.

A PROJECTIVE TOOL

In contrast with other aspects of videotaping, when emphasis is placed on more subjective aspects of the medium, the tool may become an effective **projective technique**. Projective techniques may be defined as activities and methods that provide information about patients' thoughts, feelings and needs. As in finger painting and clay modeling, videotaping is pliable, leaving room for personal interpretation. At least three facets of video recording may be a part of a projective technique: soap opera, documentary and psychodrama.

The first and one of the most common video projective tools is the commercial television soap opera serial. This program can be viewed on a daily basis, or prerecorded and shown at a time that is more therapeutically appropriate. It is essential to structure the viewing and discussion so as to involve the patients in an active manner. The highly defensive person may assume an attitude of being passively entertained and be unwilling to become involved in the projective exercise.

The viewing of the program can be structured by providing the group members with carefully constructed questions in advance. Questions may focus on a particular role being portrayed or the patient's reactions to a particular event or situation. One of the advantages of prerecording the television program is that a significant segment can be replayed quickly. This technique aids in uncovering emotional material that some patients may not wish to acknowledge by insisting they do not remember what was being depicted or said. Once the discussion has covered the specific content, the next segment of the program can be viewed. The primary objectives in using this method are to explore the roles and situations the patient identifies with, support any insights gained, and enable the patient to risk a change in behavior.

The plot of the soap opera may play as important a function in the projective process as the identification of a particular role by the patient. When the patient views the program on a regular basis, the questions used to structure the experience may direct the focus to how a situation developed and what actions were being taken to alter the results, which may be healthier for the people involved. The patients may be willing to describe attempts that they have made in similar situations and discuss the degree of personal satisfaction gained from this action. In other instances, the patients will take this new information or approach and apply it to similar situations in their own lives.

By having the entire group watch the same video action, much can be learned by noting the varying perceptions of the individual group members. The leader needs to assure all members that all perceptions are acceptable and that no moral judgments will be made as to the rightness or wrongness of their perceptions. It is helpful to the group to see how differently a given action can be perceived. Gaining an appreciation of this fact may allow viewers to expand their knowledge, their communication skills, and their sense of self-worth.

The use of video as a projective technique relies heavily on the cognitive ability of the viewer. However, the technique may be adapted to various levels of maturation and functioning by the questions formulated by the OTR and the COTA who may serve as co-leaders. This adaptation begins with the careful selection of the program to be viewed, the questions to be addressed, and the methods for processing the patients' projective reactions throughout the discussion. There is no substitute for effective group facilitation on the part of the therapist and the assistant. Neither the viewing of the video nor the questions asked can, in and of themselves, bring about a therapeutic experience.

Psychodrama, a technique in which patients dramatize their daily life situations, has proven to be an effective adjunct to soap opera viewing. A patient who has just viewed a particular scene may wish to personalize it by requesting the special fellow group members to play roles. The psychodrama is also videotaped and replayed for discussion. When this method is used, patients are often more attentive and curious about viewing themselves and their personal vulnerability, rather than watching a professional actor or actress on the monitor. This curiosity is a part of assessing body image and self-image, as well as congruency and incongruency. It provides another example of how video can serve as an effective projective tool.

A second format produced by commercial television and useful to occupational therapy personnel is the news or documentary broadcast. Although the technique used is similar to the one used with a soap opera, the content of the news is more conducive to helping the patient relate to the world at large rather than being solely occupied with one's inner self. It is advisable to create a degree of structure to assist the patient in meeting the main objective of relating to the societal realities presented through discussion of current events. The use of predetermined questions or a viewing guide outline encourages involvement in both viewing and discussion. Observing the patient's responses to the news program can provide information relative to cognitive and affective levels as well as values. Such observations of responses, together with other information, may serve as measures of appropriate adapted behavior. It also may be a way of determining whether a patient is approaching the time of hospital or facility discharge.

A TOOL FOR CREATING

A vital part of most occupational therapy programs is facilitating the patient's needed behavioral changes. The key to making these changes in behavior is the internal motivation of the individual. Creativity is individual and requires a certain freedom of space and time. When the elements of change and creativity are combined in treatment planning, the patient can be involved in the therapeutic process. Through such involvement in a creative endeavor, verbal and nonverbal communication takes place among the patient, the activity and the therapist.

Occupational therapy personnel are often challenged to introduce activities that will motivate the patient to become actively involved. Creative activities are attractive to many because they offer the creator total control of the materials used as well as a tangible product. If external limits are imposed, creativity can be stifled or lost.

Using the activity of making a videotape as a medium for creative expression may communicate information about how the patient sees the world. The impressions of a paraplegic individual who will be in a wheelchair for the rest of his or her life can be very different from those of a neurotic patient who has many unresolved societal and environmental fears. The simplicity of operating many types of video equipment makes this activity feasible for most age groups except the very young. Although staff instruction and supervision are generally required, once initial learning has taken place, the individual can often proceed with a fairly high degree of independence, focusing energy on the creative process and product rather then on the equipment. When the videotape is completed, it may reveal significant information about the patient that can be used as a communication tool to affect the behavioral changes needed to achieve a more productive and meaningful life.

Goldstein[11] describes the use of video production by individuals and groups. The staff members served as consultants in the use of the equipment and provided structure in the activity process as need arose. The communication that resulted during the production of the video recordings provided important information for therapeutic intervention. Each patient was experiencing a different level of self-confidence; some were intimidated by the equipment, whereas others wanted to control the camera. Several of the adolescents in this group were able to use the taping experience to better adapt to the treatment institution and eventually make some behavioral changes. The staff also gained insight into some hospital procedures that were improved as a result of this treatment project.

An elderly population that may not have "grown up" with television increasingly depends on it to meet social needs. The Mount Sinai Medical Center received grant funding to assist in addressing the problem of isolation felt by the elderly, such as those living in an apartment complex in East Harlem.[12] By means of a cable television system, each resident's television set was connected to a service that accessed an unused channel exclusively for the tenants in the 20-story high-rise apartment building.

The grant program provides a number of television services, one of which is resident-produced programs. Residents were involved in the overall program early in its development by videotaping group discussions about the living conditions and social activities of the apartment complex. The initial shyness of some participants was overcome, and soon about 100 residents had appeared on camera. It should be recognized that it often takes longer for the elderly to become comfortable with handling the equipment, as they did not have exposure to this technology at a young age.

One group project featured several residents demonstrating their favorite recipes, and another focused on discussion of growing up in early America. As involvement increased, so did the number of residents viewing the special channel. By becoming regular viewers, many also participated in the health care program offered under the grant sponsorship. This program was designed to reduce the health care costs of the elderly through televised and other mass media health care education.

During the next stage, resident involvement was individual. Because videotapes featuring the elderly were not that readily available for rent or purchase, the taped programs were designed to show individual residents engaged in interviews, leisure time activity demonstrations, tenant news broadcasts, and a health tips program. Once the recording was made, the resident could watch it in the privacy of his or her own apartment. Residents could also visit the studio during the recording sessions.

The elderly have many lifetime experiences to share, and this sharing enhances the quality of their life within their environments. Video recording provides a vehicle that the elderly can use to communicate to others the social riches and skills they have gleaned throughout their lives.

The use of video recording for creative purposes need not be restricted to patient or client populations. This media has great potential for the student in the classroom. Many educators who previously required that all assignments be prepared in either an oral or written form are recognizing the value of making a videotape. Since increasing numbers of curricula have access to video recording equipment, students may be given the option of making a videotaped presentation as a creative approach to completing assignments such as case studies or research projects.

Case study video productions may dramatically contrast normal and abnormal behavior and conditions. Role plays may be used if actual patients are not available to participate. The effective production and use of a short, ten-minute video presentations can often convey a stronger and more accurate message than a 10- or 15-page paper.

Researchers are finding that videotape is a valuable method for documenting their findings. This medium has helped to demonstrate specific research methods and assists those conducting research to duplicate previously completed studies. Information that may have been overlooked in studying the written research report is often found when the video recording is viewed.

FUTURE TRENDS

As the communication industry makes even more rapid advances, technology continues to have a strong and everchanging impact. For example, in the past ten years competition in the marketplace has caused the demise of the Beta format for videocassettes and the videodisk system. What has emerged is the VHS video cassette format, the camcorder, and a "sleeper"—the video laser disk system. The technology for recording video laser disks is not yet available to the general consumer, but it will soon be in great demand as the process doubles the video resolution, producing a much sharper image, and it has superior audio reproduction.

In the not too distant future, the increased development and expansion of video technology will provide the general population with many new services that are seen now in their early stages of development at mass media and technology fairs. For example, communication systems for every household may include video-telephones connected directly to frequently used services such as the bank, supermarket, department store, and primary health care provider. When considering the latter, it is feasible to predict that the annual physical examination by a physician may be conducted in the privacy of one's home by means of a combination of video, telephone and a microcomputer system connected to a health center. Medical history, current symptoms if any, and other pertinent data can be entered into the computer. Simple electronic devices will automatically record temperature, heart rate and blood pressure and interactive video will allow the individual to talk with the physician. If additional diagnostic tests or services are required, the monitor will display these along with times they can be scheduled, thus automatically making appointments and printing a list of them for the individual.

The home health care delivery system may be dramatically different in the future. For example, occupational therapy personnel could gather some screening and evaluation data through a computerized questionnaire and an interactive video system that would allow discussion of work, play and self-care skills and problems. The individual could move a small video camera about the house that would assist the occupational therapist in making an initial evaluation of the environment. Other health professionals will also be using video techniques and "video visits" as a supplement to actual home visits. Such measures should ultimately result in reduced health care costs and increased efficiency in service delivery.

As more and more families find that economic pressures require both parents to be employed, the responsibility for day-to-day child care will be placed in the hands of people other than the parents. As this trend increases, young parents are increasingly concerned that they do not have sufficient influence on their children during their formative years. Occupational therapists and assistants may become much more involved in the well community in the areas of normal child development and child care. Their services could include the use of videotape and computer programs that address topics such as the roles of parents and ways to develop "quality time" activities with their children. Programming may enable the parents to view the current relationships they have with their children and contrast them to other approaches and options. This technique may provide one method to individualize the child-parent relationship and offer resources when problems occur.

Another aspect of child development that could be addressed is the lack of quality commercial television programming for the toddler and preschool child. There is a good market for occupational therapy personnel to apply their knowledge of child development and related developmental life tasks and activities to create new programs. Programming that engages the child in active viewing and learning, some-

what like that presented on public television, is needed. Adding a parent education and interactive video discussion segment to each presentation would allow both the parents and the child to gain from the viewing experience.

The development of sophisticated satellite relay systems for video signal transmission has aided in the advancement of space science. It has made a particular impact on mass media coverage of events worldwide, which are presented regularly to the public. Of equal importance is the way this technology can be used to improve the quality of life for the handicapped. Resourceful individuals asking the question "how" will continue to find new applications when assessing individual patient needs.

SUMMARY

Each of the functions of video recording described can play an important role in the delivery of occupational therapy services. Assessing the patient's situation, treatment planning and implementation, reevaluation, and discharge planning provide numerous opportunities to use this medium. The ways that video recordings can be used—as an historical reference, a spontaneous feedback mechanism, a projective instrument or a creative experience—all address the components of the occupational therapy process. The examples of specific uses of video recording are intended to challenge occupational therapists and assistants to adapt the techniques to fit the needs of the populations they are serving.

The future of video recording applications for occupational therapy is virtually unlimited at this time. As technologic advances are made, it is imperative that members of the profession seek this new knowledge and develop the skills necessary to help the physically and emotionally handicapped to maximize their potential and improve their quality of life.

Related Learning Activities

1. Discuss some of the positive and negative influences on patients' needs when using video recordings.

2. What are some of the problems inherent in using video equipment? What preventive maintenance measures can be taken to eliminate these problems?

3. Outline factors to be considered when deciding whether an occupational therapy department should purchase new video equipment.

4. Plan a video tape production for the purpose of orienting physicians, residents and interns to the goals and objectives of occupational therapy. Outline all of the taped segments that should be included and write a script to be used with each.

5. Practice using a camcorder or other video camera to make a short film. Have someone experienced in this medium critique your work.

References

1. Fletcher D: Video: Is it too technical for occupational therapists? *Br J of Occup Ther* 30:272-274, 1987.
2. Lewis R: *Home Video Makers' Handbook.* New York, Crown, 1987.
3. Bauer BA: Tactile sensitivity. *Am J Occup Ther* 31:357-361, 1977.
4. Holm MB: Video as a medium in occupational therapy. *Am J Occup Ther* 37:531-534, 1983.
5. Rudolph M: Lights! Camera!—OT collaboration produces video for stroke patients. *OT Week* (February 16): 16-17, 1989.
6. Miller P: Life skills video produced at Columbia U. *OT Week* (May 6): 3 1986.
7. Milner N: Rehab foundation's videos are aids for OTs. *OT Week* (May 21): 12-13, 1987.
8. Cater D: The intellectual in videoland. *Saturday Review* 12: 12-16, 1975.
9. Smith A: Videos instruct care of at-risk infants. *OT Week* (July 23): 6, 1987.
10. Heilveil I: *Video in Mental Health Practice.* New York, Springer, 1983.
11. Goldstein N: Making videotapes: an activity for hospitalized adolescents. *Am J Occup Ther* 36:530-533, 1982.
12. Wallerstein E: Television for the elderly—a new approach to health. *Educational and Industrial Television* (April): 28-31, 1975.

Small Electronic Devices and Techniques

Mary Ellen Lange Dunford, OTR

INTRODUCTION

Patients with severe physical handicaps and multiple disabilities often have limited interaction with others and with their environment. Modern technology and advanced technical aids have revolutionized many areas once restricted for persons with handicaps. Powered wheelchairs and adapted automobiles provide independent mobility. Communication aids allow independent oral and written communication. Environmental control units offer access to the operation of lights, radios, coffee makers and other electrical appliances. Sophisticated instructional devices for teaching educational skills to the severely physically and cognitively disabled are now available.

Technologic advances have provided versatile opportunities for the disabled to exercise control within their environment, to live and work semi-independently, to communicate, to learn, and to be constructive, contributing members of the community. Technology has created new avenues of therapeutic intervention for health care professionals and educators who work with the handicapped. The use of electronic aids is a relatively new phenomenon in occupational therapy. It presents a challenging treatment modality as well as a valuable evaluation tool.

One of the electronic components being used to adapt devices for the handicapped is the **microswitch.** A microswitch is a small on/off lever switch. When combined with the appropriate circuitry, it can be used to replace common on/off switches found on battery-operated devices such as toys and tape recorders. Instructions for the construction and therapeutic use of a Plexiglas pressure switch operated by a microswitch are described later in this chapter.

KEY CONCEPTS

Evaluation process

Selection of control site and switch

Switch effectiveness factors

Interface and assistive device selection

Basic technical procedures

Specific switch construction techniques

Safety precautions

Treatment applications

EVALUATION PROCESS

Traditional occupational therapy skills must be the basis for a practical approach to using technical aids in treatment sessions. An assessment of each patient and his or her individual needs is essential and the first step toward incorporating electronic devices into the practice of occupational therapy.

A patient's needs can first be assessed through a brief and informal interview with the patient and his or her family. An interview will identify the needs and establish objectives to be accomplished with microswitch technology. For instance, a patient with a spinal cord injury may want a switch fabricated to operate a microcomputer or an environmental control unit, whereas the parents of a handicapped child may want to have their child use switches to play with toys that he or she is not able to operate with conventional switches.

The patient evaluation also includes an assessment of physical limitations and functional abilities such as mobility, communication and object manipulation skills. Sensorimotor components that include range of motion, muscle tone, reflex integration, gross and fine motor coordination, developmental skills, strength, endurance and sensory awareness are also assessed. Other aspects of the evaluation include the cognitive and psychological areas such as intelligence, cognitive development, motivation and attitude.

Positioning and seating considerations for the patient are important in the evaluation process. Secure and stable positioning is necessary to enhance learning and skill development.

Patient evaluations should be a team effort. Input from other health and educational professionals working with the patient can provide valuable information and insight. Ideally, a team should include an electrical engineer or a rehabilitation engineer to provide consultation about electronic aids, devices and systems. While this practice may be rare in most occupational therapy work settings today, engineers will play a major part in the therapeutic application of electronic technology in health care professions in the immediate future. Currently, it is recommended that the registered occupational therapist (OTR) be responsible for the overall evaluation procedures, whereas either the therapist or the certified occupational therapy assistant (COTA) could be responsible for the fabrication and use of electronic devices in treatment sessions.

Control Site

When the evaluation of the patient is completed and it has been determined that a microswitch adaptation is an appropriate measure, a control site for switch activation must be selected. A control site is defined as an anatomic site with which the person demonstrates purposeful movement.[1] The location of control sites can be divided into three general anatomic areas: the head and neck, the trunk and shoulders, and the extremities.

Individual control sites from the head and neck include the head, chin, lips, tongue, mouth, eyes and isolated facial muscles. The trunk and shoulders, when used as control sites, offer gross movements such as rolling; lateral tilting; and shoulder elevation, depression, retraction, and protraction. Specific control sites for the extremities include elbows, arms, hands, fingers, legs, feet and toes.

Each site being considered for switch activation is assessed for range of motion, strength and ease, and amount of control. Once the site has been chosen, the method of activation is determined. The **method of activation** is defined as the movement or the means by which a control site will activate a switch.[1] For instance, elbow extension, lateral head movement, or some type of external device such as a headstick or a mouthstick may be used.

Selection of a Switch Control

Commercial and handmade switches can be extremely simple or highly complex. Switches vary greatly in their versatility. The following are some of the general characteristics to consider when choosing a switch: feedback, weight, size, shape, safety, mounting and positioning, stability, durability, adaptability, portability, reliability, appearance, simplicity, warranties, and availability and ease of part replacement.

Three types of **feedback** are provided from a control switch:[1]

1. *Auditory feedback*—the noise the switch makes when it is activated
2. *Visual feedback*—the movement of the switch when it is activated
3. *Somatosensory feedback*—the texture of the surface of the switch, the force required to activate the switch, and the position of the patient's body when the switch is operated

The feedback provided can enhance training and the patient's successful use of the specific switch.

The weight and size of a contol may also need to be considered. Small, lightweight controls are easier to mount and to transport from place to place. Large and heavy controls can be awkward, but they also offer the advantages of having more surface area, thus requiring less motor precision for activation. These larger switches might be used by children with cerebral palsy.

Safety is a critical factor in the use of switches. They *must* be both physically and electrically safe to operate. Physical safety refers to the materials used to make the switch. Sharp edges and rough materials that irritate the skin must be avoided. Electrical safety is not a significant concern when the switches are connected to low-voltage, battery-operated toys and devices; but it is a concern when they are connected to commercial electrical outlets such as those found in the home or treatment facility. When using handmade switches with electrical outlets, it is important to be sure they are properly grounded. An electrical or rehabilitation engineer should check the switch, the mounting, and the grounding before using it with a patient. If the patient drools frequently, a common problem with children, be sure to keep the switches well covered or mounted in a position that will prevent them from becoming wet.

Mounting and positioning of the switch are as important as the positioning of the patient for the most effective use. Frequent documentation of positions and mounting techniques used during the assessment can be useful during later training sessions. Specific patient responses such as spastic movements also should be recorded, as they may interfere with the switch placement.

Stability and **durability** are also important characteristics to consider. A switch must be sturdy and able to withstand reasonable use. In some instances, modifications will need to be made to protect the switch. A switch that is adaptable can be modified as the patient's needs change. This is especially important when working with children as they grow and change.

The degree of portability of the switch is another important consideration. If a patient operates several devices or uses the switch in different seating arrangements, the switch may need to be moved from one place to another, or multiple switches may need to be constructed.

A switch must work when the patient needs it. To help ensure reliability of the switch, standard and easily replaceable components should be used in constructing handmade controls. It is a good idea to make a second switch for use as a "back up" in emergencies.

The physical appearance of a switch is an important element for many patients. It should be cosmetically pleasing and not overly noticeable. Handmade switches should be as simple as possible and not "over designed." Consider warranties and the availability of repair services for commercial switches used.

Evaluation of Switch Effectiveness

Technical research documents the need to evaluate the **effectiveness** and **efficiency** of a switch.[1] Evaluative measures include the speed of response, accuracy of response, fatigue and repeatability.

Speed of response can be assessed related to two performance components: tracking time and selection time. **Tracking time** is the amount of time needed for a patient to move from a resting position to activation of the switch. **Selection time** is the time needed to operate two switches or two functions of a switch. An example would be the amount of time required to activate a dual switch system for a Morse code communication device. Special computer software programs that come with an "adaptive firmware card" are available that will assist in tracking of progress.

Accuracy of response is estimated from the percentage of errors and correct responses recorded during the tracking and selection times. These percentages and the speed of response provide crude estimation of the degree of accuracy. Poor speed or accuracy are generally related to one or more of the following factors:

1. Switch feedback
2. The weight and size of the switch
3. Positioning of the individual
4. Mounting and positioning of the switch
5. The individual's inability to respond and manipulate the switch

Reevaluation, making the appropriate modifications, and monitoring are necessary to improve the patient's performance.

Fatigue is assessed by making comparisons between the speed of responses and the accuracy percentages recorded at the beginning of a training session and at the end of the session. **Repeatability** refers to the ability of the patient to repeat the performance over a specific period of time. It can be assessed by making comparisons between the speed of responses and the accuracy percentages documented at different training sessions over a designated time period.

Case Study 12-1

The following case study illustrates the use of evaluative measures to select a switch for a boy with cerebral palsy, a spastic quadraplegic. An initial interview with his parents identified the child's need for a microswitch. The parents wanted a means for their child to communicate, to play with toys, and to have some control over his environment.

Since the child attended a public school, various evaluations were administered by speech, psychology, education, and physical and occupational therapy personnel. The child was nonverbal with normal intelligence. An occupational therapy assessment indicated severe physical limitations. Increased muscle tone and neurologic impairment significantly delayed motor development. The patient lacked functional use of his extremities, and trunk and head control were very limited.

The child was positioned in a customized seating system built by a local carpenter. His head was chosen as the control site for the switch. The patient had minimal side-to-side head movement, and thus head turning to either side was determined as the method of switch activation.

Two commercial microswitches (round pressure type, DU-IT Control Systems Group, Appendix D) were chosen as the most desirable. They were lightweight, small in size, easy to mount, durable, and provided a "click" for auditory feedback. Mounting was accomplished by gluing pieces of Velcro to the back of the switches and attaching strips of counter Velcro to the headrest of the child's wheelchair. The switches were positioned so that as the child turned his head to either side, his cheek bone brushed against a switch and activated it.

The switches were interfaced with two battery-operated toys and tracking time trials were taken for each switch. The first four trials required 30 to 35 seconds for each switch activation. Selection time, the time needed to operate both switches, was approximately 95 seconds. Accuracy of response (the correct number of switch activations) was 60% (six activations in ten trials) for the switch mounted on the right side. The switch mounted on the left had an 80% accuracy of response. Speed of response increased and accuracy of response decreased after the first four trials, indicating that fatigue interfered with performance.

On the basis of this information, adjustments were made in the position of the headrest angle, and the position of each switch was changed slightly. Records of speed of response and accuracy percentages were compiled during the next six treatment sessions. Speed of response decreased and accuracy increased, indicating that the switches appeared to be working efficiently for the child.

Repeatability was seen as the patient was able to improve and repeat his best performance level over several weeks. Eventually, the child was able to use the two switches to operate a computer, an environmental control unit, and a Morse code system for written communication.

Selection of Interfaces and Assistive Devices

Completion of the evaluation process should result in a recommendation for a switch that can be operated efficiently by the patient, based on performance abilities and limitations. Assistive devices and switch interfaces are determined after the switch has been selected, and the patient has been trained to use the switch.

The operation of electronic assistive devices requires the use of switch interfaces. **Interfaces** are electrical circuits that connect switches to the assistive devices. With the appropriate interface, switches can be used to operate microcomputers, environmental control units, communication systems, and battery-controlled devices.

Various interfaces may be purchased through manufactur-

ers or handmade interfaces can be fabricated. Purchasing controls for assessment and training can be expensive, as numerous products are available, and it is difficult to know exactly what to buy to get started. When doubtful about purchasing a particular switch, it may be beneficial to make one first for experimentation. A resource list of supplies, equipment and related information appears at the conclusion of this chapter.

BASIC PRINCIPLES OF ELECTRICITY

Electricity needs a pathway of circuits to conduct energy. The pathway of circuits for the operation of battery-operated devices consists of a power source (the batteries); an on/off microswitch; and the toy, light, tape recorder or other device.[2]

When the microswitch is closed or turned on, it completes the electrical pathway and allows the electricity to flow from the battery to the device, thus turning it on, as illustrated in Figure 12-1. When the microswitch is open or off, the electricity is not allowed to flow from the battery so the device is not turned on, as shown in Figure 12-2.

To construct a Plexiglas pressure switch, three basic electrical components must be purchased: the subminiature microswitch, the subminiature jack, and the subminiature plug. The subminiature microswitch is the on/off lever switch, and the subminiature jack and plug are the two counterparts that make up the electrical connection between the switch and the interface. Either subminiature or miniature jacks and plugs can be used; however, the different sizes are not interchangeable and must match in size to fit together correctly. Subminiature components are not as readily available as miniature parts. It should be noted that when using a tape recorder, the subminiature plug will fit directly into the remote control jack on the recorder, and an interface is not necessary. Detailed instructions for making a switch will be provided later in this chapter.

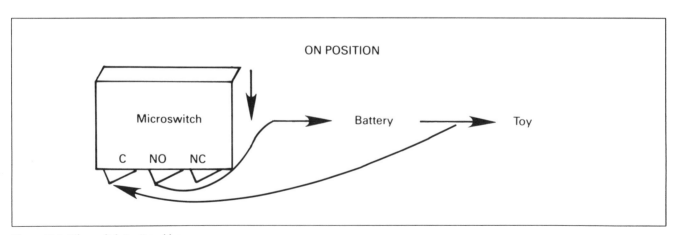

Figure 12-1. Microswitch "on" position.

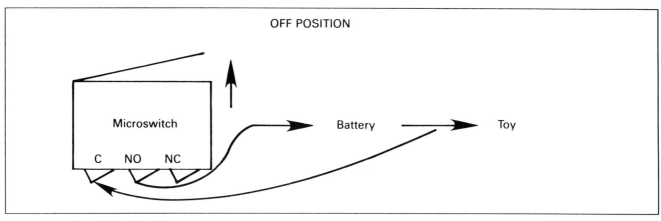

Figure 12-2. Microswitch "off" position.

TECHNICAL PROCEDURES

The technical procedures necessary to construct switches include splitting a wire, stripping a wire, and soldering.

Splitting a Wire

To **split a wire** means to separate the two strands of the wire. Each strand is coated in plastic. With either wire cutters or scissors, the two strands are cut and separated as shown in Figure 12-3. Care must be taken to avoid penetrating each plastic strand so as not to expose the wires.

Stripping a Wire

To strip a wire means removing the plastic coating from a segment of the wire. If wire gauges are marked on the wire stripper, both strands of the wire are placed in the 22-gauge hole, which is the size recommended for projects described in this chapter. The jaws of the stripper are placed about three inches down from the end of the wire. The wire stripper handles are gently squeezed together and quickly pulled up to remove the plastic coating. Care must be taken, because if the wire stripper is squeezed with too much force, the wires may be cut off. If this should happen, the procedure should be tried again.

Several varieties of wire strippers may operate differently from the one just described. The wire gauge is not marked on some, and it is necessary to adjust a bolt and set the cutter for the size of the wire. Once the plastic coating has been cut, the wire is placed in a separate hole marked on the stripper to pull off the plastic coating.

Soldering

Soldering is the process of fusing two pieces of metal together to facilitate the passage of electricity between them. The following procedure should be followed:

1. Some wires, plugs, jacks and other electrical terminals may need to be cleaned with steel wool.
2. After the wire is threaded to the terminal, hold the parts with pliers or tape them to the table. A small table vise may also be used if the components become very hot and it is difficult to hold them while soldering.
3. To solder, first heat the wire and terminal parts at the same time by holding the soldering iron tip firmly against them. (Be patient until both the wire and terminal are hot.) When both parts are hot, touch the

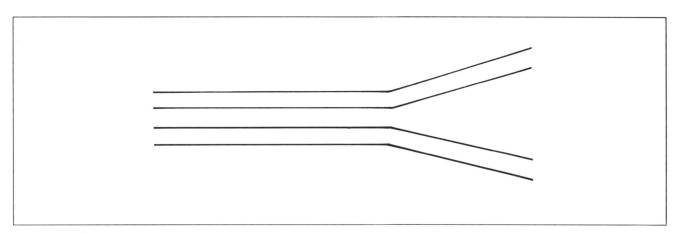

Figure 12-3. Splitting a wire.

rosin core or electrical solder to the connection. The solder should melt and flow evenly to coat the surfaces. Hold the soldered parts in a stable position until cool. If the parts have not been heated enough, the joint will lump. This is known as a cold solder joint and will make a poor electrical connection. If this occurs, simply reheat.

4. Use caution. The soldering iron must be used carefully. It becomes extremely hot and can cause severe burns and ignite fires. Avoid overheating the switch itself, as high temperatures can damage internal parts.

Instructions for Making a Plexiglas Pressure Switch Using Subminiature Components*

Basic Materials
- 2 pieces of Plexiglas each cut to $5^1/2 \times 3$ inches
- 2 sheet metal screws, No. 6 diameter and $3/4$-inch long
- 3 wooden strips cut from $1/2$-inch thick pine stock: one piece cut to $5^1/2$ inches in length by $1/2$-inch width and two pieces cut to 2 inches in length $\times$ $1/2$-inch width
- 1 spring that will fit under the screw head and is 1-inch in length; the tension of the spring is the individual's choice depending on the amount of strength the user can exert (it's a good idea to have a variety of springs on hand)
- 1 lever-type on/off microswitch
- 1 subminiature plug (miniature can be used)
- 1 22-inch piece of 22-gauge speaker wire

Other Supplies and Equipment. Rosin core or electrical solder, soldering iron, super glue, masking tape, electrical tape, hand drill, screwdriver, wire stripper/wire cutter, knife or taped, single-edge razor blade, needle nose pliers, awl, needle file, varnish, and sandpaper. The assembled switch is shown in Figure 12-4.

Instructions
1. Sand the edges and corners of the Plexiglas until smooth.
2. Sand all surfaces of the wood strips until smooth.
3. Varnish the wooden strips and allow to dry overnight.
4. Glue the $5^1/2$-inch strip of wood along the $5^1/2$-edge of one of the pieces of Plexiglas with super glue.
5. Split 2 inches from both ends of the 22-gauge speaker wire with a knife or a taped, single-edge razor blade.
6. Strip about $1/2$- to $3/4$-inch of plastic coating off each strand on both ends of the wire.
7. Unscrew the cap from the subminiature plug.
8. Thread the wires through the metal holes of the plug. Thread from the inside through the holes to the

*Instructions ©1986 by Mary Ellen Lange Dunford. Used with permission.

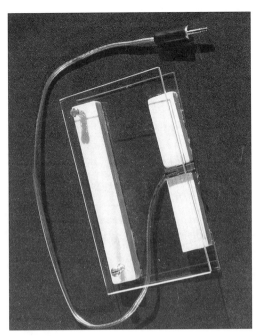

Figure 12-4. Plexiglas pressure switch.

outside. Bend the wires back and trim to $1/8$-inch. Be sure to pull through so that the plastic coating touches the inside of the metal hole as shown in Figure 12-5.

9. Solder the wires to the plug. Use only a small amount of solder so that the cap will screw back on. If too much solder is used, the excess can be removed with a needle file.
10. Using a needle nose pliers, bend the two metal prongs at the end of the plug around the plastic coating of the wire passing through that hole. This maneuver helps to hold the wire securely.
11. Screw the cap back on.
12. Test the plug by plugging it into a subminiature jack adapted to a battery-operated toy, or plug it into the remote jack of a tape recorder. The toy or tape recorder needs to have the existing switch mechanism turned to "on." Touch the two wires at the opposite ends together; if the toy or tape recorder turns on, the plug is working properly (Figure 12-6). If the plug does not work, unscrew the cap and check to see if the wires soldered are touching each other. If they are, put electrical tape around one wire and metal prong to keep them separated.
13. Twist and thread the strands of wire on the opposite end of the plug onto the lever microswitch. Thread them from the back of the switch, one through the terminal labled "C" (common) and one through the terminal labled "NO" (normally open), as shown in Figure 12-7.
14. Solder the wires to the switch and trim off any excess wire.

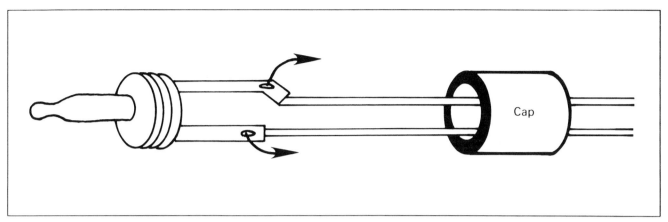

Figure 12-5. Threading wires to plug.

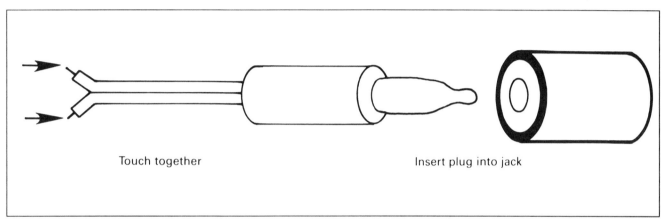

Figure 12-6. Testing the plug.

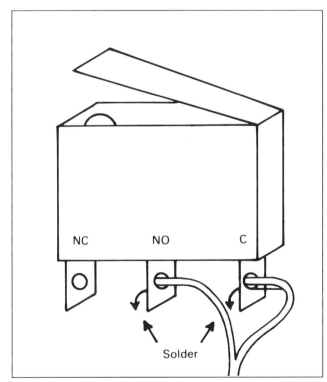

Figure 12-7. Threading wires to microswitch.

15. Test the circuitry again with a battery-operated toy or a tape recorder.

16. Glue the 2-inch strips of wood, one on each side of the switch lever and placed on the opposite edge from the 5^1/$_2$-inch strip glued earlier. It is best to glue one piece, let it dry 30 seconds, place the lever switch snugly against the glued piece, and glue the second 2-inch strip next to the switch. It is important to note that the microswitch is placed with the "C" terminal facing the inside of the switch as illustrated in Figure 12-8.

17. Drill two ^{5}/$_{32}$-inch holes in the second piece of Plexiglas, ^{1}/$_2$-inch from each edge of the 3-inch side, and ^{3}/$_8$-inch from the 5^1/$_2$-inch edge as shown in Figure 12-9.

18. Place the Plexiglas with the holes over the glued 5^1/$_2$-inch strip of wood. Use an awl or a nail to mark the screw holes on the wood.

19. Cut the spring in half with a wire cutter.

20. Put the screws through the holes in the Plexiglas, slip one piece of spring on each screw (springs under Plexiglas), and screw them into the wood. Tighten the screws so that the tension of the springs keeps the top piece of Plexiglas above and not touching the microswitch.

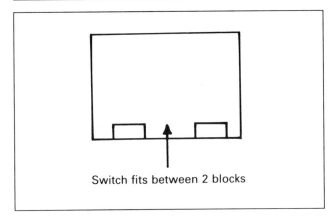

Switch fits between 2 blocks

Figure 12-8. Placement of microswitch.

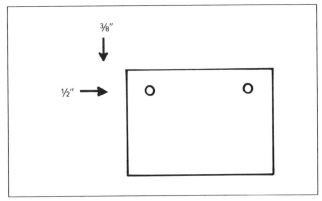

Figure 12-9. Plexiglas hole placement.

21. Retest the microswitch for operation.

This switch can be made either larger or smaller than the specifications given.

Instructions for Making an Interface for a Battery-Operated Device Using Subminiature Components*

Basic Materials
- 1 12-inch piece of 22-gauge speaker wire
- 1 subminiature jack
- 1 small piece of double-stick tape, $1/2$-inch by $1/4$-inch
- 2 small pieces of copper tooling foil, cut slightly smaller than the double-stick tape.

Other Supplies and Equipment. Wire stripper/cutter, knife or taped single-edge razor blade, soldering iron, rosin core solder or electrical solder, scissors and ruler. Figure 12-10 shows a completed device.

Instructions
1. Using a knife or a taped single-edge razor blade, split 2 inches from one end of the 22-gauge wire and split $1/2$-inch from the other end.

*Instructions ©1986 by Mary Ellen Lange Dunford. Used with permission.

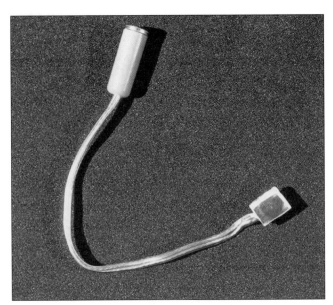

Figure 12-10. Interface for a battery-operated device.

2. Strip about $1/2$- to $3/4$-inch of the plastic coating off each strand on both ends of the wire. Twist the strands of each separate split piece of wire.
3. Unscrew the cap from the subminiature jack.
4. Thread one end of the split and stripped wire through the metal holes in the jack. Thread from the inside through the holes to the outside. Bend the wires back and trim to $1/8$-inch. Be sure to pull the wires through the holes so that the plastic coating touches the inside of each hole as illustrated in Figure 12-11.
5. Solder the wires to the jack; file off excess solder if necessary.
6. Using a needle nose pliers, bend the two metal prongs at the end of the jack around the plastic coating of the wire passing through the hole. This helps to hold the wire securely.
7. Thread the wire through the cap and screw on the cap.
8. Cut a small $1/2$- by $1/4$-inch piece of double-stick tape.
9. Cut two pieces of copper tooling foil slightly smaller than the $1/2$- by $1/4$-inch piece of double-stick tape.
10. Place the copper tooling foil pieces on either side of the double-stick tape. The tape acts as insulation and is necessary because the two pieces of copper must not come into contact with each other.
11. Place the $1/2$-inch split and stripped wires, one on each side of the copper chip, and solder each wire to it. Be sure that the plastic coating on each touches the end of the copper chip. This keeps the wires from touching each other, as shown in Figure 12-12.
12. Test the interface by using a battery-operated device in this manner: Remove the the cover from the battery compartment and place the copper chip

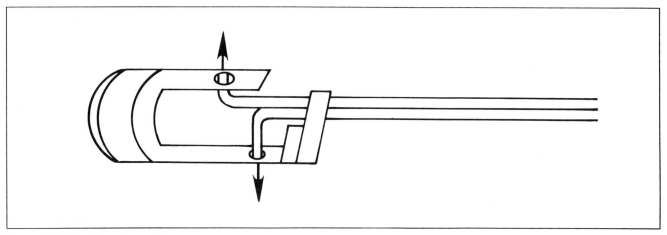

Figure 12-11. Threading wires to jack.

between the two batteries or between a battery and its contact. Turn on the device. It should not run. Connect a microswitch with a subminiature plug to the subminiature jack. Activate the microswitch. The device should work.

Variation. An insulated copper circuit board, cut to the same specifications, can be used to replace the copper foil and double-stick tape. If this option is selected, the wires are soldered to each side of the circuit board. It should be noted that chips made from circuit board are thicker and often more difficult to fit into a battery compartment. Foil-constructed chips are more flexible and fit compartments more easily, but they often break and will wear out faster than chips made from circuit board.

SELECTION OF TOYS AND BATTERY-OPERATED DEVICES

Toys provide valuable learning and growing experiences for children. Switches combined with toys encourage and motivate handicapped children and provide opportunities for them to play alone or with peers and actively participate in learning situations.

When purchasing battery-operated toys, it is important to select the ones with on/off switches. Check the battery box to be sure there is room for insertion of the copper chip from the interface. Some battery boxes are so small that once the batteries are inserted, there is not enough room for a small copper chip.

Toys that provide movement are very stimulating for children. Some action toys have a "bump and go" movement; they accelerate forward until they bump into a boundary or object and then reverse direction. Toys that are safe, durable, and colorful; make noises; and have lights are good choices for handicapped children. Some favorites

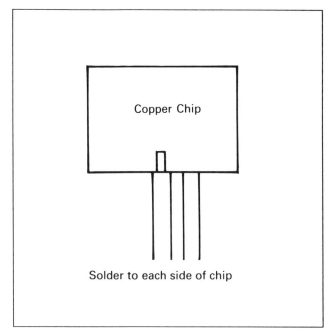

Figure 12-12. Placement of wires.

include small trains or engines, police cars with sirens, and animal characters that play musical instruments.

In addition to toys, small battery-operated fans and vibrators can provide sensory stimulation. Flashlights and other battery-powered light devices can be used for visual tracking and visual stimulation activities.

Tape recorders are also useful. Favorite songs and tunes, voices, and noises can be recorded and used as a play activity or as a reinforcement for correct performance. For example, a handicapped child who correctly moves an electronic car through a simple maze might be rewarded with a short taped segment of a favorite song, which is activated when the car reaches the final point. When using a tape recorder with a switch that has a subminiature plug, an interface is not necessary. The subminiature plug fits directly into the remote control jack on the tape recorder.

Toys that have more than one control switch and radio-controlled toys are difficult to adapt and require sophisticated wiring. *More Homemade Battery Devices for Severely Handicapped Children with Suggested Activities* by Linda J. Buckhart is an excellent resource that provides detailed information on complex toy adaptations. Toys that perform stunts or require a track to run on are not recommended for use with switches because the wires become twisted and break.

SAFETY PRECAUTIONS

When using microswitches and battery devices, it is important to consider the patient's responses and needs. Watch for seizures and signs of boredom, fear or annoyance. Change or stop the activity in response to the patient's behavior.

Low voltage battery-operated devices will not cause an electric shock. They do, however, contain battery acid, so care must be taken to ensure that patients do not put them in or near their mouths.

The type of solder commonly used to join electrical connections contains lead; therefore, never let patients put these soldered parts in their mouths. Exposed soldered areas can be easily covered with electrical tape or electrical solder that is 100 per cent tin can be used.

The switches discussed in this chapter are to be used with battery-operated devices only. When using a tape recorder, run it on the batteries, *not* plugged into an electrical socket. When in doubt, always consult with an electrician or someone with electrical expertise before using a device with a patient.

TREATMENT APPLICATIONS

The successful use of microswitch controls and other technical devices as treatment activities depends on the abilities and ingenuity of the occupational therapist and the assistant. Hundreds of controls are available, and not all are operated by a microswitch. Joysticks, mercury, toggle, grasp, breath control and voice-activated switches are examples of controls that are not operated by a microswitch. Treatment activities vary depending on the type of switch being used. A joystick can be used to assess a patient with quadriplegia for operation of a powered wheelchair. A mercury switch attached to a patient's head can be used to facilitate head control. The following discussion provides treatment suggestions for the Plexiglas pressure switch.

Tactile stimulation can be provided by placing different textures over the Plexiglas switch. Sandpaper, terry cloth, burlap, lamb's wool, felt and carpet pieces provide an assortment of textures for both stimulation and discrimination.

Battery-operated fans and vibrators provide sensory stimulation. When a pinwheel is placed in front of a fan, it spins and provides a stimulating visual activity. Brightly colored toys and lights can be used to encourage visual localization, tracking and discrimination. Auditory stimulation can be provided by toys that make noise, radios, and tape recorders.

By combining switches with therapeutic handling techniques, positioning of a patient can be maintained or inhibited. To encourage sitting, "on all fours," kneeling or standing, a patient may be placed in the position and required to place weight on the switch. The activity provided through activating the switch diverts attention and motivates the patient to maintain the position. To inhibit excessive or abnormal movement, the switch can be placed so that it turns on when the patient is positioned correctly and turns off with the undesirable movement, thus reinforcing the proper motor response.

Stacking blocks or various objects on the surface of the switch encourages prehension patterns. Squeezing the switch with the fingers to turn it on and off facilitates pincer grasp patterns. Switches can be used to train patients in developing headstick and mouthstick skills. Target areas can be placed on the surface of the Plexiglas and graded in size as skill develops.

Combined with specific interfaces, switches can be used with microcomputers. Computer software programs written to use the technique of scanning must be used with microswitches. **Scanning** is a technique that bypasses use of the keyboard and provides input directly to a cursor or an arrow that appears on the computer monitor. The user activates the microswitch to select specific characters. Microswitches combined with scanning techniques allow computer access for severely handicapped patients. See Chapter 13 for more information on this topic.

The use of switches also can provide leisure and entertainment. Adapted computer software games and modified toys are both enjoyable and educational. These activities offer the opportunity for patients to entertain themselves as well as a means to interact and socialize with others.

In many educational systems, the use of switches is included in the curriculum to teach cognitive skills. Concepts such as cause and effect, object permanence, and other early learning skills can be taught to children with handicaps. For example, a child learns cause and effect by understanding that if a switch is touched the toy will be turned on. Shape discrimination can be taught by placing a switch in a formboard. If the child places the shape in the correct spot, the switch is turned on, activating a reinforcement for the right answer such as a ringing bell.

GOALS AND OBJECTIVES

Switches combined with various devices offer enjoyable, motivating and rewarding activities. As with all other therapeutic activities, the use of switches must be included in the treatment goals and objectives. They must be used with a therapeutic purpose. The following are four examples of goals and behavioral objectives that incorporate switches and devices into treatment sessions for children with severe handicaps.[3]

1. *Goal:* Patient will improve gross motor skills.
   Behavioral Objective: Patient will bear weight on extended arms for at least 30 seconds.
   Procedure: Assist patient into a prone position over a large bolster or ball. Rock slowly forward and place arms and hands on floor. Encourage weight bearing on arms by having patient push pressure switch with both hands. Record length of time for weight bearing on switch.

2. *Goal:* Patient will increase fine motor skills.
   Behavioral Objective: Patient will reach for and activate a pressure microswitch without assistance at least three times out of five trials given.
   Procedure: Position patient in a prone position over a body wedge. Place a toy and switch in front of patient. Encourage activation of the switch.

3. *Goal:* Patient will improve gross motor skills.
   Behavioral Objective: Patient will walk up one step with the assistance of a handrail for three out of five trials.
   Procedure: Place patient's hand on railing. Stand close but offer no physical assistance.
   Alternate Activity: Place large flat microswitch on a step. Encourage patient to step on the step and switch using railing and wall for support. The switch should be attached to a toy and be activated by stepping up.

4. *Goal:* Patient will increase fine motor skills.
   Behavioral Objective: Patient will place four objects into a container on request four of five cosecutive days.
   Procedure: Place a switch in the bottom of a container (dishpan, can, basket, etc.) and attach switch to toy, computer or tape recorder. Give patient a weighted object to place in the container, which is heavy enough to activate the switch. After patient places one object accurately, offer objects of lesser weight so that two, three, or four objects are needed to activate the switch.

SUMMARY

The application of small technical devices in the evaluation and treatment of individuals with severe handicaps is becoming a significant part of health care. Combined with the traditional skills of assessment; use of functional, meaningful activities; and the ability to evaluate performance through the achievement of goals and objectives, this new array of therapeutic intervention techniques offers challenging opportunities for the profession of occupational therapy. There appears to be an increasing need for this technology in many segments of the treatment population. Basic principles of electricity were presented, together with specific instructions for constructing a switch and an interface. Safety precautions and examples of treatment applications were also discussed. Since the role of occupational therapy personnel is not well defined in this area, it is open for expansion and exploration of new ideas and applications. The resource list in Appendix D details sources of supplies and other related information.

Editor's Note

The construction and/or use of the devices mentioned in this chapter may result in harm or injury if not used properly. The Author, Editor and Publisher recommend close supervision and extreme care in working with these materials and cannot accept responsibility for the consequences of incorrect application of information by individuals, whether or not professionally qualified.

Related Learning Activities

1. Construct a Plexiglas pressure switch and an interface.

2. Use the interface and the pressure switch with at least three different toys or devices.

3. What major safety factors must be considered when constructing and using switches and interfaces?

4. How can microswitch devices be used to assist in achieving gross motor goals?

5. How can microswitches assist in teaching cognitive skills?

References

1. Williams J, Csongradi J, LeBlanc M: *A Guide to Controls, Selection and Mounting Applications.* Palo Alto, California, Rehabilitation Engineering Center, Children's Hospital at Stanford, 1982, pp 5-7.
2. Wethred C: *Toy Adaptations.* Toronto, Ontario, Association of Toy Libraries, June, 1979, p 1.
3. Bengtson-Grimm M, Snyder S: *Daily Goals and Objectives Written for Severely Handicapped Using Microswitches.* Clinton, Iowa, Kirkwood School, 1984.

Computers

Sally E. Ryan, COTA, ROH
Brian J. Ryan, BSEE
Javan E. Walker, Jr., MA, OTR

INTRODUCTION

This chapter provides a basic understanding of computers. Large, central computers are discussed; however, emphasis is placed on the microcomputer because of its many uses in occupational therapy management, evaluation and treatment. These small machines have been described as enhancers or amplifiers of human ability.[1] They can assist in many areas such as increasing attention span, developing communication skills, mastering eye-hand coordination tasks, improving sequencing and memory abilities, performing auditory and visual discrimination tasks, problem solving, and controlling their environment. The computer also provides creative outlets through the use of word processing and graphics programs. Both cognitive and creative abilities are used when patients learn to develop their own programs. In many instances, adults with handicaps are finding that their computer skills are creating many new job opportunities and careers that were previously unavailable to them.

Occupational therapy departments are increasing their use of computers in providing patient assessment and treatment, as well as for performing tasks such as maintenance of patient records and generation of reports, budgets, and other word processing and data management projects. Use of the computer also allows access to vast quantities of health care information worldwide.

Microcomputers, also referred to as personal computers or PCs, are small machines that are relatively inexpensive, serve a variety of general purposes, and are easy to learn to use.[2] They do not require a controlled environment or highly specialized installation, and the space requirements are minimal. Many are capable of interfacing with large central computers. Battery-powered, portable microcomputer units can be operated in practically any location.

KEY CONCEPTS

Basic and auxiliary equipment

Relationship of input and output devices

Fundamental programs

Applications for individuals with handicaps

Evaluation and treatment implications

Precautions

ESSENTIAL VOCABULARY

Hardware

Firmware

Software

Byte

Disk drive

Modem

Joystick

Paddles

Mouse

Input

Output

Bulletin board

Networking

Environmental control unit

Central computers, also called *mainframes* or *macrocomputers,* are used primarily in large corporations, health care facilities, educational institutions, and government systems that must process great amounts of data and information. These computer systems can handle hundreds of input/ output terminals at the same time. For example, a corporation might install a terminal at the desk of all supervisors and managers and provide several for the secretarial group in each division. All of these people could be using a terminal at the same time, a system called time sharing. Engineers doing research and statistical analysis at home or at another location would also have terminals connected to the same system by telephone lines.[3]

COMPUTER TERMINOLOGY

To develop an understanding of how a computer works, it is necessary to know the meaning of the following basic terms. Terms and their definitions are presented in an order that identifies relationships among them, rather than in alphabetical order.

Hardware
Hardware refers to the computer and all of its electronic parts. It includes the keyboard, the wires and the electronic components inside the computer case. Hardware is the "brain" of the computer.[1] It is the central processing unit or CPU.[2]

Firmware
The flat electronic cards that occupy slots inside the computer are called **firmware** or boards.[2] They perform functions such as connecting the disk drive to the computer, expanding the computer's memory capacity, and increasing the number of characters that can be displayed across the screen. For example, a computer might come from the manufacturer with a 40 column standard display. By adding an 80 column board, the display potential is increased to 80 characters across the screen which is a great advantage in using work processing programs.

An adaptive firmware card (ACF) allows the use of a variety of different input devices, besides the keyboard, with standard software programs.

Software
Programs that send messages to the computer telling it to perform specific functions are known as **software.** They allow the user to communicate to the computer what needs to be accomplished. Software is stored in the computer's memory on both a permanent and nonpermanent basis. Software program operations are described using the acronyms RAM meaning *random access memory* and ROM or *read only memory.*

RAM refers to the part of the computer's memory that receives information and data. The greater the RAM capacity, the greater the amount of information and data that can be stored. When someone describes a computer as "64K" they are talking about RAM. The literal message is that the computer has a random access memory of 64 kilobytes or thousands of bytes of RAM. **Byte** is a term used to measure units of computer memory storage capacity. Another way to think about software is that it gives ideas to the brain in the hardware, the computer.[4] When the computer is turned off, all RAM memory is lost. It is regained by reloading information from a software program (see Disk Drives).

ROM is a permanent part of the computer. Examples of ROM include mathematical computations and programming language such as BASIC (Beginner's All-purpose Symbolic Instruction Code),[2] which are built in to the computer's ROM memory. When the computer is turned off, ROM always remains.[4]

Disk Drives
The **disk drive** is a piece of peripheral equipment controlled by the DOS (disk operating system). It may be mounted directly above the computer in the computer case or it may be a separate "box" connected to the computer with an electrical cable. One of its main purposes is to send messages from a software program to the microcomputer's RAM memory. Some software programs may require the use of two disk drives. The disk drive is also used to save work on disk for future use. A tape recorder may be used in place of a disk drive; however, it is a much slower process and increasingly fewer software programs are available in this format.

Disks or Diskettes
Personal computers currently use hard disks, "floppy" disks, or diskettes for software programs. The latter are circular and made of plastic with a special magnetic coating that allows information to be recorded. The coating is protected by a vinyl envelope. The disk is placed in the disk drive and is activated to send information to the computer memory. This process is called *booting.* If the computer is turned off, the disk must be rebooted to continue the program. Floppy disks must be handled very carefully. Never bend them or touch the "oval window." Be sure that they are not exposed to excessive sunlight, heat, or magnetic sources.[5] Hard disks are made of rigid metal that has been magnetically coated. Although they are more costly than the plastic disks, they are capable of storing much larger quantities of information and allow faster access. Always make an extra copy of all program disks and store them in their protective envelopes in a secure place away from the computer work area.

Monitors

A monitor is another piece of peripheral equipment that is needed to see a display of computer information. The three main types are green screen, black and white, and color. The green shows green characters on a black background and is frequently used for word processing as well as other programs that do not require color. The black and white monitor is used in the same way. Color monitors are the most expensive but are very useful for graphics, games, and a variety of educational programs. A monitor is often referred to as a CRT or (cathode ray tube). A television set may be used in place of a monitor if it is compatible with the computer. If a television set is used, the display will not be as clear as that provided by a monitor. In technical terms, a monitor has higher resolution, which means it displays more lines per inch on the screen.[4] Display peripherals are referred to as terminals or video display terminals rather than monitors when they are a part of a large mainframe computer system.

Printers

Printers are available in four basic types: dot matrix, letter quality, laser, and ink-jet, with dot matrix currently being the most popular for internal daily work and letter quality or laser used for external communication.[4] A dot matrix printer will produce text in a variety of fonts or letter sizes. Many also produce graphics. The quality of the printed material depends on the density of the dots. Printers with high density dot systems can produce printed material that is almost the same quality as that made by a typewriter.[1]

Letter quality printers are most frequently used by people who do extensive word processing and must produce written work of a professional quality. Most of these printers have a "daisy wheel" that produces characters similar to a typewriter.[4] Some models also present excellent graphics.[1] Letter quality printers are more expensive than the dot matrix type.

Laser printers use electromagnetic material and light to reproduce precise images that resemble professionally typeset work. They produce material much faster than a letter quality printer and are more expensive.

Ink jet printers also produce precise characters of a professional quality, with a considerable reduction in operating noise.

Modems

A **modem** is a device that allows computer signals to be sent to and received from other computers over telephone wires. The term modem is a blend word for *modulator/ demodulator*. It converts electronic signals received from a computer so that they can be sent through a personal telephone.[1] It also converts information sent from another computer so that it can be received by the initiator. Use of a modem requires a special firmware card in the computer.[4]

Joysticks

A **joystick** is another peripheral device that allows the user to interact with the computer. It basically sends six messages: on, off, up, down, right and left, which are often used with games and elementary educational programs. It operates in the same manner as the computer's arrow keys and can easily be adapted for patients who are unable to control the handle. Methods used include increasing the size of the handle with foam rubber, placing a rubber ball over the handle, or constructing a specialized adaptation with plastic splinting material or plastic pipe fittings available at most hardware stores. A joystick is shown in Figure 13-1.

Paddles

A paddle or a set of two **paddles** may be used in place of a joystick. The paddle uses rotational movements that the computer recognizes and has an on/off switch. Paddles may be adapted in many of the ways described for joysticks.

Mouse

Another common peripheral input device is a **mouse.** This mechanism rolls on a small bearing that electronically guides the cursor on the screen. Its simplistic design often allows individuals with limited strength and dexterity to access the computer.

RELATIONSHIP OF INPUT AND OUTPUT EQUIPMENT

Operation of a microcomputer system requires correct electrical connections and a power source, most commonly a regular commercial current of 110 volts. Follow the directions in the manual *exactly* as they are described when setting up a computer. Figure 13-2 shows a typical work station and the relationship of input and output equipment. **Input** refers to the ways the computer can receive information or how it can be "put in." **Output** refers to the

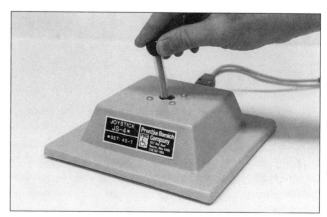

Figure 13-1. A joystick.

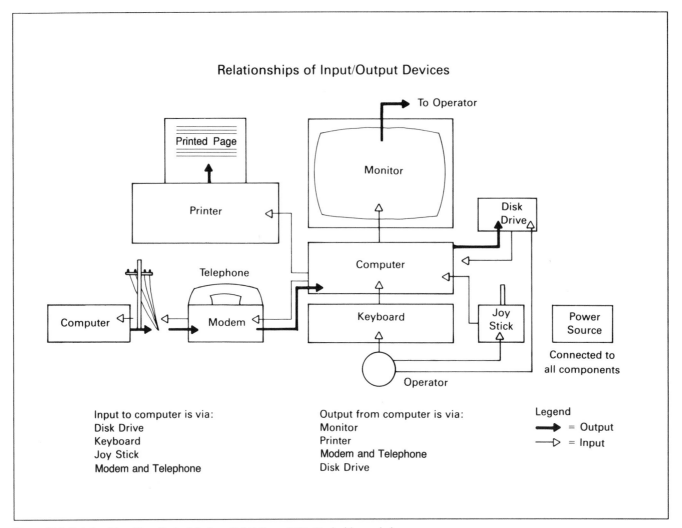

Figure 13-2. Relationships of input/output devices. © S.E. Ryan, 1985. Used with permission.

information that is sent from the computer or "put out."

Input on a microcomputer can be accomplished in a number of ways, including the activation of the disk drive to load a software program and use of a keyboard, joystick, mouse or a modem. In addition to being stored on a disk in the disk drive, output can also be produced by the monitor, the printer and the modem.

HOW COMPUTERS WORK

A complete description of the many aspects of how computers work would require several chapters; therefore, only very basic information on this subject will be discussed as it applies to microcomputers. Computers are versatile machines that perform a variety of functions when they are instructed to do so by a software program. These functions include playing games as well as operating file, spreadsheet, database, and word processing systems. The electronic mecha-

nisms within the computer respond to input from a number of sources and translate the information received into a binary system comprised of zeros and ones. For example, if the user types "MARY" on the keyboard, small electronic components, referred to as microchips, will convert the letter "M" into a binary code of zeros and ones and store it, together with the other input information, in the RAM or random access memory of the computer. The computer's memory might be compared to a block of post office boxes, where "slots" exist to save and categorize information.

To illustrate more clearly some of the computer's functions, the use of a word processing program written in BASIC in a diskette format will be used as an example. The first step is to put the word processing program into the disk drive and turn on, or boot up, the computer and monitor. The program is then "loaded" into the computer's RAM memory. Next, the user removes the word processing diskette from the disk drive and places an initialized "file" diskette in the drive. At that point, information can be entered via the keyboard or another type of input device.

Periodically, as the information is put in, the user can "save" it on the diskette by inputing the correct "save" command and entering a short title so that the information can be easily retrieved if needed. If the computer is turned off before the "save" command is entered, all of the information will be lost. If the user also needs a printed copy or "printout" of the material then the "print" command is used.

If it is necessary to add to the information at a later time, the user simply reloads the word processing program by placing the disk in the disk drive, turns on the computer, replaces the word processing disk with the file disk, and enters the "load" command. Once the information is loaded, additions, deletions and other modifications can be made. As the user continues working on the document, the "save" command must be entered so that all of the revisions are saved on the diskette. More information on the use of word processing is presented in the next section.

FUNDAMENTAL PROGRAMS

Certified occupational therapy assistants (COTAs) who are prepared to practice for the rest of this century and into the 21st century will find using a computer no more of a chore than dialing a telephone or driving an automobile. The "mystery and awe" that sometimes surround use of the microcomputer is gradually disappearing, and it will soon be a tool as common as a video cassette recorder or a microwave oven.

Much of the mystery has revolved around the differences between the concepts of the computer programmer and the computer operator. In the early days of computing, one had to be a programmer because of the relative complexity of computers and the lack of "user friendly" software programs. With the advent of more powerful microcomputers and the tremendous increase in available software, most occupational therapy assistants will be computer operators rather than computer programmers. This change opens up a wide variety of opportunities.

As a computer operator, the COTA may have access by terminal to either a large mainframe computer, such as one used by a hospital, or a microcomputer at a desk or departmental work station. Both can be linked to other computers for information sharing.

Information management is one of the most important features that the computer offers to occupational therapy service programs. With access to an electronic bulletin board or database, occupational therapy personnel will have instant access to information about a variety of health care subjects.

Currently, occupational therapy departments use a computer primarily for administrative purposes; however, use as a therapeutic tool in patient evaluation and treatment is becoming more widespread. The following four basic computer software programs are in the repertoire of the COTA who is a literate computer user:

1. A word processing program
2. A database manager (DBM)
3. A spreadsheet program
4. A terminal program

Word Processing

A word processor is software that allows a computer to function somewhat like a typewriter. It permits one to compose and edit text; move, duplicate or delete entire blocks of text; check for proper spelling; identify poor writing style; and print the document with data inserted from the keyboard, from files and from a database manager or a spreadsheet.[6]

The word processing program has become one of the most popular programs for occupational therapy personnel. Many of the routine forms necessary for evaluations, progress notes, and discharge summaries can be placed on a computer to avoid unnecessary repetition. Either through the use of a terminal program to access a mainframe computer, or a microcomputer and a printer, the therapist and the assistant can manage more efficiently the information that must be completed for every patient receiving their services. In addition to patient information, letters, reports, patient education documents, public affairs information, and other routine pieces of frequently used printed material can be stored on diskette or in the computer's main core, and quickly called up for easy revision and printing.

Many word processing packages offer added features that may be helpful such as a spelling checker for the poor speller or typist, a thesaurus; a way to link parts of different documents together; or reproduction of forms and mailing labels that are frequently used.

One of the authors worked on a psychiatric ward at Walter Reed Army Medical Center during the 1970s, which allowed all pertinent staff members to record patient chart data on a computer using a word processing program. The individual patient charts were literally maintained on the mainframe computer and hard copies were printed only when necessary. The occupational therapy staff wrote their weekly progress notes at the terminal and were able to have instant access to all data relevant to the patient. Although this program was experimental, it is becoming the norm in many hospitals, nursing homes, and other treatment facilities.

The advantages of using a word processing program over pen and paper or a typewriter become obvious when the use of the program becomes routine. One of the problems with writing a note for a chart is that many therapists and assistants are not gifted writers, and they would like to revise their notes from time to time. Using a pen and a blank progress reporting sheet, the result can sometimes be a sloppy note with error markings or a recopied note. With the typewriter, revisions require either the judicious use of "white out" or the retyping of the entire note. In contrast, the word processing program allows instant revision. By merely moving the cursor—a visual electronic position indicator symbol—back a letter, a word, a line or a paragraph, revisions can be easily made. In addition, entire paragraphs or blocks of information can be moved, edited or deleted before the final note is saved for later storage or retrieval.

Database Manager

Database managers (DBMs) maintain a file or a group of items that are related. A recipe file on small index cards is an example of a noncomputerized database management system.[7] The DBM is another software tool that is being used increasingly in occupational therapy settings. It was created due to the demand for a system to efficiently manage the volume of information created on the computer. A DBM allows access to that information in a predetermined way.

The easiest way to conceptualize a database management system is to think of a personal address and telephone directory. When there is a need to recall the telephone number of an individual named Smith, one goes to the book and looks under the "S" listing. Assuming there are not hundreds of Smiths, the individual is quickly able to gain access to the correct number.

A DBM allows the same type of access, but with considerably more power and speed. For example, if the therapist wants to identify all of the patients in the hospital records with a diagnosis of myocardial infarction who have received occupational therapy services during the last six months, using the more traditional file card or file drawer system, he or she would review all of the occupational therapy records for that period and select or note those patients who met the criteria. Obviously, this task could be long and tedious in a large hospital. On the other hand, if the departmental records are a part of the hospital's mainframe computer system, or if the department has computerized its own files and maintained that information in a database management program, access to the needed data is relatively simple.

A COTA who is seeking this specific information merely enters in the required search parameters:
1. Hospitalization during last six months
2. Treatment given by occupational therapist
3. Diagnosis of myocardial infarction

Depending on the program, such a computer search could take a matter of seconds but no more than several minutes. The information could then be printed out on paper to provide a hard copy. If patients needed to be contacted to obtain information on a posttreatment questionnaire, the computer program would print the mailing labels. If a form letter was being sent, the computer could integrate the names and addresses of each individual in the selected group and repeat the patient's name in the body of the letter, thus personalizing each one.

The database manager can be used to maintain inventories, patient information files, mailing lists, bibliographies, routine treatment techniques, and other collections of data that may be too large to maintain in a simple office filing system. It should be noted, however, that a basic, old-fashioned file card system sometimes may be more efficient. For example, if the database contains fewer than 20 or 30 files, with minimal information in each file, it is much easier to open an address book and get the needed information than to boot up the computer, load the program, call for the data, and read the CRT or wait for a printout.

Spreadsheet Programs

A spreadsheet is a software program that manipulates numbers in the same way that a word processor manipulates words. Electronic spreadsheets organize data in a matrix of rows and columns. Each intersection of a row and column forms a cell that holds one piece of information. The cells are linked together by formulas. When the user enters data to change one cell, the spreadsheet uses the power of the computer to automatically recalculate and alter every other cell linked to the original cell.[8] With the increased emphasis on accountability in health care service delivery, particularly in hospitals, a spreadsheet program can be an invaluable tool for handling the day-to-day maintenance and analysis of numerical data.

The spreadsheet allows the computer operator to perform "what if" scenarios. The program makes it quite easy to project the budgetary effect of adding or eliminating an item or a category or items. Using traditional methods, this information could be obtained only after the time-consuming task of recalculating all of the budgetary figures had been completed.

Information typically needed in occupational therapy departments, such as daily treatment count, staff time sheets, budget, inventory, and other numerically based records, can all be easily maintained on a spreadsheet program. Once the initial format, or template, is established, it can be saved and used repeatedly for subsequent calculations.

Integrated Programs

Advances in technology have produced a variety of integrated software programs that combine a word processor, database, and spreadsheet in one package. Programs may be used simultaneously and information from one mode can easily be transferred to another. This feature is particularly helpful when writing reports that require the insertion of statistical information and other data.

Terminal Programs

A terminal program is a communications program that allows the computer to "talk" with the outside world. It is responsible for instructing the computer to send the characters that are typed through the telephone line to another computer, for establishing and maintaining the connection between the two systems, for making certain that incoming information is displayed correctly on the screen, and for performing other functions to enhance communications.[9] The capability for occupational therapy personnel to communicate with others through a computer system is perhaps the most promising aspect of computing.

One of the problems in a profession such as occupational therapy is that there is an ever-increasing volume of information. Maintaining access to this data through traditional methods can often be a cumbersome and time-comsuming task. The combination of a computer, terminal program, and modem, however, can open up the "whole world" of information on topics such as rehabilitation medicine. The modem, as described earlier, modulates and demodulates the computer's digital signals. Modulation occurs when the modem converts the information coming from the computer into audible sound signals that can be sent over a telephone line. Demodulation occurs when the modem takes the sound signals coming in from a correspondent's modem, converts them into digital pulses, and sends the pulses to the host computer.[9]

Bulletin Boards. Computers are frequently being used for information access. The information can be contained on an electronic **bulletin board.** Much like the corkboard in the office, computerized bulletin boards are established to relay information or send and receive electronic mail between computers. They exist as both private and commercial operations.

These two fundamental uses, gaining or exchanging information, are the primary reasons for using a terminal program. The former is frequently accomplished by contacting commercial networks such as COMPUSERVE, DIAGLOG or the SOURCE. Each of these boards allows one access to a variety of separate electronic databases. Most offer an on-line encyclopedia, the ability to track stocks, access to various news wire services, the ability to select flights and order airline tickets, or shop and do banking electronically. Researchers and consultants have compiled a large database of literature on scientific, medical and engineering subjects. More detailed information on bulletin boards may be obtained through most local libraries or computer centers at colleges and universities.

O.T. SOURCE was established by the American Occupational Therapy Association in 1989. It has three key components: databases, bulletin boards and electronic mail.

Features include a bibliographic search system, product catalog, personnel resource file, calendar of continuing education programs, association meetings and events, and a member question and answer service. More information can be obtained by contacting the AOTA.

Networking. The second use of a terminal program involves **networking,** or electronic interfacing of individuals via their computers to share information, seek answers to specific questions, or just talk with someone electronically. This feature is accomplished either by sending an electronic message to someone (electronic mail) or by simultaneously exchanging information from keyboard to keyboard.

COMPUSERVE, for example, has an online interest section for professionals and consumers interested in medicine. One can send a message to individuals or the general public, which will be answered by anyone accessing the special interest section. On many bulletin boards, conferences have been established to deal with specific subjects. Individuals who happen to be on-line at the preestablished time are able to comment and exchange ideas.

Several bulletin boards have been established specifically for health professionals. Some are operated by universities and medical schools and are quite costly, whereas others are being developed by professional associations or private groups and have very reasonable rates.

With access to a commercial or private board, there is little information that cannot be obtained. The sharing of information among individuals is helping to limit the isolation that occupational therapists and assistants often feel when working in small communities or within highly specialized treatment areas.

When a consultant or a supervising therapist is not on site on a daily basis, a combination of the word processor and a terminal package offers some unique options as illustrated in the following example:

An OTR is employed as an occupational therapy consultant and direct service supervisor at a nursing home. Because she travels to several communities to evaluate patients, communication with the COTA that she supervises at this home is sometimes difficult. The OTR and the COTA have found that using computers makes communication much more efficient. They use electronic mail to send each other messages and other information. For example, when the therapist has completed an evaluation, she sends it to an assistant for downloading and later inclusion in the chart. The COTA can request additional information or provide updates on the patient's progress at any time, and the OTR can access it at home or through her portable computer when away.

COMPUTERS AND THE HANDICAPPED

Small microcomputers offer great opportunities for people with a wide variety of disabling handicaps. In recent years, occupational therapy personnel have been collaborating with rehabilitation engineers and others to develop electronic systems that will permit individuals with handicaps to achieve independence in areas never before thought possible.[10] This is a problem-solving process, based on a comprehensive needs assessment, which results in the design of a system or systems that provide patient-controlled decision making and solutions that assist in achieving many goals. Table 13-1 shows some of the areas of patient rehabilitation that may be addressed.

Environmental Control

The **environmental control unit** (ECU) is an electronic system with sensors that monitors and performs a variety of tasks. This ever-changing technology usually includes a microcomputer and is capable of greatly increasing the independence of even the most severely handicapped individual. A person with a high spinal cord injury is now able to control the position of an electric bed or the operation of

---

Table 13-1
Suggested Justification and Uses of a
Microcomputer in Occupational Therapy

A. Motor Training
   1. Games/programs to train severely handicapped in using specific motor functions
B. Fundamental Skills
   1. Basic cognitive functions such as attention, visual and auditory perception, differentiation and memory
C. Assessments
   1. Test batteries to assess memory functions, intelligence; several standardized assessments are now being computerized
D. Basic Educational Skills Training
   1. Preschool skills building
   2. Pre-reading
   3. Reading
   4. Typing tutors and keyboard skills
   5. Mathematics
E. Basic Living Skills
   1. Money management
   2. Buying and shopping
   3. Foods planning
   4. Job readiness and assessment
   5. Leisure (games designed to enhance motor coordination and learning as well as just fun)

From Rooney JA: Management information systems (MIS): Requesting the system. In Clarke EN (Ed.): *Microcomputers: Clinical Applications.* Thorofare, NJ: SLACK 1986, p 16.

---

a television set, telephone, intercom system, light switches, and electronic door locks through the use of a properly designed environmental control system.

Instead of using the computer keyboard for input, a "suck and blow" tube may be connected that allows the user to send messages consisting of Morse code dots and dashes, which are converted to a form that is recognized by the computer.[11] The computer then relays the message electronically and a task is performed such as dimming a lamp. Voice-activated input systems are also available.

Environmental control systems can greatly enhance patients' independence, as they no longer have to rely on another individual to carry out some of the everyday tasks of living. In many instances they can remain in their own home instead of moving to a nursing home because around the clock care is no longer necessary. This increased independence results in renewed self-confidence and self-esteem.[12] Figure 13-3 illustrates the components of an ECU system.

Enhanced Communication Skills

The microcomputer, coupled with a voice synthesizer, can allow a patient with expressive aphasia to speak. A software program allows the person to simply type in such statements as "I am hungry" or "I want to go to bed" and they will be spoken audibly by the synthesizer so that they can be heard by others in the room. If an intercom system is in place, these messages can also be heard in other rooms. The voice level can be muted for conversations.

A voice synthesizer may also be used to facilitate communication for the blind. Braille "caps" can be placed over the keyboard keys, and the written material is then typed one character at a time and relayed audibly to the user. A Braille printer may also be connected to the system to allow the blind person to go back and review work that has been completed.

Communication does not require use of the alphabet. A young child with cerebral palsy who is unable to spell can interact with others by using a special keyboard overlay that has symbols and pictures. Messages can be sent to the screen and the voice synthesizer by pressing just one key.

For the person who has some knowledge of the alphabet, programs are available that allow programming of complete sentences of up to 250 characters that can be recalled with one or two key strokes. For example, a message that states "I would like to have a hamburger and french fries" could be assigned a simple letter code of "HF"; "I would like to go outside" could be assigned "GO."

People with hearing impairments are able to overcome their communication handicaps by using a microcomputer and a **speech analyzer** device with a special microphone input system. This device allows them to learn correct pronunciation, accent, and other subtleties of speech patterns. These systems literally allow the user to see the words they are saying by producing a graph on the monitor. The

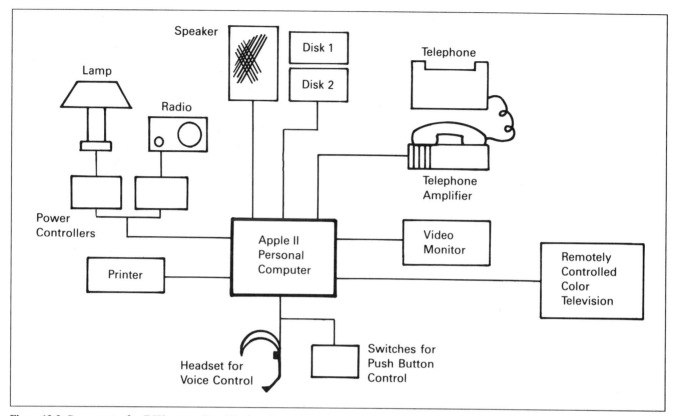

Figure 13-3. Components of an ECU system. From Wambott JJ: Computer environmental control units for the severely disabled: A guide for the occupational therapist. *Occup Ther Health Care* 4:156, 1984. Used with permission.

person repeats the word and tries to duplicate the graph pattern. When the graph pattern has been reproduced exactly as it appears on the screen, correct pronunciation has been achieved. People who do not have hearing deficits are using these programs to assist in learning foreign languages. Programs are also available that teach sign language.

Patients with amyotrophic lateral sclerosis (ALS), or Lou Gehrig disease, can become so disabled in the later stages of the disease that the only motor movements they can perform are swallowing, eye rolling, and raising the eyebrows. Through the development of an electronic eyebrow switch mounted on a special headband that is connected to the microcomputer, the patient can communicate. A software program directs the cursor to scan a group of letters on the monitor screen. When the cursor is on the desired part of the screen, the switch is activated and it becomes the first character in the message. While this is a time-consuming process in the beginning, after some practice, the patient is able to reproduce several words per minute. It is possible for him or her to write informal messages, letters, grocery lists, and other communications and have them reproduced on the computer's printer.

These are but a few examples of the many possible applications. Every day, advances are being made that offer a great variety of both basic and complex communication aids and systems.

Increased Employment Opportunities

People with handicaps are finding that microcomputer skills are "door openers" in the employment market. The ability to use a simple word processing program has allowed the previously unemployed to work at home as typists and free-lance writers and editors. The spreadsheet programs open up many opportunities for work in areas such as accounting, tax preparation and financial planning. Skill in using file programs allows many to fill positions that involve management of inventory systems and other data processing tasks for business and industry. Others who are skilled in the use of graphics and creative applications are finding jobs with advertising agencies and public relations firms.

Shadick[13] wrote about a woman with advanced multiple sclerosis who was able to continue her career as a loan investment advisor at home with a microcomputer, a printer, and a software program that had a spreadsheet and the capability of processing data to predict or forecast future trends. Crystal[14] provided a recent account of a deaf young man who had cystic fibrosis. He developed programming skills in seven different computer languages and is well on his way to a career as a free-lance computer programmer. An article in the *Washington Post* profiles a blind stock broker who uses a microcomputer with a synthetic voice system; *Information Thru Speech* (ITS) allows this account executive to carry out all of his job responsibilities.[15] As technologic advances increase, so will the employment opportunities for individuals with performance deficits.

New Leisure Pursuits

The opportunities for developing new leisure-time pursuits using a microcomputer are virtually endless. The great variety of games that involve one, two, or more players can provide many hours of entertainment and challenge. Programs such as bridge, chess and conversational foreign languages offer education as well as entertainment. Creative abilities can be expressed through the use of word processing and graphics programs. For example, the adolescent with a learning disability who would never have considered creative writing or drawing as a pastime is now able to use a word processing program and a graphics program to write and illustrate original poetry.

OCCUPATIONAL THERAPY EVALUATION AND TREATMENT IMPLICATIONS

Occupational therapy personnel now have a challenging opportunity to use microcomputers for evaluation and treatment of a wide variety of patients. The key to the successful use of computer activities depends on the skill of the therapists and assistants using them.[16] Care must be taken to match the best hardware, peripherals, adaptations and software programs to the needs and goals of the patient. Costs must also be carefully considered, particularly when complex systems are needed.

The following case studies give some specific examples of the effective use of microcomputers in occupational therapy [*Editor's Note:* Please see the information presented in the section on Precautions for Computer Use in this chapter]:

Case Study 13-1

Computer Assisted Rehabilitation for a Patient with Head Trauma. A 26-year-old man suffered a closed head injury in a motor vehicle accident. After treatment in an acute care hospital, he was transferred to a custodial facility with a diagnosis of severe vegitative state based on the Glascow Coma Scale.[17] Two years after the injury, he was admitted to the University of Texas Medical Branch Adult Special Care Unit with left hemiparesis. The patient was then classified as level two severe disability and was oriented to person but was disoriented to the environment. His attention span was less than five minutes. He was without problem solving skills, had severe left-sided neglect, and exhibited an inablility to cross the midline. He had incoordination $1^1/_2$ inches past pointing and poor dexterity, and all responses were severely delayed. He used a wheelchair for ambulation.

The occupational therapy program included peg and block

designs, range of motion, perceptual tasks, right and left discrimination activities, orientation to time and environment, and activities of daily living. Modalities were used to increase right upper extremity strength and to inhibit hypertonus of the left upper extremity. The patient began to learn bathing, dressing, basic cooking and laundry tasks. He was oriented to the hospital environment, played simple games, and joined in group activities.

Seven months later, computer-generated tasks were added to the treatment plan. A stimulus/response and discrimination software program, which measures latency of response times in averages of computer cycles as well as variance and number of errors, was used for an evaluation tool because of its concrete database. The computer indicates correct responses with an auditory tone so that the patient can receive immediate feedback, and after 15 trials a cumulative score is given.

One discrimination task requires the patient to respond to a 1-inch yellow square and to inhibit a response when a blue square appears. The randomly presented stimuli require the patient to cross the midline visually and to scan the screen, along with eye-hand coordination required to use the keyboard or the joystick. The patient was not trained on these programs to prevent overlearning and thus to ensure an objective evaluation tool.

The computer programs used for training were *Search,*[18] *City Map,*[19] *Driver,*[20] *Sequential,*[21] *Baker's Dozen,*[22] and *Stars.*[23] The cognitive skills required for these programs involve planning, organization, decision making, simple problem solving, attention to details, logical thinking and sequencing. Treatment goals focused on these areas.

On admission the patient had severe deficits in concentration and attention span, which interfered with his functional performance and self-care activities. The computer programs selected for him provided a mechanism for developing his attention span and increasing coordination. A year and a half after admission, the patient was independent in bathing and dressing and required only stand-by assistance for transfers. He was able to integrate visual field information, move his wheelchair through an environment with distractions, and had marked improvement in his ability to delay gratification.

Many computer programs are available for training patients. The programs selected for this patient have resulted in his improvement in activities of daily living as well as cognitive and perceptual skills. Originally diagnosed as severe vegetative state, the patient was reclassified as between severely and moderately disabled.[24]

Case Study 13-2

Computer Assisted Learning for the Child with Cerebral Palsy. Computer assisted learning was used with an 11-year-old boy with cerebral palsy (quadriplegic athetoid type) who is completely dependent for all activities of daily living. His head control, trunk control, and graded movements are all poor. He is nonverbal and uses a Bliss communication system, pointing to the symbols with his index finger. His cognitive abilities are age appropriate and he is a highly motivated person. For mobility, he uses a powered wheel-chair (Figure 13-4).

To address his educational plan objective, "improve written communication skills," the child used a microcomputer, a word processing program, an interface for the computer, and a single switch. The interface converts the input from the switch into audible Morse code signals that provide feedback to the user. A brief activation of the switch results in a single "dot," or "short," of the code heard as a one tone output. A longer activation results in a tone change, and the child can hear by the two tones that he has entered a "dash," or "long" of the Morse code. This code input is converted by the interface and displayed on the computer screen as keyboard characters.

The occupational therapist working with this child has used two types of switch placement. One consists of a plate strapped to his chest, at the top of which, directly below his chin, the pressure switch is placed. He activates the switch by depressing his chin while his arms are secured to his lapboard to provide stability and limited extraneous movement. The other method uses the same switch mounted on his wheelchair lapboard. His right forearm is strapped to a board that elevates his hand approximately two inches to the same height as the surface of the switch. In this manner, flexion of the wrist operates the switch.

Formerly using a head pointer, keyguard, and keyboard input, the child was capable of inputing one word per minute with a large number of errors. Through the use of Morse code, he is now capable of four words per minute with few errors. It is anticipated that his performance will improve as he memorizes the Morse code, as switch operation is mastered, and as input simplification methods (through the use of special interface codes) are introduced.

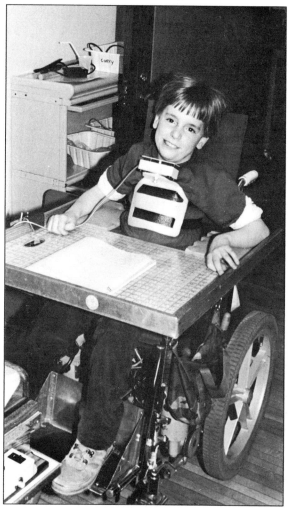

Figure 13-4. Child with cerebral palsy.

PRECAUTIONS FOR COMPUTER USE

Many individuals become so absorbed in the use of computer technology that it can literally consume their waking hours. Such people are often referred to as "hackers." It is important for occupational therapy personnel to carefully monitor the time periods that patients spend working on a computer. Since the lower extremities, trunk and neck often remain in a static position for a considerable length of time, it is necessary to make certain that work breaks are taken at frequent intervals and that proper positioning is maintained while the patient uses the computer. The computer and peripheral equipment should be placed on an adjustable height table to accommodate the individual needs of a variety of users. Adequate lighting must be provided, with glare reduction devices used as needed. Failure to take these measures may result in patients experiencing general fatigue, eyestrain and body aches, particularly in the neck and head.

According to Breines,[25] care should be taken when using computer programs for patients with cognitive and percep-tual disorders. Overemphasis on this treatment medium should be avoided. She has recommended further analysis and points to the problems inherent in using ". . .a two-dimensional tool for the resolution of a problem which derives from a three-dimensional dysfunction requiring peripheral (vision) input. . ."[25]

Breines also notes that furthur investigation is needed regarding the effects of computers for those individuals who are cataract prone or neurologically impaired. She has stated that since bifocal glasses are commonly used by the elderly as well as others, special near vision glasses may need to be substituted for these lenses when doing computer work.[25]

RESOURCES

The wide availability of computer resources may seem overwhelming to the new user. Among the many books on the market, one that is particularly useful to occupational therapy personnel is *Independence Day: Designing Computer Solutions for Individuals with Disability* by Peter Green and Alan J. Brightman.[26] In addition to specific recommendations for particular patient problems, an array of excellent resources are provided. Closing the Gap (see Bibliography) offers publications that are useful to both the new and experienced user of computers. It is also recommended that the reader refer to the "Software Review and Technology" column, a regular feature in the *American Journal of Occupational Therapy*. The bibliography at the end of this book lists additional information sources.

FUTURE DIRECTIONS

As technologic advances continue, opportunities for occupational therapy personnel to use computers will surely expand. The demands of the "information age"[26] will increase our reliance on computer systems to generate the information necessary to carry out everyday management and organizational tasks. For example, the use of bar code scanning, now common in grocery and department stores, will be used in health care settings to input data more quickly and to monitor varying changes more closely.

The Technology Assistance program, established by Congress in 1989, provides funds for states to help "establish programs for education, training, and delivery of assistive devices and services to disabled individuals of all ages."[27] Funding was authorized for $15 million for 1990. The availability of this money will certainly have an impact on our profession and those we serve.

Modern-day inventors, such as Raymond Kurzweil, are providing society with major innovations. Of particular note is Kurzweil's work on voice recognition as a means of computer input.[28] By simply speaking key words to the computer, a report or message can be quickly generated at the rate of 600 words per minute. Originally used by physicians for documentation purposes, this system is now available for health care professionals and their patients.[29] As the demand increases, costs are likely to drop. Kurzweil has stated that the Massachusetts Insurance Commission has ruled that physicians "who use the system are entitled to a reduction in malpractice insurance rates, since a study of reports showed them to be superior from a risk management point of view."[28]

Voice recognition systems are available also for individuals; however, the cost is currently quite high, resulting in limited access.[29]

The use of computer technology as a treatment modality will become even more widespread, as research studies continue to validate its effectiveness. Future research must also focus on identifying precautions and contraindications for specific problems. Work must continue to identify ways in which the use of computers and related devices can serve as a meaningful, goal-directed activity for recipients of occupational therapy services. We must establish standards for practice in all areas of technology as well as in quality assurance.

SUMMARY

Computers have numerous applications in occupational therapy departments. Once the user learns basic operations and related terminology, initial fears are replaced with new challenges. The variety of input and output equipment and devices and software programs available offer numerous opportunities for occupational therapy personnel to use computer technology in administrative tasks as well as patient evaluation and treatment activities. Word processors, databases, spreadsheets, and terminal programs offer ways to accomplish tasks in a much more efficient manner, thus increasing the overall productivity of the department. Small microcomputers offer many new opportunities to individuals with a variety of disabling handicaps. They are often an important tool to enable patients to control elements of their environments, enhance their communication skills, increase their employment opportunities, and develop new leisure pursuits. A great variety of computer systems and software are currently available.

Since use of computer technology is relatively new in the profession, care must be taken to exercise certain precautions, particularly with patients who have cognitive, neurologic, or certain visual impairments. Research must be conducted to further validate the use of computers in rehabilitation in general and in occupational therapy specifically.

Editor's Note

Only the most elementary terminology has been presented to acquaint the reader with basic information. Once one begins using the microcomputer and the many peripheral devices and software programs, efforts should be made to expand one's computer vocabulary and knowledge.

Acknowledgments

Case Study 13-1 was prepared by Ruth Garza, BS, COTA, former employee at the Occupational Therapy Department, University of Texas Medical Branch, Galveston, Texas. Case Study 13-2 was prepared by Mike Meyers, MA, OTR, Michael Dowling School, Minneapolis, Minnesota.

Related Learning Activities

1. Evaluate your skills in using the following programs: word processor, database, spreadsheet, and terminal. Identify areas in which more skill is needed, and enroll in the necessary classes or locate a knowledgeable person who can teach you.

2. Visit an occupational therapy department where microcomputers are used for evaluation and treatment. Prepare a report detailing the following information:
    a. Type of equipment used, including peripherals and input devices.
    b. Diagnostic groups or problems being treated.
    c. Goals being achieved
    d. Precautions and limitations

3. Visit a computer store and try out at least six demonstration programs. Identify programs that might be used in an OT program and specific goals that might be addressed.

4. What are some of the ways a computer could be used (or usage could be increased) in your classroom or clinic?

5. How could a computer be used with patients in a psychiatric setting?

References

1. Gerstenberger L: *The Apple Guide to Personal Computers in Education.* Cupertino, California, Apple Computer, 1983.
2. Doerr C: *Microcomputers and the 3 Rs: A Guide for Teachers.* Rochelle Park, New Jersey, Hayden, 1979.
3. Edwards J, Ellis A, Richardson D: *Computer Applications in Instruction: A Teacher's Guide to Selection and Use.* Hanover, New Hampshire, Timeshare, 1978, p. 13.
4. Sanders WB: *The Elementary Apple.* Chatsworth, California, Datamost, 1983.
5. Poole I: *Apple Users Guide.* Berkeley, California, Osborne/McGraw-Hill, 1981.
6. Robinson D: Word processing guide. *80 Micro Anniversary Issue.* 1983, pp. 28-31.
7. Keller W: The database explained. *80 Micro Anniversary Issue.* 1983, p. 32.
8. Ahl D: What is a spreadsheet? *Creative Computing* 10:S-2, 1984.
9. Glossbrenner A: *The Complete Handbook of Personal Computer Communications.* New York, St. Martin's Press, 1983.
10. Gordon RE, Kazole KP: Occupational therapy and rehabilitation engineering: A team approach to helping persons with severe physical disability to upgrade functional independence. *Occup Ther Health Care* 4:117, 1984.
11. Romich BA, Vagnini CB: Integrating communication, computer access, environmental control, and mobility. In Gergen M, Hagen D (Eds): *Computer Technology for Handicapped.* Henderson, Minnesota, Closing The Gap, 1985, p. 75.
12. Wambott JJ: Computer environmental control units for the severely disabled: A guide for the occupational therapist. *Occup Ther Health Care* 4:156, 1984.
13. Shadick M: Disease was her key to success. *Call A.P.P.L.E.* 10:66, 1983.
14. Crystal B: Computers help the deaf bridge the gap. In *Personal Computers and the Disabled—A Resource Guide.* Cupertino, California, Apple Computers 1984, p. 7.
15. Williams JM: Blind broker takes stock with a talking computer. *The Washington Post,* Monday, July 18, 1983.
16. Wall N: Microcomputer activites and occupational therapy. *Developmental Disabilities Special Interest Section Newsletter.* Rockville, Maryland, American Occupational Therapy Association 7:1, 1984.
17. Caronne JJ: The neurological examination. In Rosenthal M et al (Eds): *Rehabilitation of the Head Injured Adult.* Philadelphia, FA Davis, 1983, pp. 59-73.
18. Anonymous: Search. *Cognit Rehabil* 4:26-27, 1983.
19. Anonymous: City map. *Cognit Rehabil* 2:24-26, 1984.
20. Anonymous: Driver. *Cognit Rehabil* 4:23-24, 1983.
21. Anonymous: Sequential. *Cognit Rehabil* 5:46-52, 1985.
22. Katz R: Baker's dozen. *Cognit Rehabil* 5:42-46, 1984.
23. Katz R: Stars. *Cognit Rehabil* 6:47-50, 1984.
24. Ben-Yishay Y: Cognitive remediation. In Rosenthal M et al (Eds): *Rehabilitation of the Head Injured Adult.* Philadelphia, FA Davis, 1983.
25. Breines E: Computers and the private practitioner in occupational therapy. *Occup Ther Health Care* 2:110-111, 1985.
26. Green P, Brightman AJ: *Independence Day.* Cupertino, California, Apple Computers, 1990.
27. Somers FP: Federal report. *OT Week* 3:60, 1989.
28. Lipner M: Raymond Kurzweil invents his own success. *Compass Readings,* April, 1990.
29. Joe BE: IBM gives voice to computers in rehab. *OT Week* 5:44, 1991.

Section IV
CONTEMPORARY MEDIA TECHNIQUES

Thermoplastic Splinting of the Hand

Constructing Adaptive Equipment

Contemporary media techniques are the focus of this section, which provides the reader with numerous opportunities to acquire new skills or enhance existing ones. Thermoplastic splinting and the construction of adaptive equipment are addressed specifically. Although other topics could have been included, those here are the primary areas in which the COTA should establish competency. Whatever media technique is used, the practitioner must be certain that the procedures are goal directed and are carried out properly and safely to ensure that the patient will derive the maximum benefit.

Chapter 14

Thermoplastic Splinting of the Hand

Patrice Schober-Branigan, OTR

INTRODUCTION

The role of the certified occupational therapy assistant (COTA) in the area of splinting may be as varied as the environments in which assistants works. Hand splinting is certainly a technical skill; yet the judgment and knowledge of hand anatomy, biomechanics, and pathology that is required when determining what type of splint to use and for what period of time is considerable. Just as an appropriate splint can *enhance* function, an inappropriate splint cannot only fail in this respect, but may cause *harm*. Therefore, the COTA must work closely with a registered occupational therapist (OTR) to assure that the appropriate splinting is accomplished for an individual patient.

This chapter provides a basic introduction to hand splinting, including historical perspectives, basic principles and purposes, assessment considerations, techniques, and materials. With this background, the entry-level COTA will have some understanding of the many complexities of work in this area of practice. Once necessary knowledge and skills

have been demonstrated, the COTA may be assigned to make static splints, such as those presented in this chapter.

The patient with a relatively *unaltered* hand (anatomically) would be best suited for splint construction by an entry-level COTA; making even a simple resting splint for a hand that has been moderately affected by spasticity, injury or rheumatoid arthritis can challenge even the most experienced therapist.

A COTA who works in a setting where a high volume of hand splinting is performed may become particularly adept in this skill. Continuing education, both formal and on-the-job, is essential, as new materials and techniques become available.

HISTORICAL PERSPECTIVES

Splinting has become a commonly used treatment in most physical disability clinics during the past 25 years, in part because of the availability of low-temperature **thermoplastic**

KEY CONCEPTS

Purposes and types

Biomechanical design principles

Construction principles

Construction techniques

Specific fabrication procedures

Impact on role performance

ESSENTIAL VOCABULARY

Thermoplastic

Memory

Functional position

Static splints

Dynamic splints

Joint creases

Deformity prevention

Anatomic arches

Bony prominences

Patient education

materials. These materials are extremely "user friendly," when compared to the old metals, fiberglass, plaster of Paris, and high-temperature plastics.[1-3] Before 1965, when Johnson & Johnson introduced Orthoplast®, therapists and assistants using high-temperature plastics, such as Royalite™, had to use ovens and hot mitts, make repeated fittings, and possibly even use plaster of Paris molds to fabricate what still may have turned out to be cumbersome and less than satisfactorily fitting splints.[2] With the introduction of Orthoplast®, a low-temperature plastic which could be heated in 160° F water, occupational therapy personnel were able to quickly cut and shape material, often with the use of a temporary Ace bandage, directly onto a patient's extremities, with little danger of burning the skin. There was finally a high probability of good fit and appearance, with construction requiring a fraction of the time and effort needed in the past when working with high-temperature plastics.

In the 1970s, other plastics companies introduced competing, low-temperature plastics including, Polyform® and Aquaplast®. The newer materials had similarities, as well as differences, when compared to Orthoplast®. Polyform® contained no rubber, and therfore, did not require the firm stretching that certain types of Orthoplast® splints sometimes required when molding. Polyform® was also a "drapable" material that rarely required the initial Ace bandage wrappings that were commonly needed for work with Orthoplast® to assure that it would conform to contours of the extremity. Unlike Orthoplast®, however, Polyform® had no "**memory**", memory referring here to the ability of a material to return to its orginal flat shape and size when reheated. WFR/Aquaplast® introduced a material that became transparent while warm and also did have memory.

Gradually, more and more materials have been made available, including those that combine some of the qualities of the original rubber Orthoplast® and the stretchy Polyform®. Currently at least six companies produce splint products, with most offering three or more varieties of materials. Each company has competed for a larger part of the splinting market and, in so doing, has tried to develop more easily used materials than those already in existence.

Other technologic advances have helped splint fabrication develop into today's highly regarded modality. The introduction of hook-and-loop products, such as Velcro, has eliminated the need for bulky buckles and straps. Self-adhesive hook-and-loop products, adhered directly onto the splint surface, have also eliminated the need for the majority of riveting that used to be required, once again simplifying the splinting process.

Developments within surgical medicine and the therapy professions have also provided impetus for splinting technique and material development. As hand surgeons and reconstructive burn surgeons began to realize the tremendously important roles that rehabilitative therapies such as occupational therapy and physical therapy could play in assuring optimal postsurgical results, occupational therapy personnel began specializing in these fields. Due in part to the high volume of daily, often complex, and diverse splinting fabrication required of these therapists, more and more innovative designs and construction techniques developed in addition to those developed in the more traditional, long-established clinics by therapists and assistants working with patients having central nervous system dysfunction and arthritis.

In the 1990s and beyond, OTRs and COTAs will find splint fabrication to be not only useful and challenging, but also a highly approachable and effective modality when treating their patients.

BASIC CONCEPTS, TYPES AND PURPOSES

Why Do We Use Splints?

Occupational therapy personnel have always been concerned with the individual's ability to function, and hand use is a critical element. What, in particular, must a hand do to be functional? Perhaps the easiest way to answer this question and to illustrate the components of hand function is to observe your hand as you reach to pick up an object. The majority of the time, your *thumb* will *oppose* your fingers, and your *fingers* will be partially *flexed*. Although we also use our hands for other types of grasp (ie, you may flex your wrist as you reach behind your back, or you may flatten your hand as you smooth blankets on a bed), most of the time this **functional position** is the most critical position in daily activities. Figure 14-1 shows the functional position of the hand.

When individuals experience any kind of disease or injury that threatens their ability to use their hands, we must try to assure them that they will still be able to assume the position of function. A flat hand is not functional for performing *most* activities and neither is a hand that has stiffened into a severely flexed position. The use of splints, together with exercise, engagement in purposeful activities, and rest, is part of a comprehensive rehabilitation program aimed at assuring maximal function. More specific examples are provided later in this chapter.

Types of Splints

Although a wide variety of splints are available, they can be divided into two basic types: *static* and *dynamic*. **Static splints** place and maintain the body part in one position. A static wrist splint does not allow wrist motion. It *holds* the wrist in a functional position as shown in Figure 14-2, which depicts a wrist cock-up splint. These splints may be fabricated from materials, such as plastic, metal, elastic

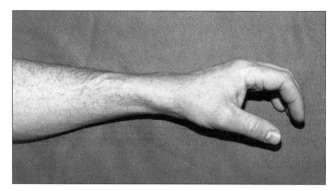

Figure 14-1. Functional position.

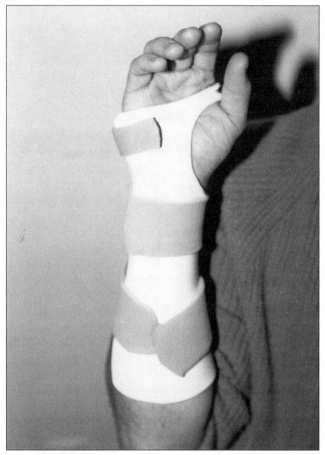

Figure 14-2. Wrist cock-up splint.

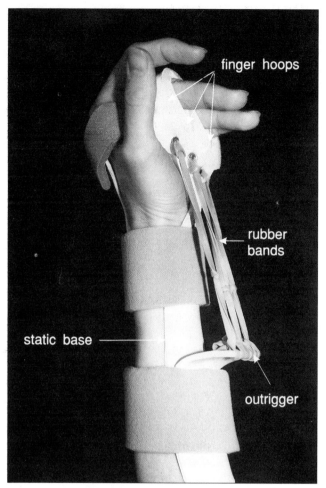

Figure 14-3. Dynamic MP flexion splint.

reinforced with metal, or leather. In contrast, **dynamic splints** allow for movement of the involved part. Usually, a force creates tension on a joint, encouraging extension, flexion or opposition. The part acted on is allowed to move instead of being held in one position. For example, rubber bands attached to leather or cloth loops may pull the metacarpophalangeal (MP) joints into a flexed position as shown in Figure 14-3. Another example is the use of a small spring-activated splint, which may assist in stretching the proximal interphalangeal (PIP) joint that has a flexion contracture into an extended position. Dynamic splints may combine any number of elements, such as a static splint used as a base, an "outrigger" of plastic or wire (see **Figure 14-3**), rubber bands, finger loops, elastic, rubber tubing, springs, pulleys, hinges and Velcro. Due to the complexity of dynamic splinting, which is beyond the scope of this chapter, readers are encouraged to refer to the references for further information and to consult with therapists who are experienced in this type of splinting.

In most cases, splints are named by the function they serve (ie, "wrist cock-up splint," "resting hand splint," "dynamic PIP extension splint"). Occasionally, names such as "anti-claw splint" as shown in Figure 14-4 or a "thumb spica splint" as shown in Figure 14-5 may need further explanation for COTAs who are inexperienced in working with splints.

Specific Purposes of Splinting

Splints may be used for any or several of the following purposes:

1. *Protection to allow for proper healing.* A physician may apply a bulky plaster splint to a patient's arm immediately after an acute injury such as a fracture or a tendon

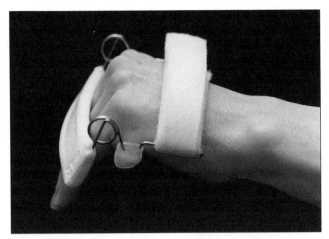

Figure 14-4. Anti-claw splint. *Product of LMB splint company.*

injury. If the physician desires a lighter weight, removable splint, however, the person may be referred to the occupational therapy department for fabrication of a thermoplastic splint. When an injury is not acute, as in the case of carpal tunnel syndrome or tendonitis, which develop over a period of time, the physician is likely to make a direct referral to occupational therapy personnel for fabrication of a splint or fitting of a prefabricated splint. An example is the Freedom Flex® splint shown in Figure 14-6.

2. *Decrease pain.* This often is also a goal of protective splints used after injury or of splints used when joints or soft tissues are inflamed or unstable, as in rheumatoid arthritis.

3. *Increase functional use.* The patient who cannot fully straighten the fingers after a nerve injury may use an "anti-claw" splint during daily activities; this splint serves roughly the same extending function as would the paralyzed muscles. Individuals with quadriplegia may also use functional splints that provide wrist extension and/or finger-thumb opposition. These are referred to as tenodesis splints.

4. *Prevention of deformity and maintenance of range of motion.* Any time a patient is unable to move a joint through its complete range of motion, the use of a splint may be indicated to **prevent deformity** and assist in maintaining range of motion. A person in a coma may have resting hand splints applied as well as lower extremity splints. An individual with rheumatoid arthritis whose MP joints are swollen, inflamed, and stiffened may use a resting hand splint, which places the MP joints in moderate extension, as this motion is typically decreased by rheumatoid disease. Figure 14-7 shows one type of resting hand splint.

Although there are a variety of approaches to splinting for spasticity, whether related to such diverse conditions as cerebral palsy or a cerebral vascular accident, a splint may be used to passively extend the fingers and wrist if the patient has overpowering tone in the flexors. In any of the preceding cases, active assisted range of motion

(ROM) and/or passive ROM exercise would be essential aspects of treatment. The splint would provide an important adjunctive function.

5. *Increase range of motion.* When a joint has limited ROM due to soft tissue tightness or contracture, static or dynamic splints may be used to correct it. Static splints that are regularly *refabricated* to provide increasing, gentle stretch are called *serial* splints. Dynamic splints that have moving parts controlled by springs or rubber bands may also be used and adjusted to provide increasing tension. Of utmost importance is that the tension be applied gently, well within the patient's pain tolerance, and that no adverse effects, such as increased swelling or stiffness, occur. The goal is never to "break loose" shortened or adherent tissue, but instead to gently stretch its fibers and allow the tissue to gradually elongate. In addition, if dynamic splints have outriggers, the line of pull from the cord or rubberband and finger loop unit to the outrigger must be at a right angle in relation to the part of the finger it is pulling (see Figure 14-3).

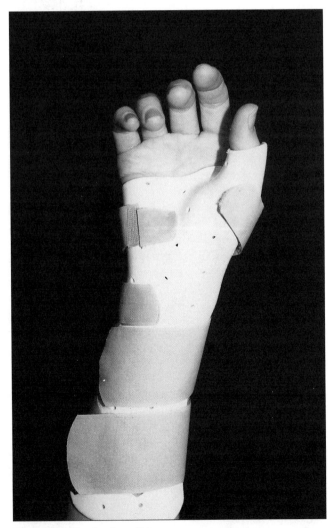

Figure 14-5. Thumb spica splint.

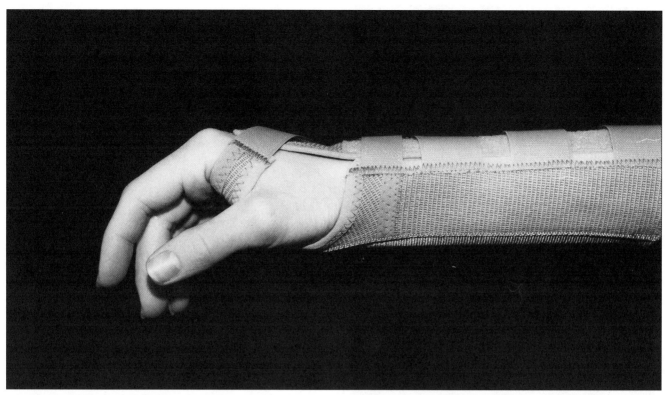

Figure 14-6. Freedom Flex® splint. *Product of Alimed, Inc.*

6. *Scar flattening.* The profuse scarring that occurs after some types of traumatic injury and severe burns may be minimized by proper pressure applied through the application of splints and pressurized elastic garments. As with dynamic splinting, readers who desire more information on this complex subject are referred to references cited in the bibliography.

ASSESSMENT PROCESS

Ideally, use of a splint is simply one part of a comprehensive rehabilitation program, so in most cases when a splinting fabrication order is received, the OTR is also completing a comprehensive assessment of the patient. The COTA may assist in some aspects of obtaining objective data, ie, measuring grip and pinch strength using a dynamometer and a tensiometer, respectively. He or she may also assist in observing and timing the patient's performance during standardized coordination testing, such as the *Minnesota Rate of Manipulation*, or measuring hand volume to monitor edema through the use of a hand volumeter device as shown in Figure 14-8. However, the patient referred to occupational therapy specfically for splint fabrication after an acute injury may be unable to tolerate this type of assessment. In addition, in some cases time and resources may be limited and

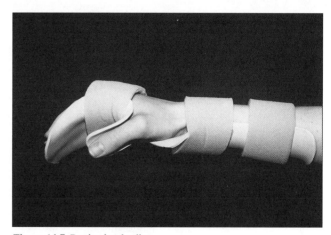

Figure 14-7. Resting hand splint.

completion of a full evaluation during the first visit will not be feasible if adequate time for splint fabrication is allowed. In these situations, the minimal assessment carried out by the OTR would require obtaining the following information:

1. Primary and secondary diagnosis
2. General health/functional status
3. Medical procedures performed, including surgery and exact dates
4. Healing status (if applicable, according to physician)
5. Goal(s) of use of splint(s)
6. Type of splint recommended

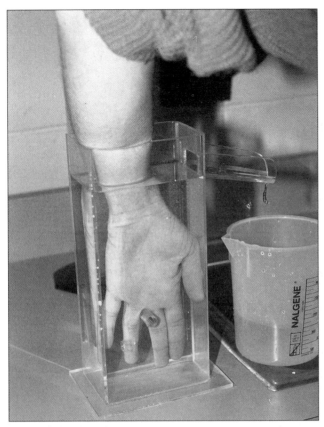

Figure 14-8. Hand volumeter for measuring edema.

7. Splint use requirements—full-time or intermittent (can splint be removed, and if so under what conditions?)
8. Precautions and restrictions
9. Is hand to be *used* with or without splint?
10. Description of location and level of pain, if applicable
11. Description of work duties, if applicable
12. Description of home duties
13. Description of sports and other leisure activities engaged in

Of equal importance, the occupational therapist needs to complete at least an informal examination of the incision (if any), skin status, degree of swelling (if present), sensation and, if possible, range of motion, muscle function, strength, endurance and coordination. If the individual is to wear the splint during specific work, home or sports and other leisure activities, an analysis of the motions required as well as particular tools, materials, and other equipment is desirable. Having the person demonstrate or describe the motions involved in carrying out these tasks is especially important to assure that the splint will interfere as little as possible with task completion.

The attitude of the patient toward wearing a splint and his or her understanding of its purpose is a critical factor. The best splint will accomplish little if the person refuses to wear it.

BIOMECHANICAL DESIGN PRINCIPLES AND RELATED CONSIDERATIONS

A splint should always be made in a way that gives primary consideration to the anatomy of the hand and wrist; the biomechanics, particularly of the involved limb; life tasks; and the abilities of the individual who must wear it. More specific biomechanical design principles are described in the following sections.

Immobilization

Any time a splint is applied to a body part, motion and sensation will be compromised and strength and function may decrease, depending on the length of time it is worn. Therefore, splints should be used only when the physician and the OTR deem them absolutely necessary and only on those parts of the arm or hand that must be immobilized.

Creases of the Hand

If full movement of specific joints is desirable, the splint must be "cut back" or folded over adequately, proximal to those specific **joint creases** (ie, grooves in the skin related to joint movement) as shown in Figure 14-9. For example, a splint that is used to immobilize only the wrist, not the thumb and fingers, should be cut back proximal to the palmar creases (proximal palmar crease for index and middle fingers, distal palmar crease for ring and little

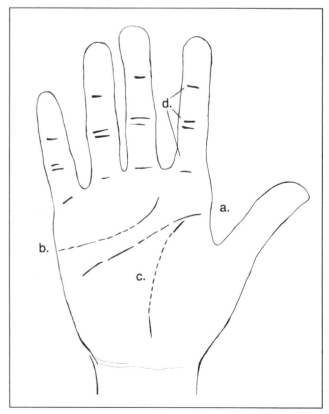

Figure 14-9. Creases of the hand.

fingers). If the thumb is to move freely, the thenar crease should be free.

Arches of the Hand

The human hand has three **anatomic arches:** the distal and proximal transverse arches and the longitudinal arch, as shown in Figure 14-10. The proximal transverse arch refers to the position of the wrist and carpometacarpal joints. This is a more rigid arch than the others and is only subtly visible externally. In contrast, the distal transverse arch refers to the more obvious and flexible arched position of the metacarpal heads that is visible as soon as the fingers are placed in any flexed position such as that shown in Figure 14-11. The long finger metacarpal head is at the highest part of the arch; the other metacarpal heads appear lower on each side. The longitudinal arch intersects the transverse arch longitudinally and is most marked centrally between the long finger MP and the wrist. When considered together, the arches assist hand function by allowing the fingers to rotate toward the thumb and providing a "deepening" of the palmar tissue to assist in securely holding objects in the palm of the hand.

When making a splint, one must be certain that these arches are preserved. The splint shape itself must be "arched" transversely and longitudinally if the patient is to use the hand when wearing it. Splints constructed from thermoplastic materials are particularly well suited to molding of this kind.

Bony Prominences

Bony prominences of the hand (the structures on the surface of bones) have little natural tissue padding and may experience skin breakdown whenever pressure is applied for long periods. The radial and ulnar styloids are two of the most common problem areas. These bony prominences are shown in Figure 14-12. Splints should provide relief over these areas. Taping padding over them before splint fabrication will provide "enlarged" relief areas when the splinting material is

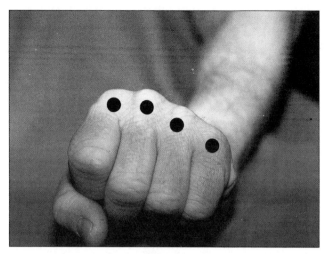

Figure 14-11. Distal transverse metacarpal arch.

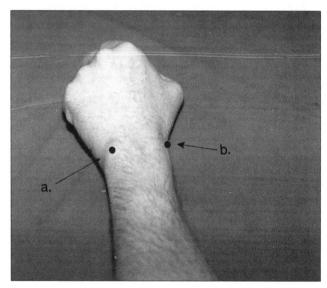

Figure 14-12. Bony prominences. A. ulnar styloid; B. radial styloid.

applied over the prominences. The padding can then be removed from the patient's arm or hand. Once the splint is completed, similar or thinner padding can be adhered to the same areas directly onto the inner surface of the splint. In many cases, however, the relieved areas themselves may provide adequate protection, even without padding.

The 2/3 Principle

Any time a splint must support the wrist or the wrist and digits, the forearm portion of the splint should extend two-thirds proximally up the forearm. This will provide adequate support for the weight of the hand and help prevent the wrist from inadvertently "popping up" out of the splint with hand use.

The 1/2 Circumference Principle

In order for straps to actually have contact with the arm or hand to *secure the splint* and to avoid slipping, the splint

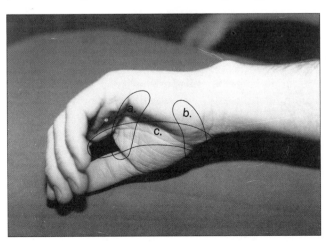

Figure 14-10. Arches of the hand: A. Distal transverse arch; B. Proximal transverse arch; C. Longitudinal arch.

material should extend only one-half the circumference of the forearm as shown in Figure 14-13. This curvature also helps provide desirable rigidity to the splint and prevents any need for extra reinforcement, making the splint less cumbersome for the wearer.

Appearance

Splints should be visually acceptable for most individuals to agree to wear them. For example, plastic and strap corners should be rounded, and there should be no fingerprint indentations or ink marks. It is important for splints to be cleaned regularly and worn parts should be replaced or repaired. If dynamic splints have outriggers, they should protrude as little as possible away from the splint, yet still accomplish their goals, ie, flexion or extension.

TYPES OF MATERIALS

With the many advances in modern splinting technology has come greater complexity for occupational therapy personnel in determining which splinting material to select. Names and characteristics of the many materials available can become so numerous that the new practitioner may become overwhelmed. For this reason the following questions must be asked and related information considered to help simplify the decision-making process.

1. *What type of materials are already available in the clinic?* If material sheets are clearly labeled, the COTA can check the chart regarding characteristics (Table 14-1) or read the manufacturer's literature. In addition, occupational therapy personnel are using "1-800" telephone numbers (see Appendix F) to gain timely information. Certainly, observing experienced co-workers and allowing time to practice

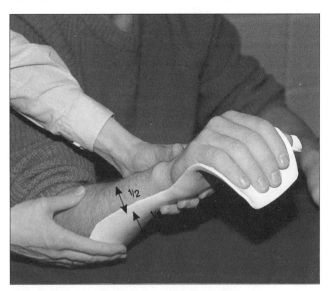

Figure 14-13. One-half circumference principle.

with an unfamiliar material would be most desirable.

2. *What type of splint is needed?* A more rubber-like* material that will not easily lose its shape or fingerprint may be especially good for:

a. the new COTA who may need to repeatedly reform the splint while fabricating it

b. an OTR who is used to stretching, pulling, and wrapping splint materials while forming them

c. an uncooperative patient or one with spasticity

d. a larger size splint with little need for intricate detail

e. a splint that may require a considerable amount of reforming over a period of days or weeks because of edema changes

In contrast, a highly conforming splint material, as described in Type C of Table 14-1, may be indicated in the following situations:

a. the therapist who is adept at draping, working with gravity, and using palms or heels of the hand to avoid fingerprinting

b. the patient is cooperative and does not require significant positioning or repositioning

c. for the burn splint or scar flattening splint when a high degree of detail is desirable

d. times when little need for reforming is predicted and no edema is present

e. construction of smaller splints such as those used for fingers

Some materials that combine rubber-like qualities with conformability are described in the Type B listing found in Table 14-1, and may provide a compromise.

3. *What other factors should be considered?*

Whenever splinting is performed it is also important to answer the following questions:

a. If the splint is to be worn for a long time over palmar surfaces (which may perspire), is perforation needed? Most splinting materials are available in perforated form.

b. Is an outrigger to be fabricated from plastic? If so, one of the more rigid materials may be needed.

c. Is long-term use probable (ie, when a patient has a chronic condition such as rheumatoid arthritis or tendonitis)? Perhaps a smooth, dirt-resistant surface is necessary to withstand frequent or near-constant use.

d. Is the splint very small or does it not require significant rigidity? Perhaps a $^1/_{16}$-inch material would be less obtrusive (check with manufacturers for availability, as standard thickness is $^1/_8$-inch for all material listed in Table 14-1).

e. Is the patient's hand particularly sensitive to touch or pressure or both? A drapable material may require the least therapist or assistant contact.

---

*The material may not necessarily contain *rubber*, but it resembles the rubber-like characteristics of Orthoplast®, which does contain rubber (see Type A in the chart shown in Table 14-1).

Table 14-1
Types of Materials

The COTA is encouraged to become familiar with the manufacturer's literature for any given material. This chart is intended to be a broad comparison of materials (see note 1).

Type A: Rubber-like materials—do not necessarily contain rubber but require stretching and tolerate handling; resist fingerprinting; minimal if any drapability

Name/ Manufacturer and/or Supplier	Material Composition	Temperature/ Time to Heat	Conformability when Heated	Memory*	Adherence to Self	Finished Product's Rigidity	Finished Product's Surface	Other Notes
Orthoplast® *Johnson and Johnson*	Isoprene rubber	150°/60 sec.	Requires stretching or wrapping with Ace bandage	Yes	Material should be dry and hot (use heat gun); solvent may enhance	Semi-flexible; requires contouring of edges and/or reinforcement to assure rigidity in finished splint	Absorbent	• Most well-known early thermoplastic • Higher priced than many thermoplastics • May shrink mildly when heated • May yellow with wear/ age
Ezeform® *Smith & Nephew/ Rolyan*	Plastic	160°/60 sec.	Requires some stretching; using Ace or firm touch may cause some indentations	Minimal	Dry and hot (may also adhere to lint and towels)	Very rigid	Absorbent	• May soil easily over time
K-Splint III® *Fred Sammons*	"	"	"	"	"	"	"	"
Synergy® *Smith & Nephew/ Rolyan*	Plastic	"	Requires stretching	Yes	Dry and hot	Mild flexibility	Smooth/non-absorbent	• Available in colors
Ultrasplint® *Polymed*	"Rubber-like compound"†	"	"	"	"	Rigid	"	
Aquaplast GS (Green Stripe)® *WFR Aquaplast Corporation*	Plastic	"	Conformable, but least of Aquaplast® products	Yes	Available either in self-adherent (original) or non-adherent, which requires scratching surface or solvent; dry and hot	Rigid	Smooth	• Transparent when heated

Table 14-1
Types of Materials (continued)

Type B: Plastic materials—combine some need for and tolerance of stretching/handling (like Type A "rubber-like" materials), yet also some drapability (like Type C plastic materials)

Name/ Manufacturer and/or Supplier	Material Composition	Temperature/ Time to Heat	Conformability when Heated	Memory*	Adherence to Self	Finished Product's Rigidity	Finished Product's Surface	Other Notes
Polyflex II® *Smith & Nephew/ Rolyan*	Plastic	150-160°/ 60 sec.	Will drape, yet less than Polyform®	Yes	Solvent or scratch finish with scissors before heating; dry and hot	Rigid	Smooth	----
K-Splint Isoprene® *Fred Sammons*	"	"	"	"	"	"	"	----
Customsplint* *Polymed*	"Combination rubber-like/ plastic compound"†	160-170°/ 60 sec.	Will drape, yet less than Precisionsplint®	Some	Dry and hot	"Semi-flexible"†	Very smooth	• A newer material
Aquaplast* Original WFR *Aquaplast Corporation*	Plastic	160°	Highly conformable	Yes	Sticky without special preparation; requires care **not** to adhere inadvertently	Rigid	Smooth	• Transparent when heated
Aquaplast T® WFR *Aquaplast Corporation*	Plastic	"	"	"	Solvent or scratch surface; dry and hot	Rigid	Smooth	• Unlike original Aquaplast®, will not inadvertently adhere to self

Table 14-1
Types of Materials (continued)

Type C: Plastic materials are highly drapable and conformable to details; do not require or tolerate more that mild stretching or handling‡

Name/ Manufacturer and/or Supplier	Material Composition	Temperature/ Time to Heat	Conformability when Heated	Memory*	Adherence to Self	Finished Product's Rigidity	Finished Product's Surface	Other Notes
Polyform® Smith & Nephew/ Rolyan	Plastic	150-160°/ 60 sec. **Do not overheat!**	Highly conformable, drapable; duplicates contours of hand/body part	Minimal	Solvent or scratch finish with scissors before heating; dry and hot	Rigid	Smooth	----
K-Splint I® Fred Sammons	"	"	"	"	"	"	"	---
Multiform I® Alimed	"	"	"	Some	Dry and hot	"	"	---
Multiform II® Alimed	"	"	"	"	Solvent or scratch; dry and hot	"	"	---
Precisionsplint® Polymed	"	"	"	Minimal	Dry and hot	"	"	---
Aquaplast BS® (Blue Stripe®) WFR Aquaplast Corporation	"	"	"	Yes	Solvent or scratch; dry and hot	"	"	• Transparent when heated

©1990 Patrice Schober-Brannigan, OTR. Reprinted with permission.
*Memory: Ability to return to original flat shape/size when reheated
†Manufacturer's description
‡Except for Aquaplast BS®, which, unlike the other materials listed under Type C, does have a memory and will return nearly to its original shape/size if reheated.

Rather than deciding that any one material is best, the experienced COTA will discover that different splinting materials require the use of different skills and that individual materials may more easily lend themselves to one type of splint construction over another. When resources are limited or when splinting is only performed occasionally, occupational therapy personnel may prefer to keep a supply of one of the materials listed under Type A or Type B in Table 14-1, as these materials more easily withstand repeated handling without a significant adverse affect on appearance, strength or splint shape.

CONSTRUCTION PRINCIPLES AND TECHNIQUES

Equipment

To ensure the efficient and timely fabrication of a splint, it is essential to have available the correct tools, materials and adequate work space. The following furniture and tools, as shown in Figure 14-14, are necessary:

1. Small table and two chairs for patient and therapist
2. Countertop or table for equipment
3. Electric frying pan or other flat-bottomed pan and a heating device that will allow water to be heated to at least 160° F
4. Thermometer
5. Tongs
6. Heat gun with a funnel (for hard to reach or small areas)
7. Fiskars®-type scissors, preferably one pair for cutting splinting material and one pair for cutting straps
8. Curved blade scissors
9. Utility knife
10. Heavy duty shears for cutting unheated thermoplastic
11. Hole punch
12. Awl

It is also desirable to have access to a sewing machine; a machinist's-type, portable, table-mounted anvil; and a ball-peen hammer.

Supplies for Static Splinting

The supplies specified in the following list should be available:

1. Thermoplastic splinting material

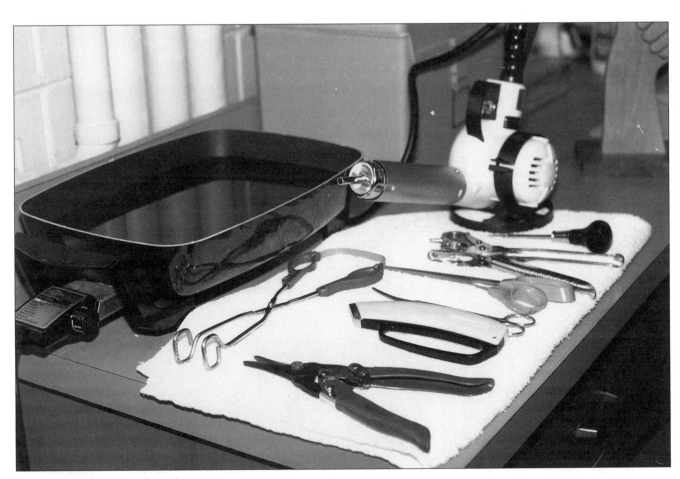

Figure 14-14. Splint construction tools.

2. Straps or rolls of 1-inch and 2-inch hook and loop Velcro
3. Padding (see note 2)
4. Paper towels
5. Ace bandage
6. Tubular stockinnette
7. Needle and thread
8. Rivets
9. Tape
10. Towels

INSTRUCTIONS FOR SPLINT FABRICATION

Resting Hand Splint (Suitable for Someone with Rheumatoid Arthritis)

Materials. The following materials and tools should be located: paper towel, pencil, pen or awl, utility knife or heavy-duty shears, scissors with a curved blade, straps, hook and loop Velcro, Ace bandage (if using Orthoplast®), electric frying pan and thermoplastic material. The author recommends a more rubber-like material that is not highly stretchy or drapable for the COTA who is learning how to fabricate splints (see preceding information on types of materials and Table 14-1). A perforated material may also be desirable (to prevent an accumulation of perspiration) unless particularly rigid support is required. In this case, it may be better to use a plain, nonperforated material for fabrication and then drill several holes as needed for ventilation.

Procedure

1. Heat water to 160° F.
2. Trace around hand to make a pattern, adding enough to extend one-half the circumference of the arm, fingers and thumb. If Orthoplast® or another material that shrinks is used, be sure to allow for shrinkage when making the pattern, as excess material can always be trimmed off. Conversely, if the material is likely to stretch, this factor must also be taken into account. The pattern will resemble a mitten. Check to be sure it extends two-thirds the forearm length (Figure 14-15).
3. Trace pattern onto thermoplastic material using a pencil or an awl. A pen is not recommended, as ink may be difficult to remove (Figure 14-16).
4. "Rough-cut" splint out of larger piece of material using heavy-duty shears or utility knife (Figure 14-17).
5. Place into pan—usually about one minute is sufficient for softening. Remove when softened and place on a counter or towel (Figure 14-18).
6. Cut out splint with scissors. If necessary, use smaller pair of scissors with a curved blade to cut thumb web space (Figure 14-19).

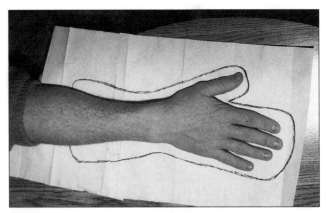

Figure 14-15. Making a pattern for a resting hand splint.

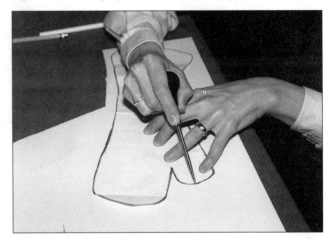

Figure 14-16. Tracing pattern.

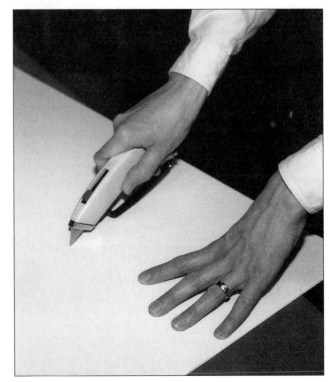

Figure 14-17. "Rough-cutting" splint.

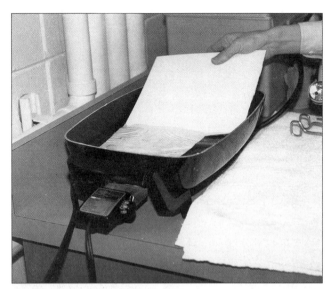

Figure 14-18. Placing material into pan.

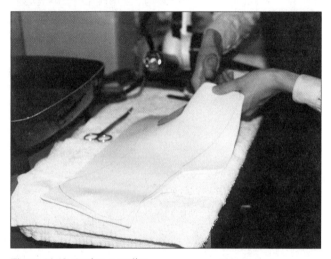

Figure 14-19. Cutting out splint.

7. Have patient assume functional hand position. Wrist should be in mild extension (15 to 30 degrees), MPs moderately extended (as close to zero degrees as is comfortable). PIPs flexed to approximately 45 to 60 degrees, and DIPs flexed to approximately 15 to 30 degrees; thumb in a gently (not maximally) abducted position from the palm. Have client supinate forearm in this position, if possible (see Figure 14-1; see note 3).

8. Place the thermoplastic material onto your own hand to assist in doing some "pre-forming," unless your hand size is vastly larger or smaller than the patient's. Remember which hand the splint is being made for (right or left)! Let the patient feel the temperature of the material before placing it onto his or her skin (Figure 14-20).

9. Place warm splint onto patient's hand. If the material drapes or stretches somewhat, the supinated position will allow gravity to assist. Work by briefly stroking this

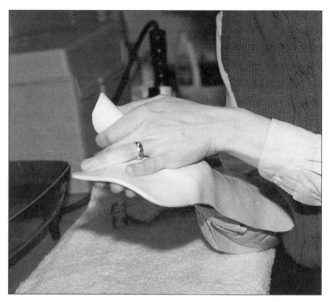

Figure 14-20. Preforming material.

type of material with several fingers or the palms of the therapist's or assistant's hands. Be sure to center it on the hand and arm so that the edge will be stretched around to make the "sides" of the splint. Avoid holding the splint on any one spot for an extended time if the material becomes fingerprinted. Check the position of the hand. Is the wrist in the desired position? Make adjustments as needed. Be sure to smooth the palmar area into the arches of the palm (Figure 14-21).

10. Optionally, gently wrap with an Ace bandage to form the splint if the material requires firm stretching as with Orthoplast®. Assure the thumb web position first; wrap throughout the palm and forearm; if necessary, return for the finger "pan" and thumb "gutter." Use another bandage if necessary. Again, be sure to mold palmar arches (Figure 14-22).

11. When the splint has cooled enough to appear formed, yet is still slightly warm (experience will develop a sense of timing regarding this step), ask patient to pronate arm. Confirm that splint is still centered on arm and adjust as needed. With a pencil or your fingernail, mark the edges of the splint material so that anything in excess of one-half the circumference of the arm will be trimmed. Splint should extend slightly beyond the fingertips and two-thirds of the forearm. Gently remove the splint when it is firm enough not to lose its shape, but still warm enough to trim with scissors. Trim. If necessary, dip edges into hot water quickly before cutting (Figure 14-23). Gently flare the proximal end of the splint so that it does not irritate the patient's forearm.

12. Assure fit on the patient. Gently stretch forearm trough by hand if it is too tight.

13. Round corners on straps near adhesive section (Figure 14-24).

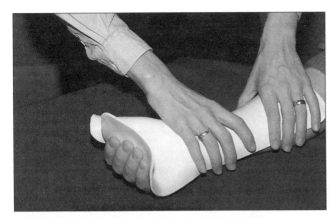

Figure 14-21. Placing of warm splinting material on patient.

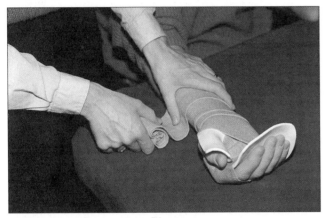

Figure 14-22. Wrapping with Ace™ bandage.

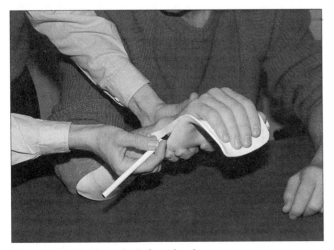

Figure 14-23. Marking splint before trimming excess.

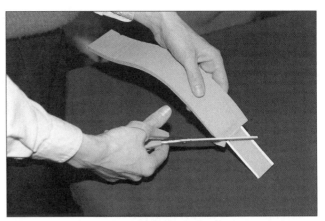

Figure 14-24. Rounding corners on straps.

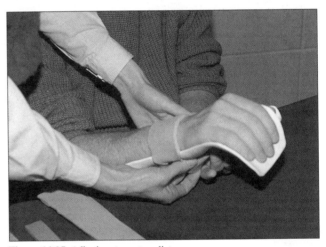

Figure 14-25. Adhering straps to splint.

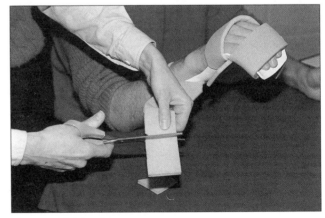

Figure 14-26. Trimming straps.

14. Adhere strap to splint (Figure 14-25).

15. Trim straps (Figure 14-26).

Figure 14-27 shows the finished splint when being worn by the patient.

16. Instruct the patient about precautions for wearing and caring for splint.

17. Check for irritating points (ie, at bony prominences, splint edges, and fingertips) and adjust as needed.

Wrist Cock-up Splint

Before constructing this splint, the reader is referred to the preceding section, "Resting Hand Splint" instructions, for a detailed discussion of fabrication. The following is an abbreviated discussion and assumes some familiarity with the splint construction process.

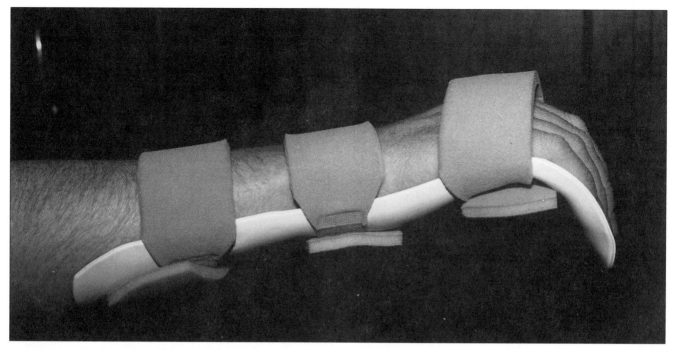

Figure 14-27. Completed resting splint.

Materials. Materials are the same as for the resting splint in the preceding section. A more stretchy, drapable thermoplastic material would be acceptable, although not necessary.

Procedure.

1. Make pattern by tracing around palmar surface of hand and forearm. Extend just distal to the distal palmar creases and lateral to the thenar crease to allow enough material for flaring splint edges. This technique adds strength and comfort (Figures 14-28 and 14-29).

2. Pre-form splint over own hand by flaring and folding over distal portion and thenar aspect (Figure 14-30).

3. Form the splint onto the patient. Be sure it is distal to the palmar creases and nearly clears (is medial to) the thenar crease; radial styloid should be free of pressure; lengths should be two-thirds of forearm. Remember to mold arches (Figure 14-31).

4. Trim edges so that one-half the circumference of forearm and two-thirds the length of forearm are covered by splint.

5. Attach straps.

6. Instruct patient on precautions for wearing and caring for the splint.

7. Check for points of irritation (ie, radial and ulnar styloids, thumb web space, dorsum of hand, and under edges of splint). Adjust as needed.

The finished wrist cock-up splint is shown in Figure 14-32.

SAFETY PRECAUTIONS

Finishing

Splints should be comfortable for the wearer. Adhering to the biomechanical principles presented in the previous sections will help assure comfort. In addition, the splint straps, the splint itself, or, if it is dynamic, its dynamic components should never cut off circulation or cause numbness. Fingertips must never be "blanched" by a splint. Edges should be smoothed.

Adjustments

Splints should be readjusted if they cause "wear" marks that remain on the skin for 15 to 30 minutes after the splint has been removed. Even if a splint is used to increase range of motion, its stretching properties must be carefully monitored and readjusted by the OTR so that stretching is done gradually.

The COTA may be involved in checking a patient's skin to assure that a splint fits properly. If adjustments are required to loosen the splint because of swelling, sometimes one is able to simply stretch the splint by hand without heating to make it wider or more narrow. With some of the more rigid materials, one may wish to use two pair of pliers to assist in stretching, being sure to protect the splint from plier marks by covering the areas with a towel (Figure 14-33).

Sometimes it may be necessary to carefully reheat parts of the splint by carefully dipping an aspect in hot water or by using a heat gun. In using the latter, the funnel may be

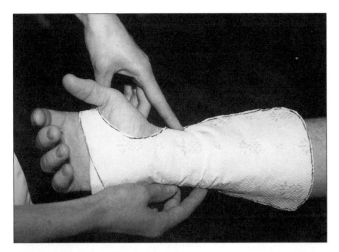

Figure 14-28. Make pattern.

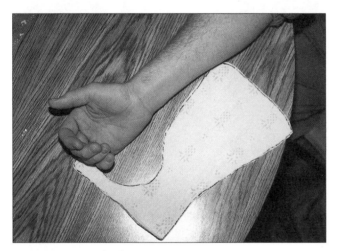

Figure 14-29. Completed pattern.

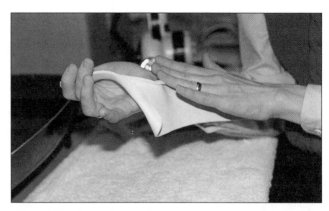

Figure 14-30. Preforming splint.

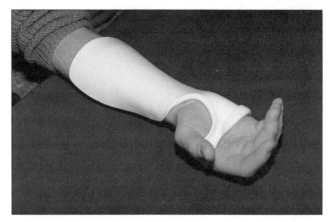

Figure 14-31. Forming splint on patient.

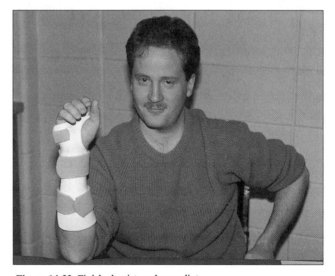

Figure 14-32. Finished wrist cock-up splint.

particularly helpful in directing heat to small areas. Splint straps may need to be repositioned to assure that the splint stays in place. If any of the these adjustments are made and problems are still evident, the splint may require refabricating, and possibly redesigning.

Problems may occur with perspiration or coldness (particularly when splints are worn outside). In these instances, the splints may require ventilation and/or the use of tubular stockinette worn under the splint. Ventilation can be achieved either by using perforated material when fabricating the splint or by punching or drilling small holes in the splint after construction. Holes should always be staggered in their placement to prevent weakening the splint (Figure 14-34).

In general, unless padding is essential for splint comfort and safety and is easily removable (does not stick permanently to the plastic or "gum" onto the plastic), it should *not* be used. Padding also may become rapidly soiled, another reason to avoid its use entirely. A 15-inch piece of

tubular stockinette, with a hole cut for the thumb and worn under the splint, may provide a better lining. If padding of more than $1/16$-inch is required, it should be applied under the thermoplastic material as the splint is formed to assure proper fit of the plastic.

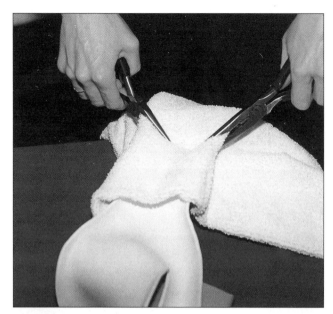

Figure 14-33. Using two pair of pliers and a towel to loosen/enlarge arm trough.

Patient Education

Both patients and their caretakers need to be shown exactly how to apply a splint properly and have opportunities to practice this skill under supervision. Written instructions should always be given, with illustrations if possible. If patients will be using the splint in a hospital or long-term care facility, instructions should be placed in the chart and also at the bedside. A sample instruction form for **patient education** is shown in Figure 14-35.

It is important to check the patient a day or several days after a splint is worn to assure proper fit and application. Even "oriented" patients have been known to experience problems with their splints when they unknowingly applied them upside down!

Patients and their caretakers should always be instructed to remove splints for cleaning and for range of motion exercises, if appropriate. If patients report increased stiffness, pain or edema, which persists after removal of the splint and exercise, the splint-wearing time, fit or design may need to be altered by the OTR.

Another important aspect of patient education is the need to caution patients about inadvertant heating of their thermoplastic splints. A splint left in a closed car on a hot day will be rendered useless if it melts into a flattened mound of plastic. Radiators, hot steam, or any intense heat source may also cause damage.

Other Considerations

No discussion of the topic of safety would be complete without including some specfic precautions that the OTR and COTA should follow in the clinic. They should develop habits of protecting their own hands by keeping sharp tools

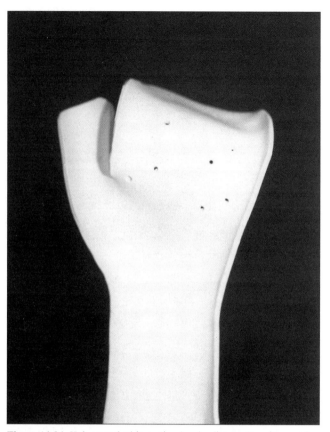

Figure 14-34. Holes punched in resting hand splint to allow for perspiration.

sharp and using them correctly. Adhesive that accumulates on scissors used for cutting strapping material should be removed routinely with a piece of cloth or gauze moistened with alcohol or a commercially made alcohol pad so that the scissors cut smoothly. Avoid touching hot materials; instead handle them with tongs.

Occupational therapy personnel also need to use good body mechanics, particularly to protect their backs. Rather than bending over to fabricate a splint, sit or kneel at the same level of the patient, as close as possible. The heating pan and cutting area should be on a countertop, to avoid unnecessary bending over a table.

Although chemical areosol sprays are available to speed cooling, occupational therapy personnel who work with splinting materials frequently should consider the risks of regular exposure to these sprays. The extra moments required for cooling without using them can be used for other purposes, such as patient education. Furthermore, if a splinting material requires use of a solvent or bonding agent, the COTA or OTR who is concerned about his or her exposure to chemicals should consider alternatives such as scratching the plastic surface with a pair of scissors before heating for adhering parts, or perhaps, choosing a more easily adhering thermoplastic. If solvents or bonding agents are used, it is important to follow the manufacturer's

NAME: _____

DATE: _____

Your splint was made especially for your hand, per order of your physician. The purpose of your splint is:

_____

_____

It is essential that your splint fit *comfortably* and *correctly*. Improper use could cause problems.

WEARING SCHEDULE

Your splint should be worn:

Daytime:

_____

_____

Nighttime:

_____

_____

PRECAUTIONS

Your hand: If your splint causes any of the following problems, contact your occupational therapist so that adjustments can be made:

- Excessive swelling
- Severe pain (pain lasting longer than one hour after splint is removed)
- Pressure areas that last for more than $1/2$-hour after splint is removed
- Excessive stiffness

Your splint: • Keep away from heat or flame. Your splint will burn or lose its shape.
- Cigarettes, hot water, or a closed car on a hot day are to be avoided.
- If any adjustments or repairs are necessary, contact your occupational therapist.

ATTACHMENTS

If your splint is equipped with an outrigger (rubber bands and slings), it is important to remember the following:

- A light, steady pull on your fingers is more effective for stretching stiff joints and safer than a hard pull.
- Slings should not cut off circulation of a finger or cause numbness.
- Rubber bands should provide a gentle stretch that you can tolerate for 20 minutes.
- If you can tolerate your slings for more than 20 minutes (without severe pain, decreased circulation or sensation), they may need to be tightened. Check with your therapist.

CLEANING YOUR SPLINT

- Clean with soap and lukewarm water daily.
- If perspiration is a problem and your hand does not have any open areas, sprinkle with baby powder before applying the splint.

If you have any questions, contact _____

Figure 14-35. Using and caring for your splint. *Developed by Patrice Schober-Branigan, OTR.*

recommendations and precautions regarding skin contact and ventilation. As health care practitioners, occupational therapy personnel should be especially cognizant of preventing occupational hazards.

IMPACT ON ROLE PERFORMANCE

The following brief case studies provide examples of how the use of splints impact on the individuals' role performance.

Case Study 14-1

Mary. Mary is a 42-year-old woman with rheumatoid arthritis affecting her hands and wrists. In addition to her comprehensive rehabilitation program, which includes rest, active range of motion (AROM) exercise, joint protection and energy saving techniques, heat and anti-inflammatory medications, she uses resting splints for her hands and wrists at night. She finds that her swollen MP joints and wrists are more comfortable, and she is able to sleep for considerably longer periods than previously. Although it has not been clinically proven, Mary is convinced that her splints are helping to minimize any deformity that is occurring due to her disease. This is particularly important for Mary's self-image, which is much stronger than when she was first seen by the occupational therapist. By carefully pacing her activities with periods of rest, using joint protection methods, and obtaining assistance for heavy household and yard work, she is able to continue to be actively engaged in her dual roles of corporate attorney and single parent of a 14-year-old daughter. She has also found time in her busy schedule to do volunteer work for the local chapter of the Arthritis Foundation.

Case Study 14-2

Bob. Bob, age 37, has a mild carpal tunnel syndrome of his right hand. His physician does not advise surgery at this time. Bob wears his wrist cock-up splint when his wrist is inflamed. In his position as a paper press operator, the condition does not interfere with his work tasks when he wears his splint, although he does use more shoulder motion with the splint than without it. Bob covers his splint with with tubular stockinette to protect it from dirt and ink. He removes it several times each day on work breaks to do gentle AROM exercises. An avid gardener, Bob has found that if he wears his splint under a work glove, he can continue to enjoy this pastime as long as he limits it to working with soft, well-cultivated soil for one hour or less. Bob continues to carry out the usual household tasks he and his wife have shared during their ten-year marriage.

Case Study 14-3

Susan. Susan, a single, retired accountant, age 63, fell on an icy sidewalk and sustained a Colles' fracture of her left wrist. The bones healed well, and she followed a regular regimen of specific exercise; however, her MP joints have remained somewhat stiff, and she is unable to bend them past 60 degrees active flexion. Her physician and the occupational therapist recommended that she use a dynamic MP flexion splint for 20 to 30 minutes, three to four times each day, followed by AROM exercises and exercises with therapy putty. She reports that the tension on the rubber bands feels gentle when she first puts the splint on, but by the end of each wearing period, her joints feel stretched. Each week, the occupational therapist readjusts the angle of pull, and after three weeks, Susan is now able to bend her joints to 80 degrees. She is beginning to resume her favorite retirement activity of golfing by practicing several times each week on a portable putting green as a part of her home occupational therapy program. In addition, she is now able to do the majority of her household tasks and shopping, the exception being lifting more than 15 pounds.

SUMMARY

This chapter provided a basic foundation of splinting for the COTA. Certainly the advances in thermoplastic technology over the past 25 years have made splinting a more approachable modality for occupational therapy assistants. Splinting principles, both anatomic and biomechanical, form the essential foundation for the assistant as he or she begins to fabricate and use splints. Careful assessment by the OTR/COTA team precedes meaningful implementation of a splinting program. Materials continue to grow in numbers and versatility; as the COTA becomes a skilled practitioner he or she will find that a variety of plastics will work well, as long as one is familiar with their properties and "feel." Furthermore, skill is developed in choosing the optimal material for individual splints and patient needs. Examples of two commonly used splints were illustrated with instructions for fabrication. Safety factors, including precautions, adjustments, and patient education were addressed. The impact of the use of splints on an individual's role performance was outlined in case study examples.

Notes to the Reader

1. Information for the Types of Materials Chart (Table 14-1) was drawn from a variety of sources including Orthoplast®, Smith and Nephew/Rolyan, K-Splint®, Polymed, Aquaplast® et al and Multiform® et al product

information; Schafer A: Splinting materials. *Alimed's O.T. Product News* 1(3):3-3, 1988-1989. Information was also provided by manufacturer's representatives; and the author's experience, which has focused primarily on work with Orthoplast® and the products of Smith and Nephew/Rolyan.

2. Numerous types of padding are commercially available. Personal preference of the therapist or assistant will determine choice. A $1/8$-inch to $1/4$-inch self-adhesive foam, which is easily removed from the splint, and/or a "loop" foam, such as Velfoam®, which can be applied to the splint with small pieces of hook Velcro, are especially practical. A thinner material, such as Moleskin® or Molestick®, may be required occasionally. All distributors of splinting materials also carry a wide variety of paddings, including those used as examples.

3. I prefer to use this "intrinsic minus" position, which gently counteracts the more common "intrinsic plus" imbalance (MP joints flexed maximally and DIP and PIP joints extended) and unstable thumb that commonly occur in rheumatoid arthritis.[4] This splint would not be appropriate for a person with the opposite type of imbalance, an "intrinsic minus" hand, because it would provide no counterbalance.[4] The COTA should confer with the OTR about goals for use of the particular rheumatoid arthritis splint being fabricated.

The modification of the resting hand splint originated at the Occupational Therapy Department of the Mayo Clinic, Rochester, MN, in the late 1970s and early 1980s. I have found this modification especially helpful for thumb comfort for patients with rheumatoid arthritis, while at the same time adding rigidity to the splint, negating the need for reinforcement, even when Orthoplast® is used.

Related Learning Activities

1. Experiment with at least one type of splinting material from each of the groups (A, B and C), as shown in Table 14-1, by making a small shoehorn. Identify problems as well as successes.

2. Construct a simple resting splint to maintain the functional position of the hand for yourself. Ask a person with experience in splinting to evaluate the splint you have constructed.

3. List at least six diagnostic groups or problems where splinting might be used.

4. Discuss important precautions that need to be considered when making splints.

5. List important points that should be discussed with the patient when presenting him or her with a new splint.

References

1. Reed KL, Sanderson SR: *Concepts of Occupational Therapy.* 2nd Edition. Baltimore, Williams & Wilkins, 1983, p. 222.
2. Shafer A: Demystifying splinting materials. *Alimed's O.T. Product News* 1(3):1, 1988-89.
3. Trombly C, Scott AD: *Occupational Therapy for Physical Dysfunction.* Baltimore, Williams & Wilkins, 1977, pp. 281-282.
4. English CB, Nalebuff EA: Understanding the arthritic hand. *Am J Occup Ther* 25:352-259, 1971.

Constructing Adaptive Equipment

Mary K. Cowan, MA, OTR, FAOTA

INTRODUCTION

The term **adaptive equipment** has been used throughout the course of occupational therapy history to describe assistive devices, aides, or pieces of equipment that allow a person with a handicap to participate in a life activity that otherwise would have been difficult or impossible. Although a variety of adaptive equipment is available for purchase, time constraints, budget limitations, and the uniqueness of the specific problem may require the construction of specialized devices.

Adaptive equipment is designed and constructed to assist with solving participation problems in activities of daily living, play or leisure, and work. Of primary importance is the development of appropriate aides that will increase independence in areas such as postural control, positioning, grasping, accessing and hand control, which will ultimately allow active participation in meaningful activities.

This participation will permit the individual to carry out important **life tasks** (activities that must be accomplished for successful living throughout the life span) and roles with a greater a degree of achievement and satisfaction.

Individually constructed equipment may be as simple as using a waxed paper box to hold playing cards or as complex as the design and use of computerized environmental control systems. Whether simple or complex, the focus of this chapter is to acquaint the reader with principles of construction and related applications for solving functional problems.

HISTORICAL USES

Early development of adaptive equipment such as page turners, card holders, and nail boards allowed the person with a handicap to read a book without using his or her hands, to

---

KEY CONCEPTS

Historical uses

Occupational therapy personnel roles

Determining needs

Precautions

Characteristics of good construction

Construction of stabilizing pillow

Equipment design priniciples

Presentation to user and follow-up

---

play cards with one hand, and to peel a fruit or vegetable when the person did not have use of a stabilizing hand. Although adaptive equipment was originally developed to provide improved ability to perform activities of daily living and participate in leisure pursuits, it also became commonly used as a term to apply to therapy equipment that helped the person with a handicap develop skills in therapy. Eventually balance boards, bolsters, standing tables, prone boards, and related equipment were designed and used by one or several therapists before they became standard pieces of therapy equipment.

Therapist-made equipment was a necessity for many years and only in recent times have many of these innovations been mass produced, marketed through catalogs, and readily available to occupational therapy personnel. However, this availability does not rule out the need for individually constructed equipment. The unique needs of the individual may require the design and construction of a device that is not commercially available or is too costly to purchase. These situations require the therapist or assistant to use **problem-solving skills** to determine the relationship between the individual's motor skill problem and the life task that needs to be accomplished and then construct a helpful tool to make participation possible. These skills include studying the situation that presents uncertainty or doubt, and arriving at the most likely solution. The process involves definition, selection of a plan, organizing steps, implementing the plan, and evaluating the results.

OCCUPATIONAL THERAPY PERSONNEL ROLES

The *Entry-Level OTR and COTA Role Delineation* describes the certified occupational therapy assistant's role in program planning as it relates to adapting techniques and media and selecting and using therapeutic adaptation (assistive/adaptive devices) under the direction of the registered occupational therapist.[1] As with other areas of treatment, however, close supervision by an OTR is required in situations where "patient conditions or treatment settings are complex (involving multiple systems) and where conditions change rapidly, requiring frequent or ongoing reassessment and modification of (the) treatment plan."[1] Designing and constructing a positioning device for a child with cerebral palsy, based on the theoretical principles of neurodevelopmental treatment, is an example where OTR supervision is required. A therapist with this specialized training should decide if the design and the final product do indeed fulfill the principles and intent of that therapeutic approach. Frequently, the COTA who works closely with an OTR in a complex treatment setting may be the individual with the most knowledge of tools and equipment and, therefore,

the one who will actually construct the needed equipment once the OTR/COTA team has determined the need and type of equipment required.

The COTA working in a setting where chronic conditions are prevalent is continually dealing with recurring functional problems that may not require the OTR's clinical involvement in the adaptive equipment decision-making process. The design and construction of card holders, book holders, and built-up handles on recreational games for people with physical handicaps are examples of situations where the COTA would not require close supervision.

Designing and constructing adaptive equipment, at various levels, can be a collaborative effort between the COTA and the OTR, but it must also be emphasized that the patient or client is the third partner in this collaboration. The individual receiving treatment will often exhibit or describe a problem that creates a need for adaptive equipment. The user gives the therapist or assistant feedback on the fit and comfort. Finally, the user determines the ultimate usefulness of the item by his or her choice to use it or not.

DETERMINING THE NEED FOR ADAPTIVE EQUIPMENT

Whether a piece of adaptive equipment is temporary or permanent, it should meet a **specific need** for the individual. Unnecessary use of specialized equipment has the potential for making any person feel additionally "handicapped." Therefore, it is important for the COTA/OTR team to be certain that the individual meets the following criteria:
1. Unable to complete the task without the use of aides
2. Understands the need for additional equipment
3. Is agreeable to trial or long-term use of the needed equipment

PRECAUTIONS

Whether a device is safe for use is determined during all three stages of the process of development: 1) design, 2) construction, and 3) use.

When designing equipment, safety must be considered so that time in construction is not wasted on a piece of equipment rendered useless later when it is discovered to be unsafe. In this context, **safety** refers specifically to the employment of measures necessary to prevent the occurence of injury or loss of function. Some questions the therapist or assistant should ask during the design phase are the following:
1. Will a breakdown of materials from ordinary wear cause discomfort or injury?

2. Will the shape of the equipment interfere with safe use of any other equipment regularly used, such as a wheelchair or crutches?

When constructing adaptive equipment, safety problems can be anticipated by eliminating rough finishes on wood, metal, or plastic and by sanding all surfaces, edges, and corners smoothly to prevent splinters, cuts, and bruises. It is also important to use nontoxic finishes, particularly for equipment used with children who might be likely to chew on it.

Instructing the patient or client in safe usage of equipment is the final step in making safe equipment. Observing the individual using the equipment and discussing with him or her where, when, and how to use it properly alerts the person to any possible misuse, therefore unsafe use, of equipment made by occupational therapy personnel.

CHARACTERISTICS OF WELL-CONSTRUCTED ADAPTIVE EQUIPMENT

Simplicity in Design

A simple design facilitates the construction of the device and increases the likelihood of it being used more frequently. An example is provided in Figure 15-1, the **Cowan stabilizing pillow,** an adaptive pillow for children who have balance problems when sitting on the floor.[2] The design's simplicity (eight sections of cloth, sewing of simple seams, filling with Styrofoam pellets) makes it possible for others such as therapists, assistants, volunteers, teachers, or parents to make more pillows when recommended for other children (Figure 15-2). The chance of the next item being made improperly is also reduced by having a simple design. Because a small, soft pillow is easily transported and easily stored in a corner of the classroom, both children and teachers will be more likely to use it. If the stabilizing seat had been made from a more complicated design (for example, a metal and leather seat with a backrest), it would be more difficult to make, move, store and use.

Size of Equipment

It is important that the size of equipment bè controlled so that it does not become awkward or cumbersome to use. An example of this might be carrying devices for wheelchairs, such as lapboards or trays, armrests, and back pockets. Although anyone in a wheelchair may want to carry large items occasionally, making the tray or pocket too large may make daily use of the wheelchair cumbersome. The **half-lapboard** for patients with hemiplegia shown in Figure 15-3 demonstrates this principle by having a surface large enough to support the person's hemiplegic arm, without having the surface extending out to either side.[3] This thoughtful consideration allows the person in the wheelchair to avoid

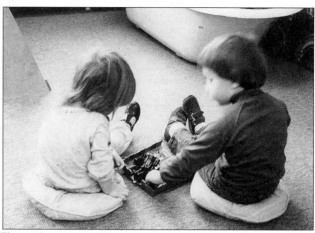

Figure 15-1. Cowan stabilizing pillow.

bumping into objects and people with extra or unnecessary tray extensions, and also allows adequate space to transfer in and out of the chair. (See reference three for specific information on how to construct this equipment.)

Cost of Materials and Construction Time

If a piece of adaptive equipment requires expensive materials, or if it takes a long time to make, the item is no longer **cost-effective.** The hourly wage of the therapist or assistant, as well as the cost of the materials, must be considered. Many hours of therapy time spent constructing one piece of equipment may increase the cost of that equipment to such a point that purchasing a similar item may prove less expensive, as well as a better use of valuable time.

The inexpensive **bolsters** shown in Figure 15-4 are designed for use with children under three years and demonstrate the use of economical materials. Mary Clarke, a COTA in Portland, Oregon, uses vinyl or oilcloth for the covering and lightly rolled newspapers for the interior.[4] The seam on the outside is closed with cloth tape. Larger bolsters can be made by taping empty three-pound coffee cans together, covering them with one-inch foam, and then adding an outside cover of vinyl.[4] She has also used large cardboard tubes from carpet rolls to provide the inner shape of the bolster, adding a layer of foam, followed by a vinyl covering to create the finished equipment.[4] All of these bolsters involve the use of economical materials and require very reasonable construction time. Because the bolsters are inexpensive, they can be provided to many families. In this way, it is possible to leave adaptive equipment in a home, a practice that is often not possible when similar, commercially made but more expensive bolsters are used.

Attractive Appearance

An unattractive piece of equipment, no matter how useful, can interfere with its potential use. People do not like to use equipment that is roughly made or battered from use or that

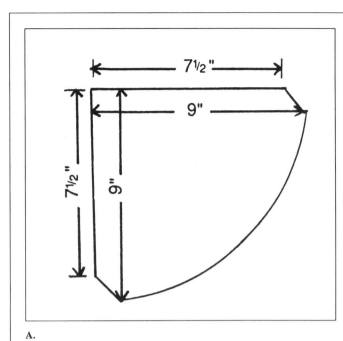

A.

Basic Materials

- 1¼ yards washable upholstery fabric
- Small Styrofoam pellets
- Heavy-duty sewing thread
- Graph paper, pencil and ruler for pattern making
- Pins, scissors and sewing machine

Instructions

1. Using paper, pencil and ruler, make a pattern as shown in Figure A.
2. Cut eight pieces of fabric to pattern specifications.
3. Using heavy-duty thread and a sewing machine, sew four pieces of fabric together to form a circle; repeat with remaining four pieces, as shown in Figure B.
4. Sew the two large circles together, leaving an opening of about four inches.
5. Reverse the pillow so that the finished outside is visible.
6. Stuff the pillow with Styrofoam pellets until it is approximately one-third to one-half filled (this makes it possible for the child to fit snugly into a "nest" of pellets).
7. Top-stitch around the edge of the pillow to finish and close the opening.

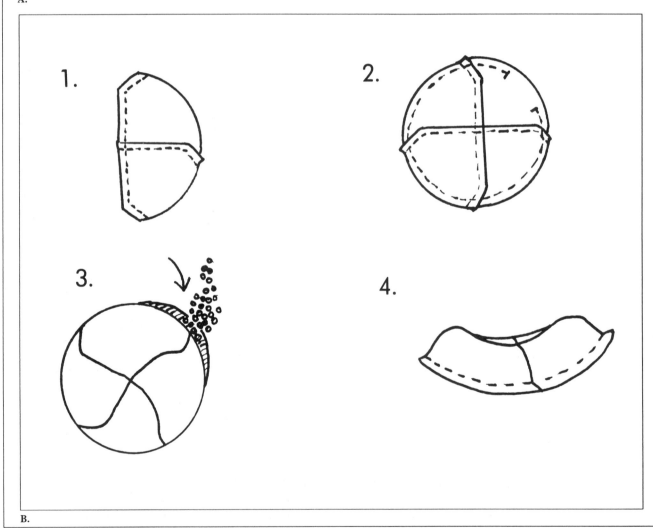

B.

Figure 15-2. Directions for constructing a Cowan stabilizing pillow for children.

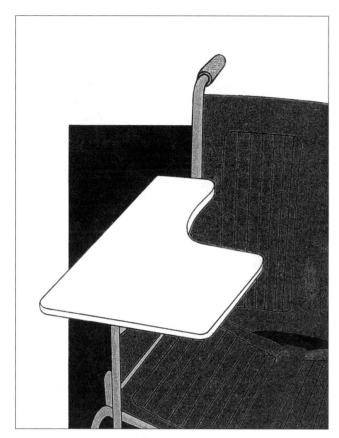

Figure 15-3. Wheelchair half-lapboard. *Adapted from Walsh.*[3]

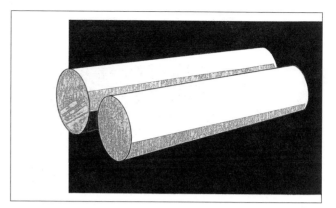

Figure 15-4. Bolsters. *Adapted from Clark.*[4]

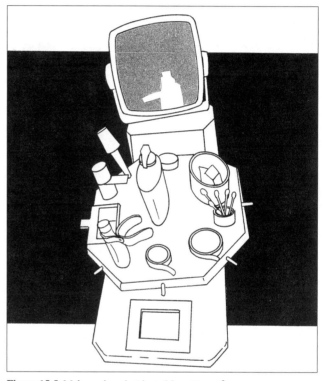

Figure 15-5. Make-up board. *Adapted from Hague.*[5]

has unappealing surfaces. For example, a waxpaper box makes a quick and easy piece of adaptive equipment for the one-handed card player. By covering the box with attractive vinyl wallpaper or other washable, durable material, it is not only useful but pleasant to look at.

Figure 15-5 shows an example of a makeup board designed for use by a women with quadriplegia.[5] It is simple in design and attractive without being medical or therapeutic in appearance and would be a natural addition to a woman's bedroom. (See reference five for specific instructions on how to make this equipment.)

Safety in Use

Although safety as a principle has already been addressed, it is an essential characteristic of well-constructed adaptive equipment that cannot be overemphasized. For example, if a stabilizer for a bowl or a pan used on the stove is not predictably stable, (ie, it can become easily detached from the surface), it serves no purpose. In fact, it complicates the already difficult task of working in the kitchen with the use of only one hand.

Comfort in Use

The comfort of the user is affected by the placement of the equipment when it is used, materials that touch the user's body in some way, and any fit that is required. A handle that requires the fit of a hand grasp or a situation where the body or extremities are resting on the equipment are examples that illustrate the need to consider user comfort. An example of this principle is the foam positioning device shown in Figure 15-6.[6] Because it uses soft foam as a basic material, it appears to be comfortable for long periods of contact with the skin, particularly when the person is immobile. (See reference six for specific instructions on how to make this equipment.)

Ease in Application and Use

The ultimate test of the ease in application and usage principle is to determine if the patient can apply the device

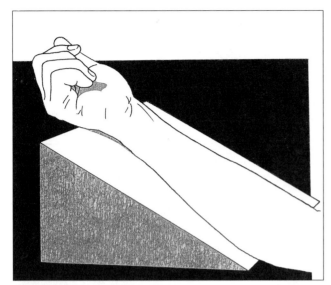

Figure 15-6. Foam positioning device. *Adapted from von Funk.*[6]

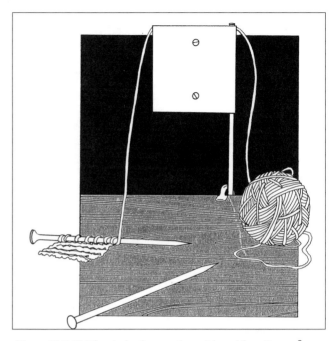

Figure 15-7. Knitting device for amputees. *Adapted from Duncan.*[7]

to himself or herself independently. If this is not the case, the individual(s) responsible for assisting the patient must be familiar with its proper positioning and use. The knitting device designed for use by a bilateral upper extremity amputee shown in Figure 15-7 is a good example.[7] The piece of equipment requires the use of a C-clamp and wing nuts (both of which the patient can manage with the bilateral prostheses) to attach the device to the table and to tighten or loosen the tension on the yarn. (See reference seven for specific information about how to construct this equipment.)

Ease and Maintenance in Cleaning

Simplicity in the design and choice of materials for any device makes it easier to maintain and to clean. A simple design eliminates corners, holes and crevices that collect debris that is difficult to remove. If the equipment is to be used with people who have infections or are highly susceptible to infection, the construction materials must withstand the intense steam or hot water required for adequate removal of bacteria. Most clinics or schools require that all equipment be washed or cleaned periodically to promote normal infection control. Nonporous surfaces such as plastic and metal are less likely to retain dirt or agents that cause infection, and heavier, porous fabrics that can be washed easily (such as upholstery fabric) are recommended.

DESIGNING ADAPTIVE EQUIPMENT

A Problem-Solving Process

The design of every adaptive device begins with a therapist or assistant and the patient facing a deficit in function together in a thoughtful, problem-solving process.

If the patient is unable to participate in an activity or to attain the position necessary for optimal work or task completion, new methods are tried and catalogs are perused for available equipment likely to alleviate the problem. In some instances, the problem will be solved only by designing a new piece of equipment.

Use of Patterns

Very early in the process of designing equipment, a pattern can be developed to guide the construction process. The Cowan stabilizing pillow (see Figure 15-1) provides a useful example. One quarter of one surface of the pillow was drawn on graph paper to establish the necessary size and shape. The paper pattern was then checked in relation to the patient's body or body part, and any necessary adjustments were made. All of the other examples shown in various figures in this chapter required a basic pattern for construction. The making of a pattern is an important step in the problem-solving process, as it guides the therapist or assistant in estimating size and shape of the piece of adaptive equipment. Errors in the construction phase will be reduced, thus increasing efficiency and reducing the cost of production.

Constructing a Model

Once a pattern has been developed, the next step is to construct the first model of the device. This step allows the patient and the therapist or assistant to discuss and experiment with changes in the design. This first model should be viewed as flexible and malleable, as well a experimental. At this point, the shape of the pattern can be changed, new materials can be tried, and dimensions can be altered.

Redesign After Trials

After any necessary redesign, the patient begins to use the piece of equipment. Some new problems may arise at this stage that inform the patient and occupational therapy personnel of changes that may need to be made. Only through a longer period of trial use can all of the patient's needs in regard to use of an adaptive device become completely clear. In **trial use,** a piece of equipment is repeatedly used in order to assure its effectiveness.

FABRICATING ADAPTIVE EQUIPMENT

Materials

This chapter does not present a complete list of materials and their characteristics for use in fabricating adaptive equipment; however, the following characteristics are examples of those that should be considered when evaluating or selecting materials:

1. *Softness and Pliability of Shape:* necessary for pillows, slings, positioning equipment. Use cloth, canvas or webbing; lamb's wool or "moleskin" for surface coverage; Styrofoam pellets, cotton batton, foam rubber or polyfoam for fillers.

2. *Resiliancy and Pliability of Shape:* needed for positioning devices. Use splinting materials such as Orthoplast™, tri-wall, acetate film, leather, rubber, vinyl.

3. *Strength, Solidity and Weight:* needed for laptrays, wheelchair arm suports, stabilizing equipment. Use wood, metal, hard plastics.

Tools

The materials chosen will determine the tools required to fabricate any piece of equipment. For example, cloth requires scissors and a sewing machine; splinting materials require scissors and a heating device; and the use of wood, metal or plastic requires hand tools or power shop equipment during the construction process. The availability of tools and the therapist's or assistant's skill in using tools contribute to the quality of the finished product.

Finishing

The final step in the construction of equipment is finishing. This step is of primary importance when one considers the emotional impact of equipment use for some patients. Rough or sharp surfaces and edges need to be sanded and rounded. Extraneous threads and uneven seams need to be trimmed and repaired. Finishes such as polyurethane varnish or nontoxic paint need to be applied to wooden objects. Colors selected may be neutral to deemphasize the equipment or bright and colorful to make equipment more attractive. The work of finishing adaptive equipment, like making furniture for a home, merits fine workmanship, with attention to important details, so that the product is both professional and attractive.

PRESENTATION TO USER

Whether or not the user of the designed and constructed adaptive equipment has been part of the collaboration process, when it is completed, the OTR or COTA should review the following information with the patient: 1) purpose, 2) uses, 3) limitations, 4) care and maintenance, and 5) any precautions. Even a young child needs to know that the stabilizing pillow "helps you sit better, or longer" (see Figure 15-1). The adult should know that the half-lapboard shown in Figure 15-3 places his or her affected arm in view to improve body awareness, control swelling, and prevent injury to an arm that lacks sensation. This review of the purposes of the equipment encourages proper use and, therefore, greater likelihood of its success. If the adaptive device is to be applied by another individual (nurse, aide, teacher or parent), the details of proper application and positioning must be presented to avoid any discomfort to the patient and to ensure safe use. On hospital and rehabilitation center wards, in classrooms, and in other community settings where several people assist the individual with equipment use, the placement of a diagram or picture of the equipment properly set up can be attached to the device as a helpful reference.

FOLLOW-UP

Follow-up is the final step of constructing adaptive equipment. Checking with the user about any problems that may have arisen gives the therapist a basis for modifying the equipment or improving its design for optimal function. If a particular device is used by many people, all of them should be followed and the fulfillment of the original purpose of the equipment validated with every patient. Questions such as the following can then be asked:

1. How many individuals have used the equipment?
2. For what length of time?
3. How successfully did it fulfill its purpose?
4. Should any modifications be made?

Compilation of this information will inform the COTA and the OTR who design and construct adaptive equipment whether the equipment is successful. If the equipment is also accepted and used by the patient or patients, it may be timely to share this information with other therapists and assistants through professional publication in journals and newsletters, as the examples provided in this chapter demonstrate.

SUMMARY

Construction of adaptive equipment is addressed within the whole continuum of design and construction that is a part of the occupational therapy process of problem solving. A definition of adaptive equipment is given, together with significant historical uses of such devices. The role of the COTA/OTR team was presented to inform the reader of the areas of supervision, collaboration and independent work. Principles are delineated for determining need, designing, fabricating, presenting the device to the user and follow-up. Important precautions and safety measures are stressed. Examples of well-constructed adaptive equipment are used to illustrate important considerations.

Related Learning Activities

1. List the criteria to consider before making adaptive equipment.

2. Study the characteristics of well-constructed adaptive equipment. Working with a classmate or peer, view at least five pieces of adaptive equipment constructed by therapists or assistants (visit clinics and use journal articles). Determine which characteristics are present and which are not.

3. Construct one of the pieces of adaptive equipment presented in this chapter.

4. Role play the presentation of a piece of adaptive equipment to a patient. Be sure to include the five factors stressed in the chapter.

References

1. American Occupational Therapy Association: *Entry-Level OTR and COTA Role Delineation*. Rockville, Maryland, AOTA, 1981.
2. Cowan MK: Pillow helps keep young OT clients "stabilized." *OT Week* 2(19):5, 1988.
3. Walsh M: Brief or new: Half-lapboard for hemiplegic patients. *Am J Occup Ther* 41:533-535, 1987.
4. Clark M: Unpublished material and personal correspondence, September, 1990.
5. Hague G: Brief or new: Makeup board for women with quadriplegia. *Am J Occup Ther* 42:253-255, 1988.
6. von Funk M: Positioning device has multiple benefits for patients. *Advance for Occupational Therapists* (August 21): 13, 1989.
7. Duncan S: Brief or new: Knitting device for bilateral upper extremity amputee. *Am J Occup Ther* 40:637-638, 1986.

Section V
PURPOSEFUL ACTIVITY AND ANALYSIS

Arts and Crafts

Activity Analysis

The last section may best be described as an integration of the preceding sections. It draws on historically significant principles, values and beliefs of the profession, as well as the core concepts of human development, the components of occupation, and occupational performance areas. Of equal importance are teaching and learning, interpersonal relationships and applied group dynamics, and the individualization of occupational therapy services, which concentrates on factors such as environment, society, change, and prevention. The analysis of activities used for evaluation and treatment requires knowledge and skill that is best drawn from experience in engaging in a wide variety of activities. Through experience one comes to know not only the properties of activities but also their therapeutic potential The chapter on arts and craft offers specific examples of how activities can be applied in therapy.

Activities are universal and are a cornerstone of the profession. As People, Ryan and Witherspoon have stated, developing skill in activity analysis allows the practitioner to "select the most appropriate activity, which is of interest to the patient, relates to his or her life tasks and roles, and provides opportunities for goal achievement."

Chapter 16

Arts and Crafts

Harriet Backhaus, COTA

INTRODUCTION

The profession of occupational therapy is concerned with the pursuit of purposeful, goal-directed activity. Among the many activities available, arts and crafts are deeply rooted in our history and continue to be an important treatment modality in many areas of contemporary practice. Just as our early predecessors used tools to construct, create, repair and modify, we continue this tradition as tool users, remembering our past and passing on our heritage to future generations by making artistic and creative objects. The building of a simple, primitive birdhouse or the creation of a magnificent oil painting hold the same degree of value to the person who created it. Each represents the unique interests, knowledge, skills and asthetic interpretation of that individual. Moreover, the completed object offers an opportunity for self-expression and provides another personal link to one's environment. Additional benefits to the patient are numerous and will be discussed later in this chapter.

The use of arts and crafts has been an area of **controversy** in the profession of occupa-

tional therapy in recent years. Some practitioners have abandoned these treatment modalities altogether, whereas others have often found a need to defend their use. Those in the latter group might quote Eleanor Clarke Slagle, an occupational therapy pioneer and founder of the profession, who firmly believed in the value of using arts and crafts. She offered an eloquent defense to those who challenged using handicrafts as a therapeutic intervention, particularly during the machine age:

Handicrafts are so generally used, not only because they are so diverse, covering a field from the most elementary to the highest grade of ability; but also, and greatly to the point, because their development is based on primitive impulses. They offer the means of contact with the patient that no other does or can offer. Encouragement of creative impulses also may lead to the development of large interests outside oneself and certainly leads to social contact, an important consideration with any sick or convalescent patient.[1]

KEY CONCEPTS

Historical considerations

Conflicting practitioner values

Contemporary trends in utilization

Activity planning goals

Redefinition of arts and crafts

Rehabilitation applications

Relationships to decision making, work, leisure and social skills

The debate over the use of arts and crafts as a method for therapeutic intervention will likely continue well into the 1990s. It will be necessary for each certified occupational therapy assistant (COTA) to examine carefully the historical significance of such endeavors, their contemporary use and interest, as well as future potential, before deciding whether to use arts and crafts as a legitimate tool of occupational therapy practice.

HISTORICAL ROOTS

Purposeful activity, defined as those endeavors that are goal-directed and have meaning to the individual, has, and continues to be, an important cornerstone of the profession. Susan E. Tracy, a nurse who has often been called "the first occupational therapist," noted the importance of activities for the mentally ill.[2] In 1910, some of her ideas were incorporated into the first book on activities titled, *Studies in Invalid Occupations: A Manual for Nurses and Attendants.*[3] It was primarily a craft book and stressed that the action of performing a craft activity was as therapeutic as the final outcome of the craft.

During World War II, occupational therapy schools trained therapists in crafts and occupations. The goal of treatment was to enable the patient to move from acute illness to vocational readiness as quickly as possible. In the late 1940s and 1950s, the profession was challenged by those who favored the medical model, which was becoming evident in other allied health professions. This approach forced traditional crafts to the background, as new treatment techniques were being developed and taught in the curriculum.

Later, some occupational therapy personnel found it increasingly more difficult to include the use of arts and crafts in treatment plans and treatment goals, due to problems with the **documentation** (written records of the patient's health care, including current and future needs) required as justification for reimbursement. As the dilemma became more pervasive, members of the profession continued to look to the sciences for increased credibility and respectability.[4]

CONFLICTING VALUES AND CONTEMPORARY TRENDS

The use of arts and crafts as an occupational therapy treatment modality has become a focal point in our professional literature and discussions. Two questions have arisen:
1. What exactly is the role of arts and crafts?
2. Why has their use decreased?

One answer might be that the therapeutic use of these modalities can be more difficult to document and justify than other structured and standardized activities with more easily reportable outcomes, such as repetition of an exercise or the amount of gross grasp that has been increased. This may be why some occupational therapy personnel view the use of arts, and crafts in particular, as giving a poor image to the profession. Some see the use of these activities as demeaning to the patient, whereas others report that there is not enough space, money or staff to support such programs.[5]

If the use of arts and crafts is indeed so difficult to justify to other members of the profession, to the public, and to third-party payers, what are some of the reasons supporting their use? The answers are complex and multifaceted. For example, many of the skills the COTA may be helping the patient to acquire through treatment can be accomplished by the careful selection of an appropriate activity, which well might include work on an art or craft project. To meet the **criteria of appropriateness,** the activity must fulfill the following factors for the patient:
1. It must be goal directed
2. It must be age appropriate
3. It must have some relevance and purpose

If these factors are not present, the patient may not comply in performing the task(s). For example, it is often difficult for an adult to accept the task of completing a peg board pattern, knowing that the activity was designed for use by a child. Although this activity may sometimes be viewed as necessary, the decision regarding its use should be carefully evaluated.

ACTIVITY PLANNING GOALS

When planning an activity to use in a treatment program, the COTA must consider the following goals/requirements for improving human performance deficits:
1. Attention to task
2. Coordination
3. Strength
4. Perceptual motor
5. Activities of daily living
6. Socialization
7. Leisure interests
8. Self-esteem
9. Time management

Two types of activities can address these goals and requirements. One activity does not produce an end product, such as completing a peg design. The other activity has a definite end point, such as constructing a project using mosaic tile. Both activities can address increasing coordination and perceptual motor skills, but only one has an end product that represents the work achieved. Making a mosaic tile project can also address a leisure interest, may improve self-esteem and time management, and, depending on the structure of the task, provide some opportunities for socialization. The need to follow detailed steps, such as grasp and release of small objects, and squeeze a substance from a bottle, are also skills needed to carry out activities of daily living. In contrast, the patient who needs to spend a large portion of occupational therapy treatment time working on a peg design repeatedly to increase certain skills may experience frustration. This frustration may be amplified if the individual observes the therapist or assistant quickly removing all of the pegs after the work is completed. Although peg board design duplication does have importance, both as a diagnostic tool and a treatment technique, care must be taken to avoid its repeated use to increase certain skills. Perhaps a more long-term project with an end product should be used, an art or a craft that can provide an alternative to the usual treatment methods.

REDEFINING ARTS AND CRAFTS

Many members of the profession immediately think of traditional projects and kits when the therapeutic medium of arts and crafts is discussed. This is a limited view; one needs to look at many possibilities, such as the art of planning and planting a rock garden, the craft of repairing a leaky fawcet, the art of writing a poem, and the craft of baking cookies. In terms of the latter, much information can be obtained by observing a patient placing cookies on a cookie sheet. For example, size and shape perception can be addressed by observing if the patient makes cookies of uniform size and shape. If the patient puts all of the cookies on one side of the sheet, there may be a visual neglect problem. The same information can be obtained by using a peg board activity, but the bigger question must be answered: Which activity is the most appropriate and will provide the greatest benefit to the patient?

REHABILITATION APPLICATIONS

As stated previously, arts and crafts can be used to complement other activities in the treatment plan. The results of a survey conducted by Barris, Cordero and Christiansen in 1986[5] indicated that crafts were used more frequently in psychosocial occupational therapy treatment programs than in physical disability programs.[6] This practice may result because physical disability

rehabilitation tends to rely on the use of strengthening modalities, such as pulley exercises and bilateral sanders and neurodevelopmental techniques. Although occupational therapy personnel in both settings offer treatment for activities of daily living, the physical disability centers tend to view arts and crafts as strictly a leisure pursuit, which is not commonly dealt with.

Once the registered occupational therapist (OTR) has completed an evaluation of the patient, both the therapist and the assistant formulate a treatment plan. The following are examples of some arts and crafts that could be used in achieving treatment goals.

Pediatric Applications

Offer activities to provide opportunities for gross motor manipulation of objects:
- Constructing simple clay slab projects
- Finger painting using palm and forearm
- Kneading and forming bread dough into loaves

Offer activities to provide opportunities for fine motor manipulation of objects:
- Stringing beads
- Constructing pipe cleaner sculptures
- Making mosaic projects with macaroni

Psychosocial Applications

Provide opportunities to make choices or decisions necessary for task completion:
- Leather stamping
- Stenciling
- Original picture painting
- Tile mosaic work

Provide opportunities to follow directions through adherence to clear procedures necessary to complete task:
- Macramé
- Cross stitch
- Basketry
- String art
- Leather lacing

Provide graded cognitive and functional directions to increase attention span and concentration:
- Embroidery
- Weaving on a harness loom
- Stenciling
- Macramé
- Wood kits

Provide opportunities for analysis and problem solving to complete task:
- Handbuilt ceramics
- Macramé
- Weaving
- Tile mosaics
- Wood kits

Provide opportunities to complete specified tasks or subtasks within established time limits:
- Painting
- Knitting or crocheting
- Mosaics
- Slip casting
- Embroidery

Physical Disabilites Applications

Provide activities graded for strengthening:
- Elevated inkle loom with wrist weights
- Sanding wood (for project)
- Handbuilt ceramics
- Leather stamping

Provide opportunites to use fine motor skills:
- Tile work
- Copper tooling
- Jewelry making
- Macramé

It is evident that some art or craft activities can address more than one treatment goal, depending on which aspect of the activity is emphasized. The COTA must always use the process of **activity analysis** to decide if the activity being considered is appropriate, given the goals of treatment and the interests of the patient (see Chapter 17). Activity analysis may be defined as the breaking-down of an activity into detailed sub-parts and steps. The characteristics and values of the activity are examined in relation to the patient's needs, interests and goals. Activities that do not relate to the interests, needs and goals of the patient are not appropriate and should be avoided.

TREATMENT CONSIDERATIONS

When the activity is introduced, the COTA must explain the **therapeutic value** of the particular art or craft to the patient to assure that he or she has a clear understanding of why active engagement in the activity will contribute to improved performance. Therapeutic value refers to the extent to which an activity or experience has potential for assisting the achievement of particular goals. Specific goals must be clearly stated. For example, if the selected activity is macramé, as a means of increasing strength and endurance, the patient should be aware that the problem of decreased strength of the upper extremities will be remedied by working on the project while it is suspended at increasing heights because work is performed against the force of gravity. The amount of time spent knotting the cord could be increased at specified intervals to increase endurance.

From time to time, patients may need reassurance. It is important for them to believe they have the necessary skills to perform the task. The COTA must assure them

that the demands of the activity are not greater than their ability to participate.

Relationship to Decision-Making Process

COTAs often treat patients who have difficulty with the **decision-making** process (the process of weighing options in order to reach the best conclusion). These deficits may be the result of head injuries, psychiatric or neurologic dysfunctions, or, at times, prolonged institutionalization. Developmentally disabled individuals may also have a delayed acquisition of skills in decision making. Activities chosen for remediation of these deficits must be graded to accommodate the patient's current level of functioning.

It is important for the COTA to analyze the art or craft to determine the number of steps required, as well as the number of choices necessary to complete the task. A good example of grading a craft for the purpose of improving or developing decision-making skills is ceramics. Molded ceramic projects involve fewer decisions than hand-built projects. Certain steps can be carried out before the patient begins the project, such as pouring the slip into the mold, removing the molded object and cleaning it. In that way only two steps remain: applying glaze and firing. The number of glazes to choose from can be limited if the patient has difficulty choosing colors. As the patient gains greater ability in making decisions, the activity can be graded in complexity accordingly. The following decision making opportunities exist:

1. Choosing the mold to be used
2. Deciding when the project should be removed from the mold
3. Determining what areas need to be cleaned
4. Selecting which glaze(s) should be applied
5. Deciding how long the project should remain in the kiln
6. Determining how the finished project will be used

Alternatively, the patient can make clay sculptures or hand-built pots. The important principle is that the difficulty level of the art or craft used for treatment should increase as the patient's ability increases. **Difficulty level** is the degree of complexity that is required to execute a particular activity or step.

If a patient lacks opportunities to use decision-making skills, due to prolonged institutionalization, an art or a craft activity can be used. Initially, the decision might be choosing the color of paint or yarn to be used from only two possibilities.

Patients may also exhibit better decision-making abilities if they are motivated to participate in the activity. Hatter and Nelson[7] found that the decision of elderly residents residing in a nursing home to participate in a cookie baking task was higher among those who were told that the cookies were a surprise gift to a preschool day-care center than among those who were told to simply join a baking group.

The COTA can provide opportunities to enhance the patient's ability to function in the treatment setting, whether individually or in a group, by knowing his or her decision-making abilities. Allowing too many choices for patients who cannot make decisions adequately can cause disruptions in the treatment session and can be frustrating for both the COTA and the patient.

Relationship to Work, Leisure and Social Skills

Occupational performance areas include work and leisure skills as well as those necessary for self-care. The amount of time devoted to work and leisure changes as an individual matures and ages. The amount of leisure time that a child has is far greater than that of a working adult. Leisure time for a child can be considered play, whereas adult leisure pursuits are considered recreational or diversional and may include arts and crafts. As people age and enter retirement, the amount of leisure time increases again (see Chapter 7).

Socialization skills are needed at each stage of life. These are the skills that enable individuals to establish interpersonal relationships and social involvement. For children, good socialization skills are necessary for making friends at school, carrying friendships over into after-school activities, and to form the basis for later socialization. Often engaging in a craft activity, such as a group finger painting or collage, will strengthen these ties.

For some adults, socialization, work and leisure skills are interrelated (eg, participation in company-sponsored bowling leagues and baseball teams). Many of these adults may find that their ability to socialize changes greatly after retirement because they have not pursued independent leisure activities during their working years. Others, often referred to as "workaholics," are so consumed by their work that they never develop any leisure interests to use in retirement.

Changes in the amount of time spent for work and leisure activities can also be the result of disability or disease. The COTA can help the patient deal with these sudden changes by using information from the initial assessment regarding the individual's work history, leisure interests and social skills to plan a program to address any skills that may have been lost or altered. An important consideration is the disruption in the patient's daily routine and the degree to which the patient can realistically return to that routine. For some, the disruption can be expected to be short-term, such as recovery from a hip fracture. For others, the disruption can be long-term or permanent, as in the case of a cerebral vascular accident, spinal cord injury, or a particular psychiatric condition. The important point is to understand where the patient is in the **work-leisure continuum** (range of activities in which one engages throughout the life span, with varying amounts of time devoted to particular pursuits). To assure a good understanding the following questions should be answered:

1. Do new skills need to be taught, or can existing skills be adapted or modified?
2. Does the patient need to return to some type of meaningful employment, or do other activities need to be found?
3. Does the patient need to improve socialization skills to allow interaction in the workplace or other settings?

COTAs work in numerous settings providing treatment to individuals with a variety of performance deficits. Regardless of the specific treatment facility, the link between work, play/leisure and socialization is an important consideration when planning art and craft activities that are meaningful and appropriate.

Case Study 16-1

Janet. Janet is a 30-year-old married woman who is the mother of two children, ages five and seven years. She has been diagnosed as having leukemia and is an inpatient in the bone marrow transplant unit of an urban hospital. Her family resides in a small town 170 miles from the facility; thus her husband and children are able to visit only on weekends. She has frequently stated how much she misses them and that she feels "very removed and out of touch." It is estimated that Janet will be hospitalized about six weeks.

At initial evaluation, Janet had good strength and endurance. Due to the course of the bone marrow treatment, however, a decrease in strength and endurance could be anticipated. It was also necessary for her to remain active during the treatments.

After receiving chemotherapy and high-dose radiation treatments, Janet did experience decreased strength and endurance, as well as some disruption in concentration skills. The physical therapy department provided a program of exercises and ambulation, and Janet was able to perform light, progressive, resistive exercises and to walk 50 feet.

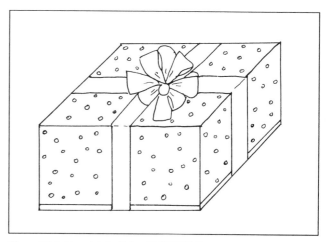

Figure 16-1. Completed gift box 2″ X 2″ X 1″.

The occupational therapy assistant, under the supervision of the occupational therapist, contributed to the planning and independently carried out a treatment program for Janet. The long-term goal was to prevent further debilitation due to the chemotherapy treatment by engaging the patient in vocational and avocational activities. Janet was encouraged to perform her own self-care activities, and she was taught energy conservation techniques to enable her to use her time more effectively and to reduce fatigue. Since she was not able to see her husband and children frequently, the assistant encouraged her to engage in a craft that would provide a meaningful gift for them and also required coordination and endurance.

Several small craft projects were presented to Janet, and she chose to make gift boxes out of wallpaper as shown in Figure 16-1. The boxes would be used to "personalize" small gifts for her family that she could readily purchase at the hospital, such as candy and hair bows. The activity of constructing the boxes would enable Janet to use both physical and cognitive skills, require sitting tolerance, and emphasize fine coordination skills and complex direction following (Figure 16-2).

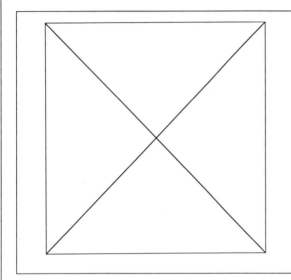

A. Steps 1-4.

Supplies and Equipment
- Wallpaper or other stiff paper
- Rule
- Pencil and eraser
- Scissors

Procedure
1. Measure and mark a square 5 × 5 inches. This is the lid.
2. Measure and mark another square 4 3/4 × 4 3/4 inches. This is the bottom.
3. Cut out the two squares.
4. Draw two diagonals from corner to corner, forming an X on the back of each square (Figure A).
5. Turn each of the four corners toward the center of the X, fold and crease firmly (Figure B).
6. With the corners made in step 5 still folded, turn each "side" of the square in toward the center line, crease firmly and unfold.
7. Completely unfold the square. The creases should correspond to those shown in Figure C.

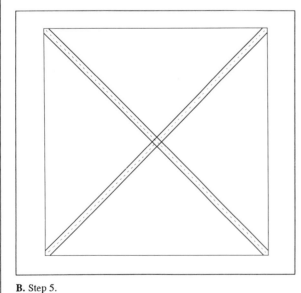

B. Step 5.

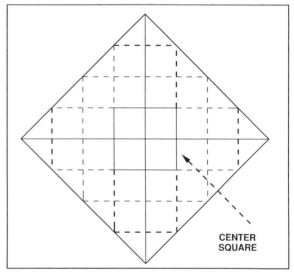

CENTER SQUARE

C. Creases (steps 6 and 7).

Figure 16-2. Directions for constructing a gift box.

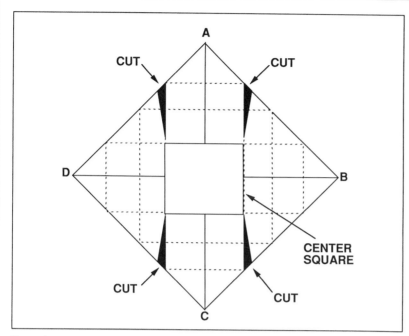

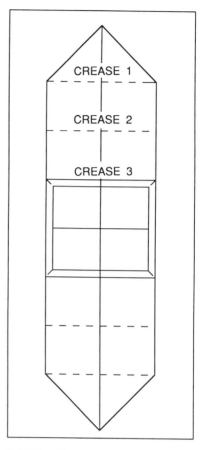

D. Cutting pattern (step 8).

8. Make cuts from the edge of the square to the corner of the center square formed by the creases. Make two cuts on one side of the box and two cuts on the opposite side of the box (Figure D). Do not make cuts on the adjacent sides.

9. Fold each crease (1, 2, and 3), as indicated by the dotted lines in Figure E, to the center. When the fold is made at crease 3, fold the paper up to form the side of the box.

10. Flip the two "wings" that have been folded up over the box and crease into the bottom. These will form the other two sides of the box. Tuck under folds on adjacent sides to secure.

11. Repeat steps 4 through 9 to complete the other half of the box. The completed box will measure 2 x 2 inches and be 1 inch deep.

12. Ribbon, lace, sequins, feathers, etc., may glued to the box top if desired.

E. Folding sides (step 9).

Figure 16-2. Continued.

DOCUMENTATION CONSIDERATIONS

In many instances, the problems occupational therapy personnel have been experiencing in justifying and being reimbursed for arts and crafts as treatment are the result of inadequate or inaccurate documentation. Accurate and thorough documentation is imperative. The goals to be achieved and the skills to be addressed must be clearly stated using appropriate, understandable terminology, consistent with the required documentation format and standards of the profession. Proper documentation of the patient's progress or lack thereof must be made at regular intervals. It is the responsibility of the COTA to inform the supervising therapist of any changes in the level of performance so that the treatment plan can be modified accordingly.

FUTURE IMPLICATIONS

During the last several years, changes in thinking about the old concepts and techniques of occupational therapy have become evident in the literature as well as at presentations and discussions. Many members of the profession feel that the foundation of occupational therapy has been forgotten.[6] It is important to remember that the use of arts and crafts served a necessary therapeutic need at one time, and that a well-chosen art or craft can still be a meaningful form of treatment in keeping with the profession's philosophy of purposeful activity.

SUMMARY

The decision to use arts and crafts in occupational therapy treatment should be made after a thorough review of the patient's history and an activity analysis to assess the appropriateness of the particular arts and crafts being considered. The activity selected should be age appropriate and purposeful; have meaning to the patient in terms of his or her particular needs, interests, and roles; and relate directly to the goals established in the treatment plan. Examples of a wide variety of art and craft activities provide the reader with further evidence of the potential use of these modalities in therapeutic intervention. The importance of relating the activity to decision making and recognizing the importance of work, leisure and social skills in relation to art and craft activities is another primary consideration. Thorough and accurate documentation is essential for reimbursement.

Related Learning Activities

1. Discuss the three criteria for a craft activity to be appropriate for a patient.

2. Make a craft project that you are unfamiliar with. List the specific decisions that you made. How could you increase or decrease the number of decisions required?

3. What other craft activities could have been presented to Janet?

4. Construct the gift box according to the directions provided. Identify areas where difficulties or problems might occur.

References

1. Slagle EC: Occupational therapy: Recent methods and advances in the United States. *Occup Ther Rehabil* 13:5, 1934.
2. Hopkins HL: *Willard and Spackman's Occupational Therapy,* 7th Edition. Philadelphia, JB Lippincott, 1988, Chap 1.
3. Tracy SE: *Studies in Invalid Occupations.* Boston, Whitcomb & Barrows, 1918.
4. Cynkin S: *Occupational Therapy: Toward Health Through Activities.* Boston, Little, Brown, 1979.
5. Barris R, Cordero J, Christiansen R: Occupational therapists' use of media. *Am J Occup Ther* 40:679-684, 1986.
6. Friedland J: Diversional activity: Does it deserve its bad name? *Am J Occup Ther* 42:603-609, 1988.
7. Hatter JK, Nelson DL: Altruism and task performance in the elderly. *Am J Occup Ther* 41:376-381, 1987.

Chapter 17

Activity Analysis

LaDonn People, MA, OTR
Sally E. Ryan, COTA, ROH
Doris Y. Witherspoon, MS, OTR
Rhonda Stewart, OTR

INTRODUCTION

Activity analysis is extremely important in occupational therapy. This process involves the "breaking down" of an activity into detailed subparts and steps, which is a necessary foundation for all activities of daily living, play/leisure and work tasks used in intervention. It is an examination of the therapeutic characteristics and value of activities that fulfill the patient's many needs, interests, abilities and roles. Without such analysis, it may be impossible to use the proper application of activity or to obtain the best treatment results. Skill in activity analysis is critical to determine the validity of the use of activities in occupational therapy assessment and treatment.

The type of activity analysis used will be determined, at least in part, by the individual therapist's or assistant's frame of reference.[1] Such analysis will also be influenced by the use of particular techniques and variations in the use of equipment. While there is no universally accepted method of activity analysis, it is useful to consider the general categories of motor, sensory, cognitive, intrapersonal and interpersonal skills, as well as adaptations.[2] Other considerations should include factors such as the supplies and equipment needed, cost, the number of steps required for completion, time involved, supervision required, space needed, precautions and contraindications. It is also helpful to think of several aspects of experience or functional requirements of the activity and then analyze them in terms of gradability.[3] **Functional requirements** may be defined as components of an activity that require motor performance and behaviors for adequate completion. **Gradability** refers to a process whereby performance of an activity is viewed step-by-step on a continuum from simple to complex, or slow to rapid.

The activity analysis yields the kind of data needed for determining **therapeutic potential** of a particular activity in relation to established

---

KEY CONCEPTS

Historical foundations

Activity engagement principles

Purpose and process of activity analysis

Development of analysis skills

Adaptation and grading of activities

Utilizing specific forms and examples

patient goals, interests and needs. Therapeutic potential is the degree of likelihood that therapeutic goals will be achieved. As specific techniques and equipment vary considerably for many activities, so will the results of an activity analysis. Once an activity is thoroughly analyzed, it can be adapted for therapeutic purposes.

HISTORICAL PERSPECTIVES

The profession of occupational therapy was founded on the notion that being engaged in activities promotes mental and physical well-being and, conversely, that the absence of activity leads at best to mischief and at worst to loss of mental and physical functioning.[4] Through their activities, human beings show their concern with how to survive, be comfortable, have pleasure, solve problems, express themselves, and relate to others. They come to know their strengths and they fulfill their roles in life. Thus the term occupation, as used in occupational therapy, is in the context of the individual's directed use of time, energy, interest and attention.[5]

Activities being the foundation of the profession, historical definitions and other accounts place a strong emphasis on occupations or purposeful activities.

When William Tuke established the York Retreat in England in the late 1800s, employment in various occupations was a cornerstone of treatment in this facility for mental patients. Review of historical accounts of Tuke's work show that he had spent some time analyzing activities. For example, activities and occupations were selected to elicit emotions that were opposite of the condition; a melancholy patient would be given activities that had elements of excitement and were active, whereas a manic patient would be engaged in tasks of a sedentary nature. The habit of attention was a key element in using activities for treatment.[6]

Among the early pioneers of our profession, history records the work of Susan Tracy in relation to the process of analyzing activity (see Chapter 1). Tracy's work with mentally ill patients led her to believe that remedial activities ". . .are classified according to their physiological effects as stimulants, sedatives, anesthetics. . ."[7] Over time, she analyzed the use of leather projects with patients and identified various components of a specific activity that would measure abilities in areas such as judgment, visual discrimination, spatial relationships, and making choices.[7] In 1918, she published a research paper, "Twenty-five suggested mental tests derived from invalid occupations."[8]

Eleanor Clarke Slagle's work in developing the principles of habit training certainly reflects her knowledge of activity analysis, as she placed particular emphasis on the gradation of activities and a balance among them.[9]

The 1918 principles, established by the founders of our profession, also address aspects of activity that imply an ability to analyze the activity's properties. Emphasis was placed on the qualities of particular activities, with crafts and work-related activities being prominent; games, music and physical exercise were also used.[10]

The terms *employment, labor, moral treatment, recreation, amusement, occupation, exercise,* and *diversion* among others have been used by different writers at various times to describe the forms of treatment used by occupational therapy personnel. The philosophy of the profession also places a strong emphasis on activities (see Chapter 3). Throughout our history, particular properties of activities were also addressed, giving strong roots to our basic belief in the activity analysis process. **Activity properties** are those characteristics of activities (eg, being goal-directed, having significance to the individual, requiring involvement, gradability, adaptability, etc.) that contribute to their therapeutic potential.

Contemporary definitions of occupational therapy are summarized in the 1981 definition of the profession, developed for licensure purposes, which describes occupational therapy as the therapeutic use of self-care (activites of daily living), work and play/leisure activities to maximize independent function, enhance development, prevent disability and maintain health.[11] It may include adaptations of the task or the environment to achieve maximum independence and to enhance the quality of one's life. Implicit in the latter statement is the ability to analyze activities. One must indeed know the particular properties and possibilities of a variety of activities to *adapt the task* to help the patient attain his or her goals. A related point, emphasized by Mosey, is that activities used by occupational therapy personnel include both an intrinsic and a therapeutic purpose.[12] This point is important to consider during activity analysis.

ACTIVITY ENGAGEMENT PRINCIPLES

Occupational therapy personnel must know various types of activities. Some of the **categories of activities** used in evaluation and treatment are the following:

1. Crafts: leatherwork, ceramics
2. Sensory awareness: music, dance
3. Movement awareness: dance, drama
4. Fine arts: sculpturing, painting, music
5. Construction: woodworking, electronics
6. Games: bingo, checkers
7. Self-care: dressing, feeding, hygiene
8. Domestic: cooking, homemaking
9. Textiles: weaving, needlecraft
10. Vocational: rock and stamp collecting

11. Recreational: sports, exercise
12. Educational: reading, writing

For activities to be considered purposeful and therapeutic, they must possess certain characteristics, which include the following:[13]

1. Be goal-directed
2. Have significance to the patient at some level
3. Require patient involvement at some level (mental or physical or both)
4. Be geared toward prevention of malfunction and/or maintenance or improvement of function and quality of life
5. Reflect patient involvement in life task situations (activities of daily living, work and play/leisure)
6. Relate to the interests of the patient
7. Be adaptable and gradable

The selection of appropriate activities for evaluation and treatment of patients must be based on sound professional judgment that is well grounded in knowledge and skill.[13] As activity specialists, occupational therapists and assistants must have strong skills in this area.[14] A thorough knowledge of and experience in analyzing a wide variety of activities is an essential element of this process. The *Essentials and Guidelines for an Accredited Educational Program for the Occupational Therapy Assistant* state that analysis and adaptation of activities is a requirement for entry-level personnel: "Activity analysis should relate to relevance of activity to patient/client interests and abilities, major motor processes, complexity, the steps involved, and the extent to which it can be modified or adapted."[15]

Mosey[12] stresses that purposeful activities cannot be designed for evaluation and intervention without analysis. Dunn[4] states that if activities are to be the core of occupational therapy they must be delineated, classified and analyzed in terms of therapeutic value.

PURPOSE AND PROCESS OF ACTIVITY ANALYSIS

The purpose of activity analysis is to determine if the activity will be appropriate in meeting the treatment goals established for the patient. To analyze an activity with knowledge and skill, it is necessary to know how to perform the processes involved. It is also relevant to know the extent to which the activity fosters or impedes various types of human performance and interaction.

The patient must be receptive to the activity selected. Patients will be more motivated and participate more if their interests, life tasks and roles are considered. In addition, the patient's **functional level** should be considered. The individual may be interested in the activity and it may relate

directly to his or her life tasks and roles, but due to performance deficits, it cannot be accomplished.

The process of analyzing an activity involves breaking it down to illustrate each step in detail that leads to the expected outcome. Consideration must be given to numerous factors that are used to achieve activity completion as shown in examples later in this chapter.

An activity analysis can be helpful when determining the use of an activity for an evaluation or for treatment. When analyzing an activity intended for evaluative purposes, it must be broken down into separate components to determine what opportunities exist to objectively measure what is to be evaluated.[16] For example, as Early[16] points out, when the purpose of engagement in an activity is to measure decision-making skills, the activity selected must provide choices, as well as decision points, to allow it to be useful. She also stresses that occupational therapy personnel must know the exact responses and outcomes that might potentially occur and how they relate to the patient's ability to make decisions. An interpretation of observations of the individual's engagement in the activity (performance) would follow. When the activity is intended to be used for treatment, it again must be broken down into small units to determine which **components** (constituent parts) of the activity will help to achieve the treatment goals, such as to increase range of motion, to improve attention span, or to decrease isolative behavior.

An accurate analysis of an activity allows occupational therapy personnel to select activities that will address the needs and goals of the patient therapeutically. This process also aids in determining the therapeutic potential of specific activities and their purposeful use. The absense of a thorough activity analysis is likely to prevent achievement of the best treatment results.

DEVELOPING SKILLS

Skill in activity analysis is critical to determine the validity of the use of activities in occupational therapy intervention programs. Prerequisite to achieving skill is the ability to understand the basic components of the activity, that is, the fundamental processes, tools, and materials required for task completion. Self-analysis of a simple, frequently engaged in activity, such as bathing, is useful as an initial step. Asking questions, such as the following, is recommended:

1. Why is the activity important to you?
2. What supplies and equipment are needed?
3. What is the procedure?
4. What other factors should be considered?

Once these questions have been answered, look at the information critically to determine if *precise* information was recorded. Recheck to be sure that no important factors were omitted. Ask a family member or peer to also answer these questions. In comparing results, differences in answers emphasize the uniqueness of the individual. Other questions can then be considered, such as how to adapt the activity for persons with various disabilities.

Experience in engaging in a wide variety of activities is also important in building skill, as it allows the certified occupational therapy assistant (COTA) to make comparisons and formulate potential applications based on several possibilities. Practice in using several forms of activity analysis and receiving objective feedback also is as a way to develop skill. Once skill is achieved the COTA can more easily select the most appropriate activity, which is of interest to the patient, relates to his or her life tasks and roles, is within the individual's functional capacity to perform, and provides opportunities for goal achievement.[17] **Goal achievement** is to the accomplishment of tasks and objectives one has set out to do.

RELATED CONSIDERATIONS

Frame of Reference

Occupational therapy personnel use many approaches to analyze activities. The type of activity analysis is determined, at least in part, by the individual therapist's or assistant's frame of reference.[1] For example, if a developmental frame of reference is used, activities are analyzed to determine the extent to which they might contribute to the age specific development and related areas of occupational performance. If gratification of oral needs was a goal of treatment, it would be important to analyze the activity in terms of opportunities for eating, sucking, blowing and encouraging independence, among other factors.[12]

Activity analysis is also influenced by the use of particular techniques and variations in the use of equipment recommended, such as in sensory integration and in the theoretical approaches of Rood, Bobath, and Brunnstrom. Additional information on theoretical frameworks and approaches may be found in Chapter 4.

Adaption

To adapt an activity means to modify it.[16] It involves changing the components that are required to complete the task. Adaptions are made to allow the patient to experience success in task accomplishment at his or her level of functioning. For example, an individual who has had a stroke, resulting in paralysis of one side of the body, will need to use a holding device such as a lacing "pony" or a vice to stabilize a leather-lacing project. A change in positioning of the project, due to loss of peripheral vision and neglect of the involved side, is another important adaption. Although few adaptions

are required in this example, all of the components of the specific activity must be considered for potential changes to increase their therapeutic potential.[16]

Grading

Grading of an activity refers to the process of performance being viewed step by step on a continuum that progresses from simple to complex. For example, a patient might begin by lacing two precut layers of leather together, using large prepunched holes and a simple whip stitch, to make a comb case. Once this is satisfactorily completed, additional challenges, such as the following, could be introduced over several treatment sessions:

1. Use of saddle stitching, followed by single cordovan, and double cordovan lacing, on other short-term leather projects
2. Use of simple stamping, followed by tooling and carving to decorate the project
3. Application of basic finishes, or more advanced techniques, such as antiquing and dyeing with several colors

Activities may also be graded according to rate of time, varying from slow to rapid. An important concept is that the grading of activities builds on what has already been accomplished in progressive stages.

FORMS AND EXAMPLES

Although no universally accepted method of activity analysis exists, the following outline, checklist, and examples are provided to assist the reader in understanding the many diverse and complex factors inherent in the process of activity analysis. Study and use of these materials provides the COTA with opportunities to gain new skills or improve existing ones. Although every effort has been made to make these examples as complete as possible, other relevant aspects could undoubtedly be included. Some of the examples are formated in such a way that they could be filled out and used as protocols for an occupational therapy clinic, thus assuring that all personnel had information about a particular activity and its potential therapeutic uses. Those with limited experience in activity analysis should focus first on the general outline shown in Figure 17-1. From time to time, unfamiliar terminology may be introduced. Definitions may be found by consulting the glossary, which appears at the end of this text.

ACTIVITY ANALYSIS CHECKLIST

The **Activity Analysis Checklist,** shown in Figure 17-2, is a faster method of determining the particular components

1. *Name of activity:*

2. *Number of individuals involved:*

3. *Supplies and equipment:*
   List all tools, equipment, and materials needed to complete the activity. Optional items should be so designated.

4. *Procedure:*
   List all steps required to complete the activity.

5. *Cost:*
   List costs of all supplies and equipment. Large equipment, such as a kiln or jigsaw, is usually not included because it is only purchased once.

6. *Preparation:*
   List any processes that must be or could be completed before the treatment session. (This may be due to dangerous or complicated procedures, or because of limited treatment time.)

7. *Time:*
   List total amount of time necessary, including preparation and cleanup, if required.

8. *Space needs or setting required:*
   State requirements relative to where the activity will take place. (Activities performed in the clinic may not be appropriate for treatment in a patient's room.)

9. *Activity qualities:*
   Consider such factors as controllability, resistiveness, noise, cleanliness, practability, problem areas, and likely mistakes. List both positive and negative aspects.

10. *Amount of supervision:*
    Can the activity be completed independently, or must it be supervised? (To what degree?)

11. *Physical requirements:*
    Consider factors such as motions used (be specific), fine motor skills, gross motor skills, dexterity, eye-hand and bilateral coordination, posture/position (standing, sitting, leaning, bending, prone, supine, etc.), strength, endurance, and balance.

12. *Sensory requirements:*
    Consider visual, tactile, auditory, olfactory and gustatory factors.

13. *Cognitive factors:*
    Consider requirements for organization, concentration, problem solving, logical thinking, attention span, direction following (written, oral or demonstration), decision making and creativity.

14. *Emotional factors:*
    Consider aspects such as degree of structure, initiative, control, dependence, impulse control, frustration tolerance, opportunities to handle feelings, and role identification.

15. *Social factors:*
    Consider degree of communication, interaction, and competition required; opportunities for assuming responsibility and cooperating.

16. *Potential for adaption or modification:*
    Consider points 9 through 15.

17. *Precautions and contraindications:*

18. *Grading potential:*
    Consider how to change (simple, complex, rapid, or slow).

19. *Type of condition or problem for which activity is recommended:*

20. *Activity category:*
    (Functional, supportive, vocational, diversional)

21. *Expected primary therapeutic goals:*

22. *Other pertinent information:*
    Consider age appropriateness, gender identification, cultural considerations and vocational implications.

Figure 17-1. General activity analysis outline.[18]

of an activity, as it requires less writing than the general activity analysis outline (see Figure 17-1). Figure 17-3 shows the same form used to analyze the specific activity of constructing a leather coin purse. Although the form and the example emphasize psychosocial aspects, they easily could be modified to include criteria with a more definitive focus on physical performance deficts as well as other areas.

Example I: Play/Leisure Activity

1. *Name of activity:* Volleyball

2. *Number of individuals involved:* 8-15

3. *Supplies and equipment:* Volleyball, net, poles, score pad, and pen. Optional: Refreshments and prizes

4. *Procedure:* Stand in designated space. Reach to hit the ball over the net when it approaches you. Move side to side and front to back within your designated space to hit the ball. Rotate to the space on your left after score is made. Optional: Start a new game after the established score is reached.

5. *Cost:* None if equipment is available; otherwise about $60.00 (see item three).

6. *Preparation:* 5-10 minutes to obtain equipment and set up

7. *Time:* 1 hour and 5 minutes:
   5 minutes to set up equipment
   5 minutes to instruct group (process, rules, scoring)
   45 minutes for actual activity participation
   10 minutes to clean up, pack, and store equipment

8. *Space needs or setting required:* Outdoor area or large room free of obstacles and furnishings

9. *Activity qualities:* High potential for noise, due to excitement and competitve behavior. Participants may need assistance with procedures and scoring.

10. *Amount of supervision:* Direct to assure proper follow through

11. *Physical requirements:* Reaching, jumping, standing, turning, grasping, eye-hand coordination, balance, strength, and endurance

Activity: Check the appropriate box:	None	Min.	Mod.	Max.	Comments
1. Initiative					
2. Technical ability					
3. Manipulative ability					
4. Creative ability					
5. Concentrated effort					
6. Mechanical repetition					
7. Constant action					
8. Fine motor					
9. Gross motor					
10. Tactile					
11. Visual					
12. Auditory					
13. Olfactory					
14. Gustatory					
15. Time					
16. Modification of equipment					
17. Noise					
18. Degree of cleanliness					
19. Equipment and tool costs					
20. Materials costs					
21. Use of surplus or scrap materials					
22. Opportunity to express constructively:					
a. Affect or attitude					
b. Creativeness					
c. Originality					
d. Frustration					
e. Hostility					
f. Aggression					
g. Anger					
h. Obsessive-compulsive feature					
i. Need to excel					
j. Need to have supervision					
k. Narcissism					
l. Expiation of guilt					
m. Dependence					
n. Independence					
o. Masculine identification					
p. Feminine identification					
q. Regressive features					
23. Structure					
24. Controllability					
25. Pliability					
26. Resistiveness					
27. Predictability					
28. Concentration					
29. Problem solving					
30. Improve competence					
31. Improve efficacy					
32. Gradability					
33. Directions:					
a. Oral					
b. Written					
c. Demonstration					
34. Precautions					
35. Other					

Figure 17-2. Activity analysis checklist.

Activity: *Leather Coin Purse*

Check the appropriate box:	None	Min.	Mod.	Max.	Comments
1. Initiative		✓			
2. Technical ability		✓			
3. Manipulative ability				✓	
4. Creative ability		✓			more if carving
5. Concentrated effort				✓	
6. Mechanical repetition				✓	
7. Constant action				✓	lacing
8. Fine motor				✓	lacing
9. Gross motor			✓		cutting
10. Tactile			✓		
11. Visual			✓		blind can lace
12. Auditory			✓		punching holes
13. Olfactory			✓		
14. Gustatory	✓				
15. Time		✓	✓		
16. Modification of equipment	✓				
17. Noise			✓		
18. Degree of cleanliness				✓	
19. Equipment and tool costs			✓		
20. Materials costs			✓		
21. Use of surplus or scrap materials			✓		
22. Opportunity to express constructively:					
a. Affect or attitude		✓			
b. Creativeness		✓			
c. Originality		✓			
d. Frustration		✓			
e. Hostility			✓		
f. Aggression		✓			stamping
g. Anger			✓		stamping
h. Obsessive-compulsive feature			✓		
i. Need to excel				✓	
j. Need to have supervision	✓				
k. Narcissism	✓				
l. Expiation of guilt		✓			
m. Dependence		✓			
n. Independence				✓	
o. Masculine identification		✓			
p. Feminine identification		✓			
q. Regressive features	✓				
23. Structure				✓	
24. Controlability				✓	
25. Pliability		✓			
26. Resistiveness		✓			
27. Predictability				✓	
28. Concentration		✓			
29. Problem solving				✓	
30. Improve competence				✓	
31. Improve efficacy				✓	
32. Gradability			✓		
33. Directions:					
a. Oral				✓	
b. Written				✓	
c. Demonstration				✓	
34. Precautions				✓	needle
35. Other					

Figure 17-3. Completed activity analysis checklist for constructing a leather coin purse.

12. *Sensory requirements:* Visual, tactile, kinesthetic; auditory helpful but loss can be accommodated

13. *Cognitive factors:* Attention span, concentration, problem solving, judgment, oral and demonstrated direction following, memory

14. *Emotional factors:* Initiative, frustration tolerance, activity tolerance

15. *Social factors:* Cooperative and competitive behavior; group interaction and potential for socialization. Nonparticipants can be encouraged to be "cheer leaders" or score keepers or to serve refreshments.

16. *Potential for adaptation or modification:* Good. May use a foam ball or a beach ball. May be played while seated. Playing for points and rotations may be omitted (also see gradation).

17. *Precautions and contraindications:* Participants with low tolerance may need frequent breaks; participants with short attention span or memory deficits may need frequent cueing. Avoid use with individuals with serious cardiopulmonary and respiratory problems. Thoroughly instruct in proper serving and other motions required to reduce potential for injury.

18. *Grading potential:* Rapid: Decrease time allocated and encourage increased participation. Slow: Decrease emphasis on time; allow game to proceed as tolerated; add breaks.

19. *Type of condition or problem for whom activity is recommended:* A wide variety. Not appropriate for the very young or those having pronounced perceptual and motor deficits.

20. *Activity category:* Functional and diversional

21. *Expected primary therapeutic goals:* Numerous; examples include those in items 9 to 13.

22. *Other pertinent information:* Prizes may be awarded for best serve, most points scored by a single person, good sportsmanship, etc.

Example II: Work Activity

This example illustrates a prevocational task used as one of the objective measurements of an individual's potential to work in a sheltered workshop environment.

1. *Name of activity:* Sorting and packaging screws

2. *Number of individuals involved:* 1 to 3 initially

3. *Supplies and equipment:* Chairs and table; 500 flathead screws (250 1-inch and 250 1$\frac{1}{2}$-inch); 1 box of sandwich size plastic bags with ties; self-adhesive paper labels; one felt-tip marking pen for each person

4. *Procedure:* Sort screws according to size. Count and place 20 screws in a bag, seal the bag, mark the label with the correct size, and apply the label.

5. *Cost:* .03 to .05 cents per screw; .99 cents for 100 plastic bags; .50 cents per marker; .99 cents for box of 100 self-adhesive labels

6. *Preparation:* Minimal: 5 to 10 minutes to gather supplies and set up; determine monitoring methods

7. *Time:* 45 minutes, approximately:
   5 minutes to set up
   2 minutes to explain and demonstrate process
   25 minutes to perform task (task completion within allocated time is a requirement)
   5 to 10 minutes to clean up work area

8. *Space needs or setting required:* Quiet room to permit concentration and minimize distractions (no television, telephone, people entering and exiting, etc.)

9. *Activity qualities:* Structured, offers fairly immediate gratification, controllable, simple instructions, clean

10. *Amount of supervision:* Good potential for independence after initial learning. Monitor for fatigue, problems and observable behaviors

11. *Physical requirements:* Sitting or standing, reaching, bending, grasping, balance, eye-hand coordination; at least fair strength and endurance

12. *Sensory requirements:* Visual or tactile discrimination and integration or both; auditory loss can be accommodated

13. *Cognitive factors:* Concentration, attention span, direction following, memory, sequencing, decision making, time management, and organization

14. *Emotional factors:* Initiative, motivation, competition if working in group; frustration tolerance, and activity tolerance

15. *Social factors:* Independence; interaction not required unless set up as a task group; if so, still limited

16. *Potential for adaptation or modification:* Good. May be performed while sitting, standing or supine; can be adapted for a prosthesis. Easily adapted to a task group format (see gradation potential).

17. *Precautions and contraindications:* Observe for fatigue that may not be voiced. Confused people may ingest screws or ties.

18. *Grading potential:* Simple: Count screws of one size and shape; eliminate time requirement. Complex: Sort and count screws of varying sizes and shapes. May be accomplished slowly or rapidly.

19. *Type of condition or problem activity is recommended for:* Young adults, adults, and geriatric patients with a variety of performance deficits who need vocational preparation.

20. *Activity category:* Functional; vocational

21. *Expected primary therapeutic goals:* Improve independence, work tolerance, and work behaviors; identify needs for environmental modifications (table height, lighting, etc.).

22. *Other pertinent information:* Same process could be used for sorting and counting other materials such as mosaic tile for kits.

Example III: Self-Care Activity

1. *Name of activity:* Donning a shirt with front buttons
2. *Type of program:* Daily living task
3. *Type of patient indicated:* Variable
4. *Number of patients involved:* One or small group
5. *Materials and equipment needed:* Shirt or shirts with front buttons
6. *Cost:* Variable: Patients can have shirt brought from home if not available in setting
7. *Preparation required:* None
8. *Time involved:* Depends on patient; usually about 3 minutes
9. *Space needed or physical setting required:* May be completed at bedside or in clinic
10. *Qualities of activity:* Quiet, clean, practical; problems may occur in buttoning shirt incorrectly
11. *Amount of supervision required:* Minimal once demonstrated and learned; practice may be independent
12. *Directions required:* Oral and demonstration
13. *Procedure:*
    Unbutton shirt
    Position shirt
    Pick up shirt
    Put arm in shirt sleeve
    Pull shirt over shoulder
    Put other arm in shirt sleeve
    Pull shirt together
    Fasten buttons on shirt front
    Straighten shirt
14. *Physical functions or requirements:* May be performed sitting or standing, if patient has adequate balance; may also be performed in a supine position; dexterity and coordination are needed for buttoning. Motions involved include shoulder flexion and abduction when picking up shirt, elbow flexion and extension when pulling the shirt over the shoulder, forearm pronation and supination, wrist hyperextension, finger flexion, and neck flexion.
15. *Cognitive, sensory, perceptual motor functions:* Ability to comprehend simple verbal and demonstrated instructions; ability to cross the midline in bringing the shirt over the shoulder; vision and hearing not required
16. *Psychological functions:* Not frustrating; short-term; some judgment needed to avoid putting shirt on inside out or buttoning incorrectly; may be performed independently
17. *Potential therapeutic goals:*
    Increase daily living independence in area of dressing
    Aid in adjusting to residual abilities
    Improve tactile abilities (buttoning) and motor coordination
    Increase reality orientation (appropriate shirt for weather or season)
    Build self-esteem (success provides gratification)
    Aid in assuming responsibility (patient encouraged to dress daily)
18. *Gradation:* Learn to button first, then don shirt
19. *Potential for adaptation:* Use of a button aid or Velcro fasteners; pullover shirt can be used to eliminate buttons.
20. *Relationship to experience:* Necessary in life activities
21. *Precautions and contraindications:* Activity not limited to any particular diagnosis; maintain proper posture
22. *Comments:* Should be initiated early in the patient's treatment

Example IV: Homemaking Activity

An activity analysis of a cooking activity, which follows, is presented as a contrast to the dressing activity to emphasize the variety of ways an activity may be analyzed and also to contrast a simple activity with a complex one. Although detailed, this example tends to explore more general aspects of the activity in five rather than 22 categories. As experience and skill are gained, less detailed formats may be used.

Rosette Cooking

Materials Needed.
Rosette iron molds (80 different ones available)
Rosette iron handle
Deep fryer or heavy saucepan
Paper towels
Oil for frying
Metal tongs
$1/2$ cup evaporated milk
$1/2$ cup water
$1/4$ teaspoon salt
1 teaspoon sugar
1 egg, beaten
1 cup flour
garnishes: powdered sugar, cinnamon, whipped cream and/or fruit

Directions. Prepare batter in order listed; slowly stir in flour and beat until smooth.

Place approximately two inches of oil in deep fryer or heavy saucepan.

Heat oil to 365° F.

Attach rosette iron mold to mold handle.

Immerse iron mold in hot oil until thoroughly heated.

Lift out mold and blot excess oil with paper towel.

Dip mold into batter until it is $3/4$ covered. Do not cover the entire mold.

Hold the mold in the bowl for a few seconds; lift it out and shake off any excess batter.

Dip the batter-coated mold into the hot oil.

Once the rosette begins to brown slightly, lift the mold and let the rosette gently drop into the hot oil.

Using metal tongs, turn the rosette over and cook for a few more seconds.

Use the tongs to lift the finished rosette out of the oil and drain it on paper towels.

Sprinkle with powdered sugar, cinnamon, or other garnishes.

Type of Group or Individual Patient for Whom This Activity Is Appropriate. This activity is appropriate for a lower functioning patient group, due to its immediate gratification and success assured qualities. Close supervision and some assistance are required. Patient groups functioning at a higher level would also benefit from this type of activity. They would require minimal supervision and encouragement. It would provide a means of moving to higher level task skills required in many areas of daily living.

The activity can be structured to enhance group cohesiveness by delineating various tasks for small groups or individuals to perform. In this way, all members can make a contribution to the end product of the project group.

Precautions. The hot oil presents the main safety hazard and should be closely monitored at all times. Ingredients may need to be substituted to accommodate special diets.

Goals.
- Upgrade both basic and higher level daily living task skills
- Increase self-esteem
- Increase attention span and concentration
- Increase motivation to carry out a single project to completion
- Provide immediate, basic gratification and fulfillment
- Increase group cohesiveness through shared responsibility (may also be used with individuals)

SUMMARY

Activities are universal and historically have remained a primary foundation for the profession. Activity analysis is a deeply rooted concept, which has withstood the test of time and continues to be an important cornerstone for accurate assessment and effective intervention by occupational therapy personnel. The basic concepts and processes have been described to provide a fundamental understanding of the knowledge base and skills necessary for activities analysis. These skills include activity engagement principles, methods for developing skills, concepts of grading and adapting

activities. Forms and examples of the analysis of specific activites were also presented.

Emphasis was placed on the need for the activity analysis process and the information that may be gained through exploration of activity properties and possibilities. Skill in activity analysis is essential to determine the validity of the activities used for assessment and treatment. A thorough and accurate activity analysis allows the practitioner to select the most appropriate activity, which is of interest to the patient, relates to his or her life tasks and roles, and provides opportunities for goal achievement.

Author's Note
Example III: Self-Care Activity and Example IV: Homemaking Activity were reprinted with the permission of the Occupational Therapy Assistant Program, Wayne County Community College, Detroit, Michigan.

Acknowledgment
The editor thanks Sr. Genevieve Cummings, CSJ, MA, OTR, FAOTA, for her editorial and content recommendations.

Related Learning Activities

1. Discuss some of the reasons occupatinoal therapy personnel use activity analysis.

2. Observe a person engaged in a work task. Identify the specific physical, cognitive and social skills required.

3. List the general categories of information that should be a part of an activity analysis.

4. Working with a peer and using the format for "Donning a Shirt with Front Buttons," complete an activity analysis for another dressing activity.

5. Using the format presented for "Rosette Cooking," complete an activity analysis for a different cooking activity and a craft activity.

References

1. Hopkins HL, Smith HD, Tiffany EC: Therapeutic application of activity. In Hopkins HL, Smith HD (Eds): *Willard and Spackman's Occupational Therapy*, 6th Edition. Philadelphia, JB Lippincott, 1983, p. 225.
2. United States Department of Labor, Employment, and Training Administration: *Dictionary of Occupational Titles*, 4th Edition. Washington, DC, U.S. Government Printing Office, 1981.
3. Tiffany EC: Psychiatry and mental health. In Hopkins HL, Smith HD (Eds): *Willard and Spackman's Occupational Therapy*, 6th Edition. Philadelphia, JB Lippincott, 1983.

4. Dunn W: Application of uniform terminology in practice. *Am J Occup Ther* 43:817-831, 1989.

5. American Occupational Therapy Association: *Reference Manual of Official Documents of the American Occupational Therapy Association.* Rockville, Maryland, AOTA, 1980.

6. Tuke S: *A Description of the Retreat: An Institution Near York for Insane Persons of The Society of Friends.* London, Dawson of Pall Mall, 1813.

7. Tracy SE: The place of invalid occupations in the general hospital. *Modern Hospital* 2(5):386, June, 1914.

8. Tracy SE: Twenty-five suggested mental tests derived from invalid occupations. *Maryland Psychiatric Quarterly* 8:15-16, 1918.

9. Slagle EC: Training aides for mental patients. *Arch Occup Ther* 1:13-14, 1922.

10. Dunton WR: The principles of occupational therapy. In *Proceedings of the National Society for the Promotion of Occupational Therapy, Second Annual Meeting.* Catonsville, Maryland, Spring Grove State Hospital Press, 1918, pp. 25-27.

11. Resolution Q: Definition of occupational therapy for liscensure. Minutes of the 1981 AOTA Representative Assembly. *Am J Occup Ther* 35:798-799, 1981.

12. Mosey AC: *Psychosocial Components of Occupational Therapy.* New York, Raven Press, 1986.

13. Hopkins HD, Smith HL (Eds): *Willard and Spackman's Occupational Therapy,* 6th Edition. Philadelphia, JB Lippincott, 1983.

14. Punwar AJ: *Occupational Therapy Principles and Practice.* Baltimore, Williams & Wilkins, 1988, Chapter 2.

15. Essentials and Guidelines for an Accredited Educational Program for the Occupational Therapy Assistant. *Am J Occup Ther* 45:1085-1092, 1991.

16. Early MB: *Mental Health Concepts and Techniques for the Occupational Therapy Assistant.* New York, Raven Press, 1987, pp. 274-275.

17. Trombly C, Scott AD: *Occupational Therapy for Physical Dysfunction,* 3rd Edition. Baltimore, Williams & Wilkins, 1989. Chapter 1.

18. Hopkins HL, Tiffany EG: Occupational therapy—base in activity. In Hopkins HL, Smith HD (Eds): *Willard and Spackman's Occupational Therapy,* 7th Edition. Philadelphia, JB Lippincott, 1988, pp. 93-101.

Appendices

Appendix A
SELECTED DEVELOPMENTAL SUMMARY

NEUROMOTOR DEVELOPMENT
Reflex Development

Reflex legend:

1. Rooting
2. Sucking
3. Incurvation of spine
4. Palmar grasp
5. Plantar grasp
6. Stepping
7. Moro
8. Placing
9. Flexor withdrawal
10. Extensor thrust
11. Crossed extension
12. Traction
13. Avoidance
14. ATNR / Asym. tonic m.
15. STNR / Symm. tonic n.
16. Neon. neck r.
17. Tonic. labyr.
18. Pos. supporting
19. Neck/Body r.
20. Laby. righting
21. Landau
22. Prot. extension
23. Tilting
24. See-saw

Reflex Development by age:

Age	Reflexes
prenatal / neonatal	1. Rooting; 2. Sucking; 3. Incurvation of spine; 7. Moro; 10. Extensor thrust; 14. ATNR; 15. STNR; 4. Palmar grasp; 5. Plantar grasp; 6. Stepping; 8. Placing; 9. Flexor withdrawal; 10. Extensor thrust; 11. Crossed extension; 12. Traction; 13. Avoidance; 14. Asym. tonic m.; 15. Symm. tonic n.; 16. Neon. neck r.; 17. Tonic. labyr.
2 mo.	20. Laby. righting; 21. Landau; 22. Prot. extension; 20. Laby. r.-pr.; 18. Pos. supporting; 20. Laby. righting; 22. Prot. extension
6 mo.	19. Neck/Body r.; 20. Laby. r.-su; 21. Landau
11 mo.	23. Tilting; 23. Tilt - pr/su
15 mo.	23. Tilt - all 4s; 23. Tilting/Hopping; 24. See-saw

Voluntary Control

Age	HEAD/TRUNK CONTROL	ROLLING/CRAWLING	STANDING/WALKING	ARM/HAND FUNCTION	WRITING/DRAWING
2 mo.	Lifts head when prone; Head lag when pulled to sitting; Falls forward in sitting position; Back rounded				
3 mo.		Rolls back-to-side		Hands to midline; Visual grasp; Hands often open	
4 mo.	Head lag slight when pulled to sitting; Lumbar curve only			Arms activate on sight of object; Crude palm grasp; Bilateral approach; Holds 1 object	
5 mo.	Sits hyperflexed; Head in line on pull-to-sit	Pivots in prone, arm propulsion movements			
6 mo.	Sits with support; Begins to use supporting reactions	Automatic rolling		Unilateral approach begins; Circuitous arm motion	
7 mo.	Sits alone momentarily	Assumes 4-point crawling posture	Sustains weight on extended legs; Bounces		
8 mo.		Belly crawling; Deliberate rolling		Holds 2 objects; Transfers object	

Age	Sitting / Crawling	Gross Motor	Prehension / Release	Drawing
9 mo.	4-point crawling	Stands holding rail	Release beginning	
10 mo.	No longer uses arms for support in sitting; Assumes sitting independently; Leans forward, re-erects; Sitting to prone	Pulls up to rail and lowers		
11 mo.	Sits and pivots	Lifts foot at rail; Cruises	Thumb and index tip prehension beginning	Marks by banging or brushing
12 mo. / 1 yr.		Walks with one hand held	Neat prehension; Places cube on cube; Casts object	Marks rather than bangs
15 mo.	Seats self in small chair	Assumes standing on own; Walks a few steps; Falls by collapse		
18 mo.	Discards crawling	Heel-toe progression in walking; Walks sideways (17m); Walks backwards (17m)	Crude release (on contact with surface)	Holds crayon butt end; Scribbles off page; Whole arm movements; One color
21 mo.		Squats in play; Down stairs hand held; Tries to stand on 6cm walking board; Kicks large ball	Tower 5-6 blocks	
24 mo. / 2 yr.		Runs well; Walks with one foot on 6cm walking board (27cm)	Less handedness shift	Overhand grasp of crayon; Wrist action; Process rather that product
2 1/2 yrs.		Jumps with both feet; Tries standing on one foot; Hops 1-3 steps on preferred foot; Attempts to step on walking board (33m); Stands on 6cm walking board with both feet (38m)	Throws ball with poor direction about 5-7 feet; Throws bean bag into 12 in. hole from 3 feet	Holds crayon in fingers; Small marks; Imitates vertical/horizontal stroke
3 yrs.		Rides tricycle; Alternates feet going up stairs; Alternates feet part way on 6cm walking board (38m); Ascends small ladder alternating feet (38m)	Towers 10 blocks; 10 pellets into bottle, 30 sec.; Catches large ball with stiff arms; Throws ball without losing balance, 6-7 feet; Handedness	Copies circle; Imitates cross; Encloses space; Simple figures; Beginning designs; Names drawing
3 1/2 yrs.		Stands on 1 foot, 2 seconds; Jumps from 8 in. elevation; Leaps off floor with feet together	Throws small ball 8-9 feet	

Voluntary Control (continued)

	HEAD/TRUNK CONTROL	ROLLING/CRAWLING	STANDING/WALKING	ARM/HAND FUNCTION	WRITING/DRAWING
4 yrs.			Propels and manipulates wagon Skips on 1 foot only Down stairs foot-to-step Balance on 1 foot, 4-8 seconds Walk 6cm board part way before stepping off Crouch for broad jump of 8-10in Hop on toes with both feet same time Carry cup of water without spilling Reciprocal arm motion in running pattern Ascends large ladder, alternating feet (47m)	Throws ball overhand Beginning adult stance throwing Catches large ball, arms flexed but rigid	Pencil held like adult, wrist flexed Crude human figures "Suns" Copies cross
4 1/2 yrs.			Hops on 1 foot, 4 to 6 steps Alternates feet full length of 6cm walking board (56m) Descends small ladder		More detailed human figures
5 yrs.			Roller skates, ice skates and rides small bicycle (5 or 6 yrs.) Skips alternating feet Stands indefinitely on 1 foot Hop a distance of 16 feet Walks long distance on tip toes Walks length of 6cm walking board in 6-9 sec. (60m) Running broad jump 28 to 35in. Runs 11.5 feet per second Descends large ladder	Adult posture distance throwing Boys 24 feet Girls 15 feet Catches ball, hands more that arms, misses Bounces large ball	Buildings and houses Animals Idea before starting Copies triangle

Age				
6 yrs.	Stand on each foot alternately with eyes closed	Walk a 4cm walking board in 9 seconds with one error	Jump down from 12in landing on toes only	Standing broad jump of 38in	Running broad jump of 40 to 45in	Hop 50 feet in 9 seconds

6 yrs.
- Finger and wrist movement
- Copies diamond
- Reach, grasp, release and body movement smooth
- Catch ball, 1 hand
- *Grip strength
  Boys 11.3 lbs.
  Girls 3.2 lbs.
- Stand on each foot alternately with eyes closed
- Walk a 4cm walking board in 9 seconds with one error
- Jump down from 12in landing on toes only
- Standing broad jump of 38in
- Running broad jump of 40 to 45in
- Hop 50 feet in 9 seconds

7 yrs.
- *Grip strength
  Boys 18.5 lbs.
  Girls 8.7 lbs.
- Motor performance continues to become more refined (running, jumping, balancing, etc.)
- Strength increases
- Learns to inhibit motor activity

8 yrs.
- *Grip strength
  Boys 26 lbs.
  Girls 14.4 lbs.
- Runs 5 yards per second
- Standing broad jump of 45in

9 yrs.
- 3-dimensional geometric figures
- Linear perspective
- Distance throw
  Boys 60 feet
  Girls 35 feet

10 yrs.

11 yrs.
- *Grip strength
  Boys 45.2 lbs.
  Girls 33.8 lbs
- Distance throw
  Boys 95 feet
  Girls 60 feet
- Runs 6 yards per second
- Standing broad jump of 60in

14 yrs.
- *Grip strength
  Boys 71.2 lbs.
  Girls 46.2 lbs.
- Boys standing broad jump 76in
- Girls standing broad jump 63in
- Boys run 6 yards, 8in per second
- Girls run 6 yards, 3in per second

17 yrs.
- Boys distance throw 150 feet
- Boys run 7 yards per second
- Boys standing broad jump 90in.

*Dynamometer norms for dominant hand (average/mean) (unpublished) Scottish Rite Hospital for Crippled Children, Dallas, Texas.

SENSORIMOTOR DEVELOPMENT

Vision

Rudimentary fixation
Reflexive tracking for brief periods
Sees light, dark, color and movement

Real convergence and coordination

Accomodation more flexible and eyes coordinate smoothly

Size and shape constancy

Depth perception
Visual tracking 90°
V and H planes
Color perception
Acuity
Discriminates strangers

Other

Sensorimotor Development (0-2 yrs.):
• Tactile functions
• Vestibular functions
• Kinesthetic functions
• Auditory functions
• Olfactory functions
• Gustatory functions

Integration of body sides (1-4 yrs.):
• Gross motor planning
• Form and space perception
• Equilibrium response
• Postural flexibility

Body Scheme

"Tummy," legs, feet, arms, hand, face parts

SOCIAL AND PLAY DEVELOPMENT

Individual—mothering person most important

Stranger anxiety

Immediate family group important

Solitary or onlooker play

DAILY LIVING SKILLS

Holds bottle
Finger feeds
Drinks from cup (held)
Cooperates in dressing

Grasps spoon and into dish

Feeds self, spills
Takes off hat, socks, mittens
Unzips zippers
Toilet trained daytime
Handles cup well

Ages (left axis)

prenatal
neonatal
2 mo.
6 mo.
11 mo.
15 mo.
2 mo.
3 mo.
4 mo.
5 mo.
6 mo.
7 mo.
8 mo.
9 mo.
10 mo.
11 mo.
12 mo.
1 yr.
15 mo.
18 mo.
21 mo.

Strong tactile sense

Discrimination in all functions (3 to 7 yrs.)

Parallel play
Imitation

Associative play

Dramatic play
Cooperative play

Competitive behaviors

Hold small glass 1 hand
Helps in getting dressed
Pulls on socks
Pulls up pants
Removes shoes
Strings beads, snips with scissors, opens jar lid, turns door knob
Feeds self, no spilling
Pours from pitcher
Puts on shoes
Removes pants
Unbuttons
Toilet training, independent
Washes, dries face and hands
Brushes teeth
Dresses and undresses with supervision
Laces shoes
Distinguishes front and back of clothes
Cuts line with scissors
Dresses and undresses without assistance
Ties shoe laces
Responsible for grooming

Planes of body related to objects

Thighs, elbows, shoulders, 1st and little fingers and thumb identified

Learns 2 sides of body (left, right); can't locate

Identifies ring and middle finger
Locates left, right; details body parts

Accurate left, right on self and in space

Age	
24 mo.	
2 yr.	Distinguishes vertical from horizontal lines
2 1/2 yrs.	
3 yrs.	Reacts to entire stimulus rather than separate parts
3 1/2 yrs.	Discrimination—notes similarities and differences (4 to 8 yrs.)
4 yrs.	Needs more perceptual information (clues) than 10 yr. old
4 1/2 yrs.	Distinguishes oblique, vertical and horizontal lines
5 yrs.	May have difficulty with spatial orientation of objects (attending may resolve)
6 yrs.	
7 yrs.	Errors for transformation in perspective, breaks and closures, transformation from line to curve, rotations and reversals resolved

SENSORIMOTOR DEVELOPMENT

	Vision	Other	**Body Scheme**
8 yrs.			
9 yrs.			
10 yrs.	Intercepts ball thrown from distance		Can move into another's R-L reference system

SOCIAL AND PLAY DEVELOPMENT

Gang interests

Cooperation and competition highly developed

Sex differences in group organization

DAILY LIVING SKILLS

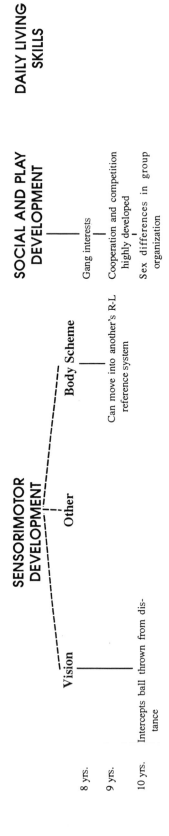

References

Ayres. (1962). Perceptual-motor training for children. *Approaches to the Treatment of Patients with Neuromuscular Dysfunction.* Third International Congress WFOT.

Barsch. (1967). *Achieving Perceptual-Motor Efficiency.*

Cratty. (1970). *Perceptual and Motor Development in Infancy and Early Childhood.*

Gesell. (1940). *The First Five Years.*

Espenschade and Eckert. (1967). *Motor Development.*

Llorens. (1970). Human development: The promise of occupational therapy. *Am J Occup Ther.* Rockville, MD: AOTA.

McGraw. (1945). *The Neuromuscular Maturation of the Human Infant.*

Mussen, Conger and Kagan. (1963). *Child Development and Personality,* 3rd ed.

Peiper. (1963). *Cerebral Function in Infancy and Childhood.*

Compiled by Mary K. Cowan, MA, OTR, FAOTA

Appendix B
RECREATIONAL ORGANIZATIONS FOR PERSONS WITH DISABILITIES

American Alliance for Health, Physical Education and Recreation for the Handicapped Information and Research Utilization Center
1201 16th Street, NW
Washington, DC 20036
Phone: 202-833-5547

American National Red Cross
Program of Swimming for the Handicapped
17th and D Streets, NW
Washington, DC 20006
Phone: 202-857-3542

Handicapped Boaters
P.O. Box 1134
Ansonia Station
New York, NY 10023
Phone: 212-377-0310

National Association of Sports for Cerebral Palsy
United Cerebral Palsy Association of Connecticut
One State Street
New Haven, CT 06511
Phone: 203-772-2080

National Park Service
Department of the Interior
18th and C Streets, NW
Washington, DC 20240
Phone: 202-343-6843

National Wheelchair Athletic Association
Nassau Community College
Garden City, NY 11530
Phone: 212-222-1245

National Wheelchair Softball Association
P.O. Box 737
Sioux Falls, SD 57101

North American Riding Association
P.O. Box 100
Ashburn, VA 22011
Phone: 703-777-3540

American Athletic Association of the Deaf
3916 Lantern Drive
Silver Spring, MD 20902
Phone: 301-942-4042

American Blind Bowling Association
150 North Bellair Avenue
Louisville, KY 40206
Phone: 502-896-8039

American Wheelchair Bowling Association
2635 NE 19th Street
Pompano Beach, FL 33062
Phone: 305-941-1238

International Committee on the Silent Sports
Gallaudet College
Florida Avenue and 7th Street, NE
Washington, DC 20002
Phone: 202-331-1731 or 447-0360

National Association of the Physically Handicapped
76 Elm Street
London, OH 43140
Phone: 614-852-1664

National Inconvenienced Sportsmen's Association
3738 Walnut Avenue
Carmichael, CA 95608
Phone: 916-484-2153

National Therapeutic Recreation Society
1601 North Kent Street
Arlington, VA 22209
Phone: 703-525-0606

National Wheelchair Basketball Association
110 Seaton Center
University of Kentucky
Lexington, KY 40506
Phone: 703-777-3540

People-to-People Committee for the Handicapped
LaSalle Building, Suite 610
Connecticut Avenue and L Street
Washington, DC 20036
Phone: 202-785-0755

The President's Committee on Employment of the Handicapped
Subcommittee on Recreation and Leisure
Washington, DC 20210

Travel Information Center
Moss Rehabilitation Hospital
12th Street and Tabor Roads
Philadelphia, PA 19141
Phone: 215-456-9900

United Stated Deaf Skiers' Association
Two Sunset Hill Road
Simbury, CT 06070
Phone: 203-244-3341

National Handicapped Sports and Recreation Association
Capital Hill Station
P.O. Box 18664
Denver, CO 80218

National Spinal Cord Injury Foundation (Marathon Racing)
369 Elliot Street
Newton Upper Falls, MA 02164

Rehabilitation Education Center (Football)
University of Illinois
Oak Street at Stadium Drive
Champaign, IL 61820

Wheelchair Motorcycle Association
(All Terrain Vehicles)
101 Torrey Street
Brockton, MA 02410

Sports and Spokes
(W/C Sports Magazine)
5201 North 19th Avenue
Phoenix, AZ 85015

The Riding School, Inc.
275 South Avenue
Weston, MA 02193
Phone: 617-899-4555

S.I.R.E. (Self-Improvement Through Riding Education)
91 Old Bolton Road
Stow, MA 01775
Phone: 617-897-3396

Winslow Riding for the Handicapped
P.O. Box 100
Ashburn, VA 22011
Phone: 703-777-3540

Vinland National Center
3675 Ihduhapi Road
Loretto, MN 55357
Phone: 612-479-3555

National Foundation of Wheelchair Tennis
3855 Birch Street
Newport Beach, CA 92660

National Recreation and Park Association
1601 North Kent Street
Arlington, VA 22209

Disabled Sportsmen of America, Inc.
P.O. Box 26
Vinton, VA 24179

Wheelchair Pilots' Association
11018 102nd Avenue North
Largo, FL 33540

American W/C Pilots' Association
4419 North 27th Street, Apt. 3
Phoenix, AZ 85105

Winter Park Recreational Association (Skiing)
Handicapped Programs
Hal O'Leary, Director
Box 313
Winter Park, CO 80482

Appendix C
ASSESSMENT FORMS

Work Skill Assessment

	Yes	No

1. Willingness to start the task
Agrees to start task without arguing ☐ ☐
Shows enthusiasm about task ☐ ☐
Starts immediately after directions have been given ☐ ☐

2. Ability to follow directions
Follows verbal directions correctly ☐ ☐
Follows written directions correctly ☐ ☐

3. Acceptance of supervision
Accepts direction without showing resentment ☐ ☐
Accepts criticism from supervisor without arguing or becoming defensive ☐ ☐

4. Ability to sustain interest in the task
Works continually without becoming distracted ☐ ☐
Tolerates small frustrations without losing interest ☐ ☐
Facial expression and posture indicate interest ☐ ☐

5. Appropriate use of tools and material
Uses familiar equipment for appropriate purposes ☐ ☐
Handles equipment skillfully and safely ☐ ☐
Uses material without wasting it ☐ ☐

6. Appropriate rate of performance
Accomplishes task successfully within the time limit ☐ ☐

7. Acceptable level of neatness
Keeps work area uncluttered ☐ ☐
Maintains personal neatness ☐ ☐
Cleans up when finished ☐ ☐

8. Appropriate attention to detail
Doesn't spend too much time or energy on unimportant details ☐ ☐
Performs accurately when necessary ☐ ☐

9. Ability to organize tasks in a logical manner
Makes sure directions are clear before starting ☐ ☐
Checks to see that all materials and supplies are ready before starting ☐ ☐
Performs steps in logical sequence ☐ ☐

10. Problem solving
Recognizes when a problem exists ☐ ☐
Attempts to solve problems without asking for help ☐ ☐
Shows creativity in solving problems ☐ ☐
Finds practical solutions to problems ☐ ☐

Adapted from Mosey, AC: Activities Therapy. New York, Raven Press, 1973, pp. 112-120.

Social Skills Assessment

Dyadic Skills				
	Yes	**No**	**Skill Components**	**Comments**
1.			Expresses ideas clearly	
2.			Demonstrates appropriate affect	
3.			Initiates conversation	
4.			Maintains eye contact	
5.			Greets and calls people by name	
6.			Manners/habits are acceptable	
7.			Responds when spoken to	
8.			Responds beyond "yes" or "no"	
9.			Expresses feelings verbally	
10.			Shows consideration to others	
11.			Remains in contact throughout conversation	
12.			Speaks audibly and clearly	
Group Skills				
1.			Participates in group discussion	
2.			Asks for information	
3.			Contributes information	
4.			Asks for opinions	
5.			Contributes opinions	
6.			Encourages others	
7.			Assumes leadership role	
8.			Suggests operating procedures	
9.			Is willing to compromise	
10.			Accepts praise comfortably	
11.			Accepts criticism graciously	
12.			Supportive of others' contributions	

Used with permission from an unpublished manual by P. Babcock.

Appendix D
SAMPLE GROUP EXERCISE

The following patients have been working on craft activities in a parallel group. After discussion with the OTR supervisor, it was decided that the COTA should plan a *project* level activity that would meet the needs of the individuals in this group.

Patient	Observation	Plan
Ms. Wisenheimer	Is not interested in crafts. Identifies with staff. Is sarcastic and irritable.	Improve self-esteem. Allow some authority.
Ms. Gloomy Thoughts	Slowed down physically and mentally. Expresses feelings of inadequacy. Has difficulty making decisions.	Increase rate of performance. Provide activities that are easily recognized as useful and have a minimal number of steps.
Ms. Jitterbug	Capable and willing to work, but is tense, agitated and restless. Socializes well with others, but sometimes annoys others with interfering behavior. Needs immediate gratification.	Increase attention span. Provide tasks that are structured and short term. Provide for release of energy.
Ms. Detached	Offers minimal conversation. Appears sensitive to the needs to others. Usually chooses to sit by herself. Is unable to make decisions without help.	Develop personal identity and decision-making skills.
Ms. Picky	Is cooperative, conscientious and a perfectionist. Works slowly and is seldom satisfied with her work. Becomes irritated with the poor performance of others. Has trouble expressing her ideas.	Improve decision-making skills. Provide tasks that are easily corrected if mistakes are made. Develop behavior that is more tolerant of others.
Ms. Finagle	Undependable and manipulative. Appears friendly but talks about the other patients. Very bright and capable.	Develop dependable behavior. Provide activities that are intellectually stimulating and absorbing.

These patients are middle class young adults. All but one have completed high school and they all have had problems with chemical dependency. Using the information regarding project groups as a reference, respond to the following:

1. What activity could the COTA choose?
2. What steps are involved in the activity and how much time would each take?
3. What tools and materials would be required to complete the activity?
4. The supervisor has also asked the COTA to develop *task*-related behavioral goals for two of the patients—Ms. Gloomy Thoughts and Ms. Jitterbug. What goals might be appropriate for these patients? Is there a specific part of the activity that could be assigned to each of these patients in order to develop the desired behavior?
5. What goals might be appropriate for these patients? Is there a specific part of the selected activity that could be assigned to each of these patients in order to develop the desired behavior?
6. How might the activity be introduced to the group?
7. How would the group goal be explained to the members?

Prepared by Toné Blechert, COTA, ROH. From Fidler G: The task-oriented group as a context for treatment. Am J Occup Ther 1:43-48, 1969.

Appendix E
SOURCES FOR MICROSWITCHES

Supplies for Handmade Switches and Battery-Operated Devices

Chaney Electronics, Inc.
P.O. Box 27038
Denver, CO 80227

Digi-Key Corp.
P.O. Box 677
Thief River Falls, MN 56701

Microswitch
A Division of Honeywell
Freeport, IL 61032

Local Radio Shack stores

Commercial Microswitches, Controls and Interfaces

AbleNet
360 Hoover Street
Minneapolis, MN 55413

Adaptive Peripherals
4529 Begley Avenue North
Seattle, WA 98103

ComputAbility Corporation
101 Rt. 46
Pine Brook, NJ 07058

Don Johnston Developmental Equipment, Inc.
1000 N. Rand Road, Bldg. 115
P.O. Box 639
Wauconda, IL 60084

DU-IT Control Systems Group, Inc.
8765 Township Road #513
Shreve, OH 44676

Prentke Romich
1022 Heyl Road
Wooster, OH 44691

TASH, Inc.
(Technical Aids & Systems for the Handicapped)
70 Gibson Drive, Unit 12
Markham, ON L3R 4C2 Canada

Zygo Industries
P.O. Box 1008
Portland, OR 92707

Appendix F
SPLINTING RESOURCE GUIDE

Alimed, Inc.
297 High Street
Dedham, MA 02026
(800) 225-2610

Polymed Industries, Inc.
Splint Products Division
9004-H Yellow Brick Road
Baltimore, MD 21237
(800) 346-0895

Smith and Nephew/Rolyan, Inc.
N93 W14475 Whittaker Way
Menomonee Falls, WI 53051
(800) 558-8633

WFR-Aquaplast Corporation
68 Birch Street
P.O. Box 215
Ramsey, NJ 07446
(800) 526-5247

Fred Sammons, Inc.
Bissell Healthcare Corporation
Box 23
Brookfield, IL 60513-0032
(800) 323-5547
Distributors of the hand volumeter

J.A. Preston Corporation
60 Page Road
Clifton, NJ 07012
(800) 631-7277
Distributors of *Minnesota Rate of Manipulation Test*
(product of American Guidance Service, Inc.)

Johnson & Johnson Orthopedic Division
501 George Street
New Brunswick, NJ 08903
Distributors of Orthoplast®

Bibliography

CHAPTER 3

Breines E: Pragmatism as a foundation for occupational therapy curricula. *Am J Occup Ther* 41:522-525, 1987.

Cassidy JC: Access to health care: A clinician's opinion about an ethical issue. *Am J Occup Ther* 42:295-299, 1988.

Hasselkus B: Discussion of "patient" versus "client." *Am J Occup Ther* 39:605, 1985.

Serrett KD: Another look at occupational therapy's history: Paradigm or pair-of-hands? *Occup Ther Mental Health* 5:1-31, 1985.

Serrett KD et al: Adolph Meyer: Contributions to the conceptual foundation of occupational therapy. *Occup Ther Mental Health* 5:69-75, 1985.

Sharrott GW, Yerxa EJ: The issue is: Promises to keep: Implications of the referent "patient" versus "client" for those served by occupational therapy. *Am J Occup Ther* 39:401-405, 1985.

CHAPTER 4

Allen CK: *Occupational Therapy for Psychiatric Diseases: Measurement and Management of Cognitive Disabilities.* Boston: Litttle, Brown, 1985.

Bruce MA and Borg B: *Frames of Reference in Psychosocial Occupational Therapy.* Thorofare, NJ: Slack Incorporated, 1987.

Christiansen C: Occupational therapy: Intervention for life performance. In Christiansen C and Baum C (Eds.): *Occupational Therapy: Overcoming Human Performance Deficits.* Thorofare, NJ: Slack Incorporated, 1991.

Cynkin S: *Occupational Therapy: Toward Health Through Activities.* Boston: Little, Brown, 1979.

Kielhofner G: *A Model of Human Occupation: Theory and Application.* Baltimore: Williams & Wilkins, 1985.

CHAPTER 5

Llorens LA: Performance tasks and roles throughout the life span. In Christiansen C and Baum C (Eds.): *Occupational Therapy: Overcoming Human Performance Deficits.* Thorofare, NJ: Slack Incorporated, 1991.

CHAPTER 6

Clark FA et al: Occupational science: Academic innovation in the service of occupational therapy's future. *Am J Occup Ther* 45:300-310, 1991.

CHAPTER 7

American Occupational Therapy Association: *Entry-Level OTR and COTA Role Delineation.* Rockville, Maryland: AOTA, 1981.

Berger B: The sociology of leisure: Some suggestions. In Smigel, EO (Ed): *Work and Leisure: A Contemporary Social Problem.* New Haven, Connecticut: New Haven College and University Press, 1979.

Broderick T, Glazer B: Leisure participation and the retirement process. *Am J Occup Ther* 37:15-22, 1983.

Cheek N, Brunch W: *The Social Organization of Leisure in Human Society.* New York: Harper and Row, 1976.

Childs E, Childs J: Children and leisure. In Smith MA et al (Eds): *Leisure and Society in Britain.* London: Allen Lane, 1974.

Clayre A: *Work and Play, Ideas and Experience of Work and Leisure.* New York: Harper and Row, 1974.

Comfort A: Future Sex Mores: Sexuality in a Zero Growth Society. London: *Current* (February), 1973.

deGrazia S: *Of Time, Work, and Leisure*. New York: Doubleday, 1962.

DePoy E and Kolodner E: Psychological performance factors. In Christiansen C and Baum C (Eds.): *Occupational Therapy: Overcoming Human Performance Deficits*. Thorofare, NJ: Slack Incorporated, 1991.

Dumazedier J: *Toward a Society of Leisure*. New York: Free Press, 1967.

Friedman E, Havighurst R: *The Meaning of Work and Retirement*. Chicago, Illinois: Chicago Press, 1954.

Fuch VR: Women's earnings: Recent trends and long-run prospects. *Monthly Labor Review* 97(May):22-26, 1984.

Gilfoyle EM, Grady AP and Moore JC: *Children Adapt: A Theory of Sensorimotor-Sensory Development*, 2d ed. Thorofare, NJ: Slack Incorporated, 1990.

Havighurst R: The nature and values of meaningful free time. In Kleemier R (Ed): *Aging and Leisure: A Research Perspective into Meaningful Use of Time*. New York: Oxford University Press, 1961.

Hinojosa J, Sabari J, Rosenfield M: Purposeful activity guidelines and position paper. *Am J Occup Ther* 37:805, 1983.

Huizinger J: *Homoludens: A Study of Play Elements in Culture*. Boston: Beacon Press, 1951.

Kimmel D: *Adulthood and Aging*. New York: John Wiley and Sons, 1974.

Klinger J, Friedman F, Sullivand R: *Mealtime Manual for the Aged and Handicapped*. New York: Simon and Schuster, 1970.

Leonardelli CA: *The Milwaukee Evaluation of Daily Living Skills: Evaluation in Long-Term Psychiatric Care*. Thorofare, NJ: Slack Incorporated, 1988.

Llorens L: Changing balance: Environment and individual. *Am J Occup Ther* 38:29-31, 1984.

Mitchell E, Mason B: *The Theory of Play*. New York: AS Barnes, 1934.

Neulinger J: *The Psychology of Leisure: Research Approaches to the Study*. Springfield, Illinois: Charles C. Thomas, 1974.

Pebler D, Rubin K: *The Play of Children: Current Theory and Research Contributions to Human Development*. New York: Tanner and Basshardt, 1982.

Piepus J: *Leisure the Basis of Culture*. New York: Partheon Books, 1952.

Reilly M: *Play as Exploratory Learning*. Beverly Hills, California: Sage Publications, 1974.

Spencer JC: The physical environment and performance. In Christiansen C and Baum C: *Occupational Therapy: Overcoming Human Performance Deficits*. Thorofare, NJ: Slack Incorporated, 1991.

Thackery M, Skidmore R, Farley W: *Introduction to Mental Health Field and Practice*. New York: Prentice Hall, 1979.

Trombly CA, Scott AD: *Occupational Therapy for Physical Dysfunction*. Baltimore, Maryland: Williams & Wilkins, 1977.

Willard HS, Spackman CS (Eds): *Occupational Therapy*, 4th edition. Philadelphia: JB Lippincott, 1971.

CHAPTER 8

Cook EA, Luschen L, Sikes J: Dressing training for an elderly woman with cognitive and perceptual impairments. *Am J Occup Ther* 45:652-654, 1991.

CHAPTER 9

Babcock PH: *The Role of the OTA in Mental Health*. Unpublished manual. Minneapolis, Minnesota: St. Mary's Junior College, 1978.

Borg B and Bruce MA: *The Group System: The Therapeutic Activity Group in Occupational Therapy*. Thorofare, NJ: Slack Incorporated, 1990.

Davis CM: *Patient Practitioner Interaction*. Thorofare, New Jersey: Slack, Inc., 1989.

Kaplan K: *Directive Group Therapy: Innovative Mental Health Treatment*. Thorofare, NJ: Slack Incorporated, 1988.

Navarra T, Lipkowitz M and Navarra JG: *Therapeutic Communication: A Guide to Effective Interpersonal Skills for Health Care Professionals*. Thorofare, New Jersey: Slack, Inc., 1991.

Ross M: *Group Process: Using Therapeutic Activities in Chronic Care*. Thorofare, NJ: Slack Incorporated, 1987.

Ross M: *Integrative Group System: The Structured Five-Stage Approach*, 2d ed. Thorofare, NJ: Slack Incorporated, 1991.

CHAPTER 10

Barney KF: From Ellis Island to assisted living: Meeting the needs of older adults from diverse cultures. *Amer J Occup Ther* 45:586-593, 1991.

English O, Pearson G: *Emotional Problems of Living,* 3rd Edition. New York: WW Norton, 1963.

Evans J (Guest Ed.): Special issue on cross-cultural perspectives on occupational therapy. *Am J Occup Ther* 46(8):675-768, 1992.

Freeman J: *Crowding and Behavior.* New York: Viking Press, 1973.

Krefting LH and Krefting DV: Cultural influences on performance. In Christiansen C and Baum C (Eds.): *Occupational Therapy: Overcoming Human Performance Deficits.* Thorofare, New Jersey: Slack Incorporated, 1991.

Knutson A: *The Individual Society, and Behavior.* New York: Russel Sage Foundation, 1965.

Opler M: *Culture and Social Psychiatry,* Part II. New York: Atherton Press, 1967.

CHAPTER 11

Bessinger C: *The Video Guide.* Santa Barbara, California: Video Info Publishers, 1977.

Fuller J: *Prescription for Better Home Video Movies.* Los Angeles: HP Books, 1988.

Kerr RJ: *Video the Better Way: A New Art for a New Age.* Yokohama, Japan: Victor Company of Japan, 1980.

Lewis R: *Home Video Makers Handbook.* New York: Crown, 1987.

Quinn G: *The Camcorder Handbook.* Blue Ridge Summit, Pennsylvania: Tab Books, 1987.

CHAPTER 12

Closing the Gap. P.O. Box 68, Henderson, Minnesota 56044.

Control Battery Operated Toys: Instructions for Constructing a Large Area Flap Switch (LAFS) to Allow Disabled Children to Control Battery Operated Toys. G. Fraser Shein, Biofeedback Research Project, Rehabilitation Engineering Department, Ontario Crippled Children's Centre, 350 Ramsey Road, Toronto, Ontario, Canada M4G 1R8.

From Toys to Computers: Access for the Physically Disabled Child. Christine Wright and Mari Nomura, P.O. Box 700242, San Jose, California 95170.

Guide to Controls, Selection and Mounting Applications. Rehabilitation Engineering Center, Children's Hospital at Stanford, 520 Willow Road, Palo Alto, California 94304.

Homemade Battery Powered Toys and Educational Devices for Severely Handicapped Children, 2nd Edition. Linda J. Burkhart, R.D. 1, Millville, Pennsylvania 17846.

Information on Communication, Writing Systems, and Access to Computers for Severely Physically Handicapped Individuals. Trace Research and Development Center on Communication, Control and Computer Access for Handicapped Individuals, University of Wisconsin-Madison, 314 Waisman Center, 1500 Highland Avenue, Madison, Wisconsin 53706.

International Software/Hardware Registry. GC Vanderheiden, LM Walsted, Editors. Trace Research and Development Center for the Severely Communicatively Handicapped, University of Wisconsin-Madison, 314 Waisman Center, 1500 Highland Avenue, Madison, Wisconsin 53706.

More Homemade Battery Devices for Severely Handicapped Children with Suggested Activities. Linda J Burkhart, R.D. 1, Millville, Pennsylvania, 17846.

Wobble Switch Toy Control Switch: A Do It Yourself Guide. B Brown. Trace Research and Development Center for the Handicapped, University of Wisconsin-Madison, 314 Waisman Center, 1500 Highland Avenue, Madison, Wisconsin 53706.

CHAPTER 13

AOTA: *Technology Review '90, Perspectives on Occupational Therapy Practice.* Rockville, Maryland: American Occupational Therapy Association, 1990.

Brecher D: *The Women's Computer Literacy Handbook.* New York: New American Library, 1985.

Brewer BJ and McMahon P: Certified occupational therapy assistants and microcomputers. In Johnson JA (Ed.): *Certified Occupational Therapy Assistants: Opportunities and Challenges.* Binghamton, New York: Haworth Press, 1988.

Christensen WW, Stearns EJ: *Microcomputers in Health Care,* 2nd Edition. Frederick, Maryland: Aspen, 1990.

Clark EN (Ed): *Microcomputers: Clinical Applications.* Thorofare, New Jersey: Slack Inc, 1986.

Cromwell F (Ed): *Computer Applications in Occupational Therapy.* New York: Haworth Press, 1986.

Green P and Brightman AJ: *Independence Day: Designing Computer Solutions for Individuals with Disability.* Allen, Texas: DLM Learning Resources, 1990.

Naisbitt J, Aburdene P: *Megatrends 2,000.* New York: William Morrow, 1990.

Okoye RL: Computer technology in occupational therapy. In Hopkins HL, Smith HD (Eds): *Willard and Spackman's Occupational Therapy,* 7th Edition. Philadelphia: JB Lippincott, 1988.

O'Leary S, Mann C and Perkash I: Access to computers for older adults: Problems and solutions. *Am Jour Occup Ther* 45:636-642, 1991.

Smith RO: Technological approaches to performance enhancement. In Christiansen C and Baum C (Eds.): *Occupational Therapy: Overcoming Human Performance Deficits.* Thorofare, New Jersey: Slack Incorporated, 1991.

Thibodaux LR: Meeting the challenge of computer literacy in occupational therapy education. In *Target 2,000 Proceedings.* Rockville, Maryland: American Occupational Therapy Association, 1986.

Viseltear E (Ed): Special issue on technology. *Am J Occup Ther* 41:11, 1987.

Workman D, Geggie C, Creasey G: The microcomputer as an aid to written communication. *Br J Occup Ther* 51:188-190, 1988.

Zaks R: *Don't (Or How to Care for Your Computer).* Berkeley, California: Sybex, 1981.

CHAPTER 14

Cannon NM et al: *Manual on Hand Splinting.* New York: Churchill Livingstone, 1985.

Fess EE, Phillips C: *Hand Splinting Principles and Methods,* 2nd Edition. St. Louis, Missouri: CV Mosby, 1987.

Kiel JH: *Basic Handsplinting: A Pattern Designing Approach.* Boston: Little, Brown, 1983.

Malick M, Carr J: *Manual on Management of the Burn Patient, Including Splinting, Mold and Pressure Techniques.* Pittsburgh, Pennsylvania: Harmarville Rehabilitation Center, 1982.

Pedretti LW: *Occupational Therapy Practice Skills for Physical Dysfunction.* St. Louis, Missouri: CV Mosby, 1985.

Ryan SE (Ed.) *Practice Issues in Occupational Therapy: Intraprofessional Team Building.* Thorofare, New Jersey: Slack Inc., 1993.

Tenney CG, Lisak JM: *Atlas of Hand Splinting.* Boston: Little, Brown, 1986.

Ziegler EM: *Current Concepts in Orthotics—A Diagnosis-Related Approach to Splinting.* Menomonee Falls, Wisconsin: Rolyan Medical Products, 1984.

CHAPTER 15

Anderson L, Anderson J: A positioning seat for the neonate and infant with high tone. *Am J Occup Ther* 40:186-190, 1986.

Dahlin-Webb S: Brief or new: A weighted wrist cuff. *Am J Occup Ther* 40:363-364, 1986.

Gesior C, Mann D: Finger extension game. *Am J Occup Ther* 40:44-48, 1986.

Hopkins HL, Smith HD (Eds): *Willard and Spackman's Occupational Therapy,* 7th Edition. Philadelphia: JB Lippincott, 1988.

CHAPTER 16

Bissell J, Mailloux Z: The use of crafts in occupational therapy for the physically disabled. *Am J Occup Ther* 35:369-374, 1981.

Cynkin S, Robinson AM: *Occupational Therapy and Activities Health: Toward Health Through Activities.* Boston: Little, Brown, 1990.

Drake M: *Crafts in Therapy and Rehabilitation.* Thorofare, NJ: Slack Incorporated, 1992.

Fidler GS: From crafts to competence. *Am J Occup Ther* 35(9):567-573, 1981.

CHAPTER 17

Bing RK: Occupational therapy revisited: A paraphrastic journey. *Am J Occup Ther* 35:499-518, 1981.

Cynkin C, Robinson AM: *Occupational Therapy and Activities Health: Toward Health Through Activities.* Boston: Little, Brown, 1990.

Fidler GS: Psychological evaluation of occupational therapy activities. *Am J Occup Ther* 2:284-287, 1948.

Kircher MA: Motivation as a factor of perceived exertion in purposeful versus nonpurposeful activity. *Am J Occup Ther* 38:165-170, 1984.

Kremer ERH, Nelson DL, Duncombe LW: Effects of selected activities on affective meaning in psychiatric clients. *Am J Occup Ther* 38:522-528, 1984.

Lamport NK, Coffey MS and Hersch GI: *Activity Analysis Handbook.* Thorofare, NJ: Slack Incorporated, 1989.

Levine RE and Brayley CR: Occupation as a therapeutic medium: A contextual approach to performance intervention. In Christiansen C and Baum C: *Occupational Therapy: Overcoming Human Performance Deficits.* Thorofare, NJ: Slack Incorporated, 1991.

Reed K, Sanderson S: *Concepts of Occupational Therapy,* 2nd Edition. Baltimore: Williams & Wilkins, 1983.

Smith PA, Barrows HS, Whitney JN: Psychological attributes of occupational therapy crafts. *Am J Occup Ther* 13:16-21, 25-26, 1959.

West WL: Nationally speaking—perspectives on the past and future. *Am J Occup Ther* 44:9-10, 1990.

Glossary

This glossary is provided to assist the reader in learning new words and acronyms and their meanings. The index of the textbook should be used to locate specific terms so that they may be reviewed within context. In addition to the individual chapter definitions of terms, the following sources were used: *Uniform Terminology for Occupational Therapy,* 2nd Edition, 1989, (AOTA); *The Random House College Dictionary,* Revised Edition, 1990; *Roget's International Thesaurus,* 4th Edition; and the *Encyclopedia and Dictionary of Medicine, Nursing, and Allied Health,* 5th Edition, 1992.

Accommodation—Ability to modify or adjust in response to the environment. The changing of an existing schema as a result of new information.

Accuracy of response—Percentage of errors and the percentage of correct responses recorded during the tracking and selection time when using a switch or other device.

Action process— Purposeful action is a process of communicating feelings and thoughts as well as non-verbal messages (Fidler).

Active listening—Skills that allow a person to hear, understand and indicate that the message has been communicated.

Activities of daily living—An area of occupational performance that refers to grooming, oral hygiene, bathing, toilet hygiene, dressing, feeding and eating, medication routine, socialization, functional communication, functional mobility and sexual expression activities.

Activity analysis—The breaking down of an activity into detailed subparts and steps; an examination of the characteristics and values of an activity in relation to the patient's needs, interests and goals.

Activity analysis checklist—A form used to document activity analysis.

Activity categories—Groupings of activities frequently used for evaluation and treatment; categories include crafts, sensory awareness, movement awareness, fine arts, construction, games, etc.

Activity properties/characteristics—Factors that contribute to the therapeutic nature/potential of a particular activity, such as being goal directed, having significance to the individual, or requiring involvement, adaptability, or gradability, etc.

Activity tolerance—The ability to sustain engagement in a purposeful activity over a period of time.

Adaptation—The tendency to adjust to the environment; modification of an activity; changing of components required to complete the task.

Adaption—*see* Adaptation.

Adaptive equipment—Assistive devices or aids that allow a person with a handicap to participate in life activities.

Adaptive response—Active responses organized below the conscious level; a progressive movement from basic relations to adaptive responses to adaptive skills to adaptive patterns of behavior.

Adaptive skills—Abilities that enable the individual to satisfy basic needs and satisfactorily perform life tasks.

Affect—One's mood and related behaviors that reflect a mental attitude exhibited by emotions, temperament and feelings.

Affective skills—Abilities to interact appropriately in relation to inner feelings, emotional tone and mood; may be characterized by body language and gestures, as well as verbal content; relates to self-esteem, the ability to develop relationships and assume responsibility, etc. (*see* Affect.)

After-care houses—Halfway homes initially established by Ellis for people released from asylums.

Aggression—A primary instinct generally associated with emotional states that prompt carrying out actions in a forceful way; often manifested by exhibiting anger and destructiveness.

Alienist—An early term for psychiatrist.

ALS—Amyotrophic lateral sclerosis.

Ameliorate—Improve; to make or become better.

Analysis—*see* Activity analysis.

Anatomic arches (hand)—The longitudinal, distal transverse and proximal transverse arches that must be supported when making splints to assure comfort and to preserve the normal anatomic structure.

Approach—A method of treating or dealing with something.

Assimilation—The ability to absorb; to make information a part of one's thinking; a process by which experience is incorporated into existing knowledge. Incoming information is perceived and interpreted according to an existing schema that has already been established through previous experience.

Association—The ability to relate experiences from the past to present experience.

Asylums—Institutions often referred to as refuges for individuals who are unable to live independently in the community; historically, majority of residents were referred to as insane.

Attention span—The ability to focus on a task or tasks over a period of time.

Attitude—A pattern of mental views established through cumulative prior experiences; manner, disposition, feeling or position; may be consciously or subconsciously assumed.

Auditory—Of or relating to the reception, processing, and interpretation of sounds through the ears; includes the ability to localize and discriminate noises in the background.

Award of Excellence—The highest award bestowed on COTAs by the AOTA; recognizes the contributions of COTAs to the advancement of occupational therapy and provides incentive to contribute to the profession's growth and development.

Biopsychosocial—One of the component systems of occupation; model that illustrates how biologic, psychologic and social factors interact in an individual to affect occupational function or dysfunction.

Axiology—A branch of philosophy concerned with the study of values.

BASIC—Beginner's All-Purpose Symbolic Instruction Code; used for computer programming.

Behavior modification—A process of reinforcing desirable responses while ignoring undesirable ones; food, praise and redeemable tokens are some of the reinforcers used.

Bilateral integration—The coordination of the interaction of both sides of one's body when participating in an activity.

Biopsychosocial—One of the component systems of occupation; model that illustrates how biologic, psychologic and social factors interact in an individual to affect occupational function or dysfunction.

Body scheme—Awareness of the body and the relationship of body parts to each other.

Bolsters—Long, cylindrical, padded pieces of adaptive equipment used to assist in maintaining functional positions and to enhance activity management.

Bony prominences—Structures on the surface of the bones that have little tissue padding and must be accommodated in the construction and fitting of splints as well as in other situations.

Boot up—Turn on the computer and monitor.

Bulletin board—Computer program that is used to gain or exchange information, and send or receive messages (electronic mail).

Byte—In computer programming, a unit of information equal to one character.

Camcorder—An electronic device for making video recordings.

Career mobility—AOTA plan that allowed COTAs to become certified as OTRs after meeting specific criteria, including work experience, professional level fieldwork experiences and completion of the occupational therapist certification examination.

Categories of activity analysis (general)—Examples of components include, but are not limited to, motor, sensory, cognitive, intrapersonal and interpersonal skills, adaptions, supplies and equipment, cost, number of steps required, time involved, supervision required, space needed, precautions, and contraindications.

Categories of occupation—Occupation performance areas that include activities of daily living, work activities, or play or leisure activities.

Categorization—The ability to classify; to describe by naming or labeling; differentiating between differences and similarities.

Cephalocaudal development—Development that proceeds from the head to the lower extremities (tail).

Choice of occupation—The selection of an activity based on cultural exposure, individual values and interests, and special abilities.

Climate—Weather conditions that impact a person's external environment.

Cognition—A mental process involving thinking, judgment and perceptions to arrive at a level of knowing and understanding.

Cognitive disability—A series of functional units of behavior that cuts across diagnostic categories and interferes with task behavior.

Collaboration—Working with others in a shared, cooperative endeavor to achieve mutual goals.

Committee on OTAs—A group responsible for all developmental aspects related to the new occupational therapy assistant personnel designation in the profession.

Communication—The ability to receive and transmit messages verbally or nonverbally.

Community—Interaction among individuals; achieving a sense of union with others; interconnectedness; also refers to where an individual lives, such as a rural, urban or suburban area.

Competence—The ability to use dexterity and intelligence in the completion of tasks; (a sense of satisfaction is implied in completion); also a legal term referring to soundness of one's mind.

Components—Fundamental units or constituent parts; in relation to activities refers to processes, tools, materials, purposefulness, etc.

Concentration—The ability to focus on a specific portion of the total; to bring all efforts to bear on an activity.

Concept formation—The organization of information from a variety of sources is formulated into thoughts and ideas.

Conditioning—A learning process that alters behavior through providing reinforcements (instrumental or operant) or associating a reflex with a particular stimulus to trigger a desired response (classic—Pavlov).

Confidentiality—Maintaining secrecy regarding patient or other information; basic tenet of medical ethics.

Conflict—Opposition or competitive action relative to incompatible views.

Contraindication—A condition that deems a particular type of treatment undesirable or improper.

Control site—An anatomic site where the person can demonstrate purposeful movement.

Controversy—Dispute.

Cost-effective—Economical in terms of benefits gained in relation to money spent.

COTA Advisory Committee—Formed in 1986 by the AOTA Executive Board to replace the COTA Task Force; the group's goal is to identify COTA concerns and formulate suggestions for addressing them.

COTA Task Force—Group established by AOTA to make recommendations regarding COTA issues and concerns; later renamed the COTA Advisory Committee.

Cowan stabilizing pillow—A supportive pillow designed to assist children with balance problems to sit on the floor; an example of simply designed adaptive equipment.

CPU—Central processing unit of a computer.

Creativity—Originality of thought, process and expression.

Criteria of purposefulness—In activity, those standards by which an activity's therapeutic value is assessed; include being goal-directed, age-appropriate, and having relevance and purpose.

Crossing the midline—The ability to move the limbs and eyes across the midline (sagittal plane) of one's body.

CRT—Cathode ray tube.

Cultural environment—Characteristics common to a particular group that provide input to an individual's life; can include values, beliefs, rituals, food, apparel, etc.

Culturally sensitive—Showing awareness and appreciation of the significance of values, beliefs, rituals and traditions held by a particular group.

Custom—Pattern of behavior or practice that is common to members of a particular group.

Daily living skills—Those things performed each day that sustain and enhance life, such as dressing, grooming and eating.

Database manager—A computer software program that organizes and categorizes data.

DBM—Database manager.

Decision-making—The process of weighing options in order to reach the best conclusion.

Deformity prevention—The act of reducing or eliminating distortions or malformations of a part of the body by various means, such as the use of a splint; taking measures to avoid disfigurement orchange ina body part.

Dementia praecox—An early term for schizophrenia.

Depth perception—The ability to determine the relative distance between self and figures or objects observed.

Developmental level—Degree of achievement in an established progression; pattern of growth, development and maturation.

Developmental sequence—An established pattern of development and growth.

Differentiation—A process of altering behavior that requires the ability to discriminate which elements are necessary and those that are not in a given set of circumstances.

Difficulty level—Degree of complexity required to execute a particular activity or step.

DIP joint—Distal interphalangeal joint.

Discovery method—Involves teaching techniques such as emphasizing contrast, informed guessing, active participation and awareness; also referred to as the reflective method (Bruner).

Disruptions—Sudden changes in one's environment that require immediate attention and response.

Disk drive—Peripheral computer equipment that sends messages from a software program to the computer; also called the disk operating system (DOS).

Disorientation—Inability to make accurate judgments about people, places and time.

Disruption—A forced interruption in a person's life.

Disuse syndrome—Complications arising from inactivity; also referred to as hypokinetic diseases.

Documentation—Written records of the patient's health care that include information about current and future needs.

Doing—The act of performing or executing; a way of knowing (Meyer); a process of investigating, trying out and gaining evidence of one's capacities; potential becomes actual (Fidler).

DOS—Disk operating system of a computer.

Dualistic—A position that views humans as having mind/body separation.

Durability—Capacity of an object or piece of equipment to last for a length of time without significant deterioration.

Dyad—A relationship between two individuals in which interaction is significant.

Dyadic—Of or relating to the interaction of two individuals on a significant, one-to-one basis.

Dynamic splint—A splint that allows controlled movement at various joints; tension is applied to encourage particular movements.

Economic status—One's level of financial independence; also refers to social class, such as poor, middle class or rich.

ECU—Environmental control unit.

Effectiveness—Degree to which the desired result is produced.

Effects of occupation—Those factors influenced by engagement in various occupations; may be broadly categorized as biologic, psychologic and sociocultural; outome(s) of a purposeful, meaningful activity.

Efficacy—Power to produce intended results; effectiveness.

Efficiency—Producing the desired outcome in a timely, productive way.

Ego integrity—Acceptance of self, nature and one's life. The value of one's life is recognized and time is not spent grieving over what might have been.

Ego strength—An executive personality structure that effectively directs and controls a person's actions; requires effective evaluation of reality and impulse control and consideration of one's ethics and values.

Employment—Activity in which one is engaged; also refers to paid work.

Endurance—The ability to sustain exertion over time; involves musculoskeletal, cardiac and pulmonary systems.

Environment—All factors that provide input to the individual.

Environmental control unit—An electronic system with sensors that monitors and performs various tasks.

Epistemology—A dimension of philosophy that is concerned with the questions of truth.

Equilibration—Process whereby new knowledge attained is brought into balance with previous experience.

Ethics—Aspect of the axiology branch of philosophy that poses questions of value regarding the standards or rules for right conduct.

Evaluation tools—Tests, checklists, questionnaires, activities and other methods used to assess strengths and limitations.

Expiation of guilt—The making amends for wrong doings; may be expressed verbally or achieved through engagement in appropriate activities.

Extinction—The disappearance of a previously conditioned response due to a lack of reinforcement.

Facilitation—Techniques used to make the desired response easier.

Facilitator—An individual who assists in making a process easier; the individual who assists in helping one make progress in reaching a goal.

Feedback—Information individuals receive about their behavior and the consequences of their actions; guides future behavior.

Feeding and eating—The skills of chewing, sucking and swallowing, and the use of utensils.

Fidelity—The ability to maintain loyalties in spite of differences.

Figure ground—The ability to differentiate between background and foreground objects and forms.

Fine motor coordination/dexterity—The ability to perform controlled movements, particularly in the manipulation of objects, through the use of small muscle groups.

Firmware—Flat electronic cards that occupy slots inside the computer.

Form constancy—The ability to recognize various forms and objects in different environments, sizes and positions.

Frame of reference—A person's assumptions and attitudes based on beliefs and conceptual models.

Framework—A structure, plan or specified arrangement.

Functional communication—The ability to use communication devices and systems, such as telephone, computer and call lights.

Functional level—An individual's occupational ability based on his or her specific performance deficits and/or strengths.

Functional mobility—The ability to move from one position to another (eg, in bed or wheelchair) or transfer to tub, shower, toilet, etc.; driving and use of other forms of transportation.

Functional position—One in which the affected part or parts of the body will be able to function maximally in relation to performance requirements.

Functional requirements—Components of an activity that require motor performance and behaviors for adequate completion.

General systems theory—A method of organizing different levels and categories of information; components include open system, input, throughput, output and feedback; *see* individual headings for additional information.

Generalization of learning—The ability to apply previously learned concepts to similar, current situations.

Generativity—Concern for the establishment and guiding of the next generation; giving without expecting anything in return.

Genuineness—Characteristic evidenced by sincerity and honesty; authenticity.

Goal achievement—The completion of those tasks and objectives one has set out to accomplish.

Gradability— Refers to the process by which performance of an activity is viewed step-by-step on a continuum, moving from simple to complex, or slow to rapid.

Grandfather clause—An exemption from certain requirements based on previous experience and/or circumstance.

Gross motor coordination—The use of large muscle groups to make controlled movements.

Group—Three or more people who establish some form of interdependent relationship.

Group approach—Therapeutic intervention that focuses on meeting the needs of individuals through active participation with others (three or more).

Group-centered roles—Behavior patterns group members share and that are required for the group to function, maintain relationships and achieve group goals; example include encourager, gate-keeper, tension reliever, etc.

Group community—The desirable outcome of group member relationships; a union with others; group cohesion.

Group norms—Standards of behavior, stated or unspoken, that define what is accepted, expected and valued by the group.

Group process—The manner in which group members relate to and communicate with each other, and how they accomplish their tasks.

Guide for supervision—One collection of the teaching materials developed from the federally funded invitational workshops held between 1963 and 1968. Concepts from this document are included in the 1990 document, *Supervision Guidelines for Certified Occupational Therapy Assistants*.

Gustatory—Of or relating to the reception, processing and interpration of tastes.

Habit of attention—Tuke's key element in the use of occupations that required concentration, limited undesirable stimuli and expanded positive feelings.

Habituation—An individual's habits and internalized roles, that help to maintain activity and action.

Half-lapboard—Device that provides a table surface for people in wheelchairs.

Hand creases—Volar surface anatomical landmarks that must be considered when constructing and fitting splints; include distal and proximal palmar, thenar and wrist.

Hardware—The computer and all of its electronic parts.

Heterogeneous group—A group of people members vary in age, sex, values, interests, socioeconomic background or cultural background.

Holism—View of the human mind and body as being one entity.

Holistic view—*see* Holism.

Home health— Area of occupational therapy service delivery that focuses on therapeutic intervention in the home environment.

Homeostasis—The tendency of the system, especially the physiologic system, to maintain internal stability.

Homogeneous group—A group of people in which members share similarities such as age, sex values, interests, socioeconomic background or cultural background.

Hostility—An opposition in feeling or action; antagonistic attitude.

Human activity—Occupations including those necessary to satisfy basic needs such as survival, productivity, a sense of belonging, etc.

Human development—Levels of growth and maturation that occur at predictable intervals.

Human needs—Physiologic, psychologic and sociocultural requirements for one's well-being.

Hypokinetic disease—Complications arising from inactivity; also called disuse syndrome.

Immunity—The possession of biologic defenses against illness.

Individualized—Adapted to the particular needs and interests of a person.

Initial dependence—First stage of group development in which members are dependent on the leader and concerned about their respective places in the group.

Initiative—Ability for original conception and independent action.

Input—The ways a computer or video system can receive information; how it can be "put in"; also refers to the model of human occupation process of receiving information from the environment.

Inservice training—Educational opportunities such as seminars and workshops provided in the workplace.

Integration of learning—The ability to use previously learned behaviors and concepts by incorporating them into one's repertoire and using them in a variety of new situations.

Integrative school—Psychiatric position relative to the biopsychologic nature of individuals.

Interdependent—Relationship characterized by cohesion and a sense of community.

Interests—Activities that the individual finds pleasurable; those occupations that maintain one's attention.

Interfaces—Electrical circuits that connect switches to devices.

Interpersonal skills—Communications skills that help individuals interact effectively with a variety of people.

Intimacy—The ability to commit oneself to partnerships or concrete affiliations; to develop the ethical strength to abide by the commitment made, even if compromise or sacrifice is necessary.

Intrapersonal skills—Developing a clear and accurate sense of self.

Intrinsic—From within; innate, natural and true.

Intrinsic minus—Describes a position where the hand is in a functional position—15 to 30 degrees wrist extension, MPs moderately extended (as close to zero degrees as is comfortable), thumb in a gently (not maximally) abducted position from the palm.

Intrinsic plus—Describes a position counter to intrinsic minus (*see* Intrinsic minus).

Joint creases—Grooves in the skin related to joint movement.

Joystick—An input device that bypasses the computer keyboard and moves the cursor (position indicator) up, down, right and left and turns the machine on and off.

Kinesthesia—The ability to identify the sensation of movement, including the path and direction of movement.

Laterality—The use of a preferred body part, such as the right or left hand, for activities requiring a high skill level.

Learning—A relatively permanent change in behavior resulting from exposure to conditions in the environment.

Leisure—Nonwork or free time spent in adult play activities that have an influence on the quality of life.

Leisure patterns—Use of discretionary time (non-work) to engage in particular activities of personal interest.

Level of arousal—The degree to which one demonstrates alertness and responsiveness to stimulation from the environment.

Life roles—Refers to the variety of experiences that occupy one's time, including worker, student, caregiver, homemaker, mate, sibling, peer, etc.

Life space—The total activities or ways of spending time; everything that influences a person's behavior (eg, objects, people and values).

Life tasks—Those developmental tasks that must be accomplished by each person for successful living throughout the life span (Havighurst).

Lines of readiness—Foundation for treatment developed by OBrock involving construction of things, communicating things, finding out things, completing things, and excelling in things.

Mainframe—A large central computer with numerous terminals.

Manipulation—Ability to handle objects and use with some degree of skill in activity performance.

Mechanical assistance—Describes a situation where the patient is independent in carrying out activities with assistive or adaptive equipment.

Medication routine—A procedure of obtaining medication, operating containers, and take medication at the required times.

Memory—In splinting, the ability of the material being used to return to its original flat shape and size when reheated.

Mentally ill—Persons having diseases and disabilities that result in impaired mental function.

Metaphysics—A branch of philosophy concerned with questions about the ultimate nature of things, including the nature of humans.

Method of activation—Movement or means by which a control site will activate a switch.

Microswitch—A small electronic "on/off" switch.

Milieu—A social and physical environment; one's surroundings.

Mind/body relationship—Interdependence of mental and physical aspects of humans; holism.

Misuse syndrome—Conditions that arise from a change in structure or function of a body part due to improper use (eg, tennis elbow).

Mobility—The ability to move physically from one position or place to another.

Modem—Modulator/demodulator that allows computer signals to be sent over telephone wires.

Monitor—Peripheral equipment that displays computer information on a screen.

Motor development—Acquisition of control and movement skills in a sequence that is relatively unvaried and characterized by milestones (Gesell).

Mouse—An electronic device that provides input to the computer without use of the keyboard.

Muscle tone—A degree of tension or resistance present in a muscle or muscle group.

Narcissism—Egocentricity; dominant interest in one's self.

NDT—Neurodevelopmental treatment.

Needs—Lack of things required for the welfare of the individual.

Networking—Informal communication with others having common interests; a supportive system for sharing information and services.

Object manipulation—Skill in handling large and small objects, such as keys, doorknobs and calculator.

Obsessive-compulsive—Behavior marked by compulsion to perform repetitively certain acts or carry out certain rituals to excess, such as handwashing or counting.

Occupation—The full range of activities that occupy a person; goal-directed behavior fundamental to human existence focused on activities of daily living skills, work and play in occupational therapy; includes meeting survival needs as well as those that lead to a full and productive life; a dynamic changing process influenced by biologic, psychologic and sociocultural environments (Reed).

Occupational behavior—The result of one's ability to organize and take action based on skills, knowledge and attitudes, and to function in one's life roles; thorough mastery of the environment, with work and play being key elements; occupation is an integrating factor for improving patient behavior (Reilly).

Occupational nurse—Early designation given to specialized occupational work provided by nurses trained by Susan Tracy.

Occupational performance—Participation in activities of daily living, work activities, and play or leisure activities.

Occupational role—Endeavors that define the nature of the individual in terms of achieving his/her potential and social worth as a member of society (*see* Life roles).

Occupational science—The academic discipline being developed at the University of California based on the concept of occupation and the complexities of its components, including purposeful activities and role- and age-appropriate occupations.

Olfactory—Of or relating to the reception, processing and interpretion of odors.

Ontogenesis—Biologic term meaning there is repetition of evolutionary changes of a species during embryonic development of an individual organism.

Operation—(cognitive) A mental action that can be reversed.

Opportunity—Situation or condition favorable for goal-attainment; a therapeutic technique of structuring the environment; opposite of prescription.

Oral-motor control—The ability to exhibit controlled movements of the mouth, tongue and related structures.

Organization—The tendency of a person to develop a coherent system; to systematize.

Orientation—Refers to the degree to which one is able to correctly identify person, place, time and situation.

Orthostatic hypotension—Condition caused by a rapid fall in blood pressure when assuming an upright position after being recumbent for a period of time.

Osteoporosis—A metabolic condition in which bones become porous and brittle because of inactivity.

Output—Information that is sent or 'put out' from the computer; also refers to the model of human occupation process concerned with mental, physical and social aspects of occupation.

PA—Physical assistance.

Paddles—Electronic devices that bypass the computer keyboard or video system and provide information input via rotational movements.

Palmar grasp—A position in which all fingers and the palm are in contact with an object.

Paraphrasing—Restating in one's own words a message received.

Patient education—Materials and methods for providing specific instruction to recipients of occupational therapy services.

Perception—Ability to receive and interpret incoming sensory information.

Performance—Actions produced through skill acquisition; a subsystem of the model of human occupation concerned with neuromuscular, communication and process skills.

Phobia—An abnormal fear or dread.

PIP joint—Proximal interphalangeal joint.

Play—An intrinsic activity that involves enjoyment and leads to fun; spontaneous and voluntary activity engaged in by choice.

Pliability—Easily bent or changed; flexibility.

PNF—Proprioceptive neuromuscular facilitation.

Portability—Degree to which an object can be readily moved.

Position in space—The ability to determine the special relationship of objects and figures to self or to other objects and forms.

Postural control—The ability to assume a position and maintain it; proper alignment of body parts, orientation to midline, necessary shifting of weight, and righting reactions are important elements for accomplishment.

Practice settings—specific situational contexts in which health professionals work (ie, hospitals, nursing homes, psychiatric hospitals, etc.).

Praxis—The ability to do motor planning and to perform purposeful movement in response to demands from the environment.

Prescription—A directive or injunction; opposite of opportunity.

Prevention—Taking measures to keep something from happening.

Problem-solving—A process of studying a situation that presents uncertainty, doubt, or difficulty and arriving at a solution through definition, identification of alternative plans, selection of a likely plan, organizing the necessary steps in the plan, implementing it, and evaluating the results.

Problem-solving skills—Steps and techniques applied in problem-solving.

Processing the group—A time in group session when members openly discuss observations and feelings relative to a group activity in which they have participated.

Projective techniques—Methods and activities used to provide information about one's thoughts, feelings and needs.

Proprioception—An individual's awareness of position, balance and equilibrium changes based on stimuli from muscles, joints and other tissues; gives information about the position of one body part in relation to that of another.

Proximal-distal development—Development that begins in the parts closest to the midline and progresses to the extremities.

Psychodrama—Therapeutic technique in which patients enact or dramatize their daily life situations.

Psychomotor—Refers to activity that combines both physical and emotional elements.

Psychomotor skills—Movement abilities related to cerebral or psychic activity, such as gross motor skills, fine motor skills and coordination.

Purposeful activity—Those endeavors that are goal-directed and have meaning to the individual engaged in them; significant.

Quality of life—A combination of factors that contribute to one's degree of life satisfaction, such as enjoyable work, meaningful relationships, leisure fulfillment.

RAM—Random access memory of a computer.

Range of motion—Movement of body parts through an arc.

Rapport—The establishment of a harmonious relationship with another person or group.

Recapitulation—To review through a brief summary.

Reciprocal interweaving—Principle of motor development that states that the development of immature behavior and more mature behavior alternate in a constant spiral until matue behavior is firmly established

Recreation—A re-creating or renewal through participation in activities that satisfy, amuse or relax.

Recumbent—Pertains to lying down or reclining.

Reeducation—A process of relearning a task or behavior; also used to refer to retraining of specific muscles or muscle groups.

Reflection—The act of thinking about circumstances, events, activities and relationships; a summary of the affective meaning of a message, both verbally and nonverbally.

Reflective method—*see* Discovery method.

Reflex—An involuntary, immediate and unconscious response in reaction to sensory stimulation; may involve limbs and organs. Reflex movements are precursors to basic fundamental movements.

Reinforcement—The rewarding of desired behavior.

Repeatability—Ability to repeat performance over a specified length of time.

Response—Any item of behavior.

Right-left discrimination—The ability to discriminate one side of the body from the other side.

Roles—Pertains to the functions of the individual in society that may be assumed or acquired (homemaker, student, caregiver, etc.).

ROM—Range of motion; also refers to the Read only memory of a computer.

Safety—Taking measures to assure that risk, injury or loss will not occur; the application of measures necessary to prevent injury or loss of function.

SBA—Stand-by assistance.

Scanning—A technique that bypasses use of the keyboard and provides input directly to the cursor or arrow on the computer monitor.

Script—The written text followed when producing a film or a play.

Selection time—In electronics, the time needed to operate two switches or two functions of a switch.

Self-acceptance—Recognition and acceptance of one's strengths, limitations and related feelings.

Self-actualization—The highest level of need in Maslow's theory; refers to the desire to be fulfilled and achieve one's full potential.

Self-awareness—The ability to recognize one's own behavior patterns and emotional responses.

Self-centered roles—Individuals are primarily concerned with satisfying their own needs rather than those of the group; examples include withdrawing, blocking, dominating and seeking recognition.

Self-concept—Overall awareness or "picture" one has of oneself, both physically and emotionally, and including both positive and negative qualities.

Self-ideal—The way one would like to be seen by others.

Self-image—*see* Self-concept.

Self-management—The ability to use coping skills, exhibit self-control and manage time effectively.

Self-reinforcing—A process in which each success acts as a motivation for greater effort or a more complex challenge.

Sensory integration—The ability to develop and coordinate sensory input.

Sensory processing—The interpretation of sensory stimuli from visual, tactile, auditory, and other senses; information is received, a motor response is made, and sensory feedback is provided.

Sentient—Possessing sensory capabilities; the capacity to be highly sensitive and responsive to another person's feelings.

Sequencing—The placement of actions, concepts and information in a particular order.

Shaping—The use of prompts (and sometimes reinforcement) to promote desired behavior.

Skill acquisition—Learning or relearning to do something well based on knowledge, talent, training and practice.

Skill components—Distinctive attributes that lead to successful adaptation; include perceptual motor, cognitive, drive-object, dyadic interaction, primary group interaction, self-identity and sexual identity (Mosey).

Skill environments—Those settings that maximize the acquisition of skills through dynamic interaction.

Social conduct—Refers to one's ability to interact with others appropriately; includes the use of manners, gestures, self-expression, etc.

Social environment—Elements that comprise the relationships and places where one's social interactions occur.

Socialization—Process whereby skills in establishing interpersonal relationships with others are gained; implies community ties and societal involvement; development of the ability to interact with others appropriately with consideration to cultural and contextual factors.

Society of Friends—A religious group concerned with humane treatment of those in asylums; also known as Quakers.

Soft tissue integrity—Maintenance of skin and interstitial tissue condition, both anatomically and physiologically.

Software—Programs that send messages to the computer to perform certain functions.

Sold time—Time spent in meeting physiologic needs, such as sleeping, eating, bathing, eliminating and sexual activity.

Soldering—The process of fusing two pieces of metal together.

Specific needs—Those needs related to a definite goal or set of circumstances.

Splitting a wire—Process for dividing two portions of an electrical wire in order to make modifications for other uses.

Spreadsheet—A computer software program that manipulates numbers in a matrix of rows and columns.

Stability—Firmness in position; permanence; reliability.

Static splint—A splint used to prevent motion and to stabilize or immobilize a specific part in a functional position.

Stereognosis—Ability to use the sense of touch to identify objects.

Stimulus—Any input of energy that tends to affect behavior.

Strength—Muscle power and degree of movement is demonstrated in the presence of gravity or resistive weight.

Stress—Physical, mental or emotional strain or tension that interferes with the normal equilibrium of the individual.

Stripping a wire—A process of removing the plastic coating from a segment of wire.

Subcortical—Conscious attention is directed to objects or tasks rather than specific movements.

Superstition—Beliefs and practices that result from ignorance and fear of the unknown; irrational attitudes of the mind toward supernatural forces.

Supportive personnel—OT aides, technicians and COTAs who assist in the provision of services.

Synergy—Combined action; the correlated actions of several muscles working together or combined activities of organs of the body.

Synthesis of learning—A process whereby concepts that were previously learned are restructured into new patterns and ideas.

Tactile—The use of skin contact and related receptors to receive, process, and interpret touch, pressure, temperature, pain, vibration and two-point stimulation.

Task analysis—*see* Activity analysis.

Task group—Therapeutic activity where all members make a contribution to achieving the group goals through sharing in the completion of a task, such as planning and implementing a party.

Task roles—Functions necessary for a group to accomplish its objectives; examples include initiator/designer, information giver/seeker, opinion giver/seeker, challenger/comforter and summarizer.

Teacher's role—Primary function that helps the learner change behavior in specified directions.

Teaching process steps—Ten specific points that must be addressed to assure maximal teaching effectiveness related to objectives, content selection, modifications, units, materials, work space, preparation of student(s), presentation, tryout performance and evaluation.

Teaching/learning process—An interactive strategy involving the instructor and the learner in achieving desired goals.

Temporal adaptation—The way in which one occupies time and the appropriate balance of activities within specific and general time frames.

Terminal program—A communication program that allows a computer to link up with others via a modem to gain or exchange information.

Theoretical framework—An interrelated set of ideas that provides a way to conceptualize fundamental principles and applications.

Therapeutic potential—Degree of likelihood that therapeutic goals will be achieved.

Therapeutic value—The extent to which an activity or experience has potential for assisting in the achievement of particular goals.

Thermoplastic—Type of material that becomes soft and pliable when heated, without any change in basic properties.

Throughput—Refers to the model of human occupation; pertaining to one's internal organizational processes.

Topographic orientation—The ability to determine the route to a specified location; to identify the location of particular objects and settings.

Tracking time—The amount of time needed for the person to move from a resting position to activation of a switch.

Traditions—Inherited patterns of thought or action that can be handed down through generations or developed in a singular family unit.

Trial use—Utilizing a piece of equipment or an adaptive device for a specified length of time to determine its effectiveness and whether or not modifications are needed.

Values—Beliefs, feelings or ideas that are important and highly regarded and have value to the individual.

Vestibular—Receiving, processing and interpreting stimuli received by the inner ear relative to head position and movement.

Video feedback—Objective tool that provides information regarding the individual's performance, affect, interactions, and other factors; objective information received via the camera and tape.

Video lighting—Specific procedures that must be followed in using auxiliary illumination in videotaped productions.

Video maintenance—Procedures, such as cleaning, that must be performed periodically to assure that equipment will be operating maximally.

Visual—Of or relating to the reception, processing and interpretation of stimuli received by the eyes, such as acuity, color, figure ground and depth.

Visual closure—The ability to identify objects or forms from incomplete presentations.

Visual-motor integration—The coordination of body movements with visual information when engaging in activity.

Vocational exploration—A process of determining appropriate vocational pursuits through study of one's aptitudes, skills and interests.

Volition—Exercise of the will or will power; it guides choices of the individual and is influenced by values and interests.

Word processing—The use of a software computer program that composes, edits, moves, deletes and duplicates text.

Work—Skill in socially productive activities, including gainful employment, homemaking, child care/parenting, and work preparation activities.

Work-leisure continuum—Range of activities in which one engages throughout the life span, with varying amounts of time devoted to these pursuits.

Index